Stunted Lives, Stagnant Economies

Stunted Lives, Stagnant Economies

Poverty, Disease, and Underdevelopment

Eileen Stillwaggon

Rutgers University Press

New Brunswick, New Jersey, and London

No part of this book may be reproduced or utilized in any form or by any means, electronic or mechanical, or by any information storage and retrieval system without written permission from the publisher. Please contact Rutgers University Press, Livingston Campus, Bldg. 4161, P.O. Box 5062, New Brunswick, New Jersey 08903. The only exception to this prohibition is "fair use" as defined by U.S. copyright law.

Manufactured in the United States of America

Permission of *Buenos Aires Herald* to reprint material from Eileen Stillwaggon, "Measuring Health in Argentina," *Buenos Aires Herald*, October 31, 1993, p. 16, is gratefully acknowledged.

Library of Congress Cataloging-in-Publication Data

Stillwaggon, Eileen, 1949–
    Stunted lives, stagnant economies : poverty, disease, and underdevelopment / by Eileen Stillwaggon.
        p. cm.
    Includes bibliographical references and index.
    ISBN 0-8135-2493-8 (cloth : alk. paper). — ISBN 0-8135-2494-6 (pbk. : alk. paper)
        1. Poor—Medical care—Economic aspects—Developing countries.   2. Poor—Health and hygiene—Developing countries.   3. Poor—Medical care—Economic aspects—Latin America.   4. Poor—Health and hygiene—Latin America.   5. Poor—Developing countries—Social conditions. I. Title.
RA418.5.P6S74   1998
362.1'09172'4—dc21   97–22313
                                                                            CIP

To Rosemary and Jim Stillwaggon,
whose compassion, broad horizons, and sense of humor
have always been an inspiration

Contents

Maps and Tables

Maps

Tables

Preface

One of the purposes of this book is to make the living conditions of the poor and the health problems they face understandable to people who have never seen a Third World slum. Whether the reader is an economics student or an epidemiologist, a government planner or a citizen who wants to be informed, the description of how the poor live needs to be as concrete as possible. I have relied on the usual sources for research, such as census data and scholarly reports and articles. My research benefitted even more from many interviews and visits and the hundreds of hours I spent in slums, health centers, and public hospitals.

The presentation of the work is a weaving of census data, scholarly articles from economic and medical journals, and information and insights from interviews and personal observation. The generosity and openness of many Argentines, slum dwellers, patients, nurses, and doctors have made it possible for me to describe their homes, their streets, their hospitals, their injuries, and their illnesses.

Organization

This book comprises five parts. Part I begins with an introduction to the subject of poverty and health. Argentina is used as a case study, and Chapter 1 surveys the extent of poverty in Argentina. Chapter 2 surveys Argentine economic and medical history with emphasis on the factors that contribute to Argentine underdevelopment.

Part II focuses on how poor people get sick. It examines numerous factors in the everyday life of the poor that produce illness and premature death. Nothing distinguishes the living conditions of the poor from those of the rich more than the level of protection afforded by their homes. Chapter 3 contains a detailed description of the structural conditions of poor housing—city tenements, rural houses, and suburban shanties—as well as problems of crowding, location, equipment, and neighborhood services. The health effects of poor housing are described, including respiratory, skin, gastrointestinal, and other infectious and parasitic diseases.

Chapter 4 provides a detailed look at the ecology of the rural house and farm-yard and how it contributes to the spread of Chagas' disease, an incurable de-generative illness that affects at least eighteen million people in the Americas. Chapter 5 examines the other key element in the physical environment of the poor: the availability of safe water and safe disposal of human, solid, and indus-trial waste. That chapter covers the quality of the municipal water supply and groundwater; the breakdown of an already inadequate sewage system; the haz-ards of solid waste, in particular for the many thousands of people who live in garbage dumps; and the health effects of poor sanitation, including the spread of cholera in the Western Hemisphere since 1991.

Chapter 6 discusses the institutional environment and the health and safety impact of the government's failure in its regulatory role. The chapter documents that, through corruption, neglect, and intentional dismantling of regulatory agen-cies, the Argentine government has left consumers and workers in grave danger of poisoning and other injury from shoddy products and shoddy work, in every-thing from defective condoms to nuclear waste, to hazardous elevators, to bogus medicines. It also discusses the treatment of state mental patients, the treacher-ous state of traffic, and the careless spread of acquired immunodeficiency syn-drome (AIDS) through the lack of good medical practices and the failure of the government to address the problem concretely.

Part III considers what medical resources are available to address the health needs of the poor. Chapter 7 examines the rise of private-sector medical care and its weaknesses and the collapse of the social-security and public sectors. The financial interactions of the three sectors are an important focus of the chapter and an important cause of the collapse of the public system. The decline of med-ical education and of the keeping of vital statistics and their importance in health strategies also are included. Chapter 8 discusses the central role of primary health care in a strategy of public health and the weaknesses of primary health care in Argentina. Several primary health posts are described in detail. Chapter 9 details the problems facing public hospitals in staffing, physical plant, equipment, maintenance, lack of procedural norms, and morale. Several key public hospitals are presented in detail, showing the strengths and weaknesses of the public system.

Part IV evaluates the health outcome of inadequate housing and water supply, lack of government oversight, and poor medical assistance for the poor. Chapter 10 discusses the impact of poverty and poor medical care on infants and young children. It explains the different kinds of environmental factors that affect the mortality of children at different ages. The causes of death in early infancy, late infancy, and early childhood are examined, as well as the distribution of mortality among regions and among classes.

Chapter 11 examines how poor nutrition and unhealthy living conditions produce a cycle of disease in children and adolescents, leading to stunted physical growth and retarded mental development. The chapter shows how the conditions of poverty produce children who are unable to succeed in school and who have less physical stamina, impaired small and gross motor skills, and behavioral problems. Chapter 12 discusses the health problems of adults and the contribution of poverty to morbidity, poor work performance, and the loss of productive years. The obstacles to development posed by a work force weakened by disease and injury are the focus of that chapter.

Part V summarizes the problems and presents some solutions. Chapter 13 brings together an assessment of the overall impact of poor living conditions, poor medical attention, and governmental neglect. The chapter proposes low-cost solutions to many of the medical and environmental problems of poor countries. Successful programs and individual health centers are identified, and the social environment necessary for human development is discussed.

Acknowledgments

I was continually amazed and delighted by the generosity and hospitality of countless Argentines who helped me on this research. They would hear about my project and invite me to spend hours with them at work and arrange for others to help me further. People have asked me if it was not depressing to spend almost every day in hospitals, and one-room health posts, and to slog through the muddy streets of shantytowns. In fact, it was rewarding to work alongside people who struggled against great odds to provide the very best possible care. There were many people who helped me. Those listed below gave generously of their time, and none should be considered responsible for any errors or opinions I express.

I am deeply indebted to Dra. Aprigliano of Health Center Number 6, Buenos Aires; Dra. Nilda Chávez of Hospital Materno-infantil Gregorio La Ferrere, La Matanza; Instituto Torcuato di Tella for the use of the library; Dr. Horacio Lejarraga of Hospital Nacional de Pediatría Dr. Garrahan, Buenos Aires; Dr. Raúl Mercer, director of *Mi Pueblo* Hospital, Florencio Varela; Dra. María Coruja, director of Hospital de Quemados, Buenos Aires, and Dr. Jorge Barkansky and the nursing team of Quemados; Dr. Marío Rípoli, director, and Dra. Graciela Spatz of Health Center Number 5, Buenos Aires; Jorge Sparvoli of the *cooperadora* of Hospital Materno-infantil Del Viso; Dr. Alberto Schwarcz of Diego Paroissien Hospital, La Matanza; Padre Tomás Llorente of Santa Rosa de Lima parish in Manuel Alberdi, Pilar; Gabriela Cante, librarian of the Pan American Health

Organization, Buenos Aires; Nicholas Tozer of the *Buenos Aires Herald,* who provided the cover photo; Dr. Pedro de Sarasqueta of Hospital Nacional de Pediatría Dr. Garrahan, who was extremely helpful and also lent me many books; and Dr. Pablo Muntaabski, who was a fountain of information and invited me to spend as much time as I wanted with the doctors and nurses in Villa de Retiro and Health Center Number 21.

Dr. Roque Teixidor was very generous with his time. He took me to three hospitals and three neighborhood health centers in Mendoza, enabling me to interview many people. He was a very kind host. I asked Dr. Carlos Ray, First Chair in Pediatrics of the University of Buenos Aires at Hospital de Clínicas General San Martín, for a brief interview. He told me I could not know the problems of their department unless I spent a month there, and he invited me take on the schedule of the residents in pediatrics. I stayed for six weeks in 1992 and two weeks in 1993, both in Clínicas Hospital in Buenos Aires and in the Hospital Maternoinfantil Gregorio LaFerrere. Of course, he was right; it was an invaluable experience. The faculty and the residents, the patients and their parents, and the nurses all received me with great hospitality. Dr. Ana Bernard, chief of residents in 1992, was very helpful and a wonderful teacher.

All our friends in Buenos Aires were helpful in so many ways. They made us welcome in their country, which we came to think of as our own. Cynthia Jenkins, Giselle Jenkins, and Edgardo Jenkins were great help and delightful company. María Luísa Gualco de Etiennot can accomplish anything that needs to be accomplished; she is a national resource. She and Roberto Etiennot are also great fun. Celia and Arturo Vallés-Bosch took good care of us and became surrogate grandparents for our children. Mariana Vallés-Bosch de Jorge and Fernando Jorge made sure we were housed, fed, and schooled. They made everything work for us, and we enjoyed many *asados* and political discussions.

Back in the United States, Elizabeth Sawers took care of our mail and finances. Rosemary and Jim Stillwaggon managed our affairs in the States and brought us anything we needed. Larry Sawers read the entire manuscript, some parts more than once, made helpful comments throughout and also created both maps. Brian Sawers made many useful comments on the entire manuscript. Dr. Doreen Valentine, Acquiring Editor for the Sciences at Rutgers University Press, was an enthusiastic and astute editor. The Economics Department at Gettysburg College was a supportive environment in which to prepare the manuscript. I was able to leave many tasks at school in the hands of two capable and willing helpers: department secretary, Betty Smith, and teaching assistant, Kim Schneider.

I also would like to thank my family, whose enthusiasm for the project never faltered. Robbie, a toddler when we first went to South America, took it upon himself to test gastrointestinal bugs in Venezuela, Ecuador, Brazil, Paraguay, Uruguay, and every province of Argentina. Kate broke both arms as we were beginning a bus trip to Paraguay. That enabled me to see two modest health centers in Buenos Aires province and an orthopedic practice in Asunción. Brian traveled three hours each day to and from school on packed *colectivo* buses as a human subject for in-your-face tuberculosis transmission. Larry started out doing half the housework and ended up doing it all.

Part I
Poverty and Health

Argentina

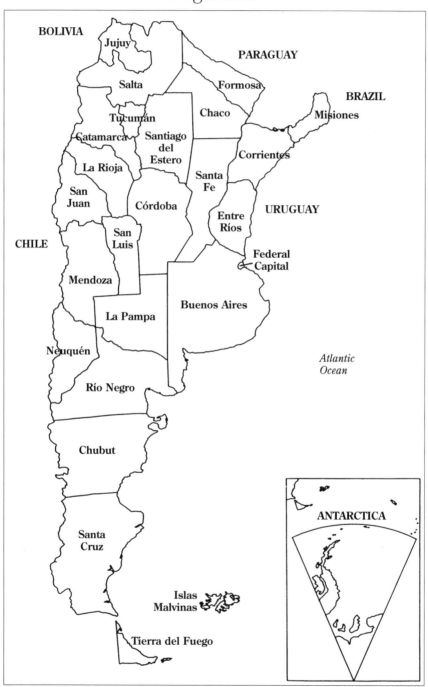

Partidos of Greater Buenos Aires

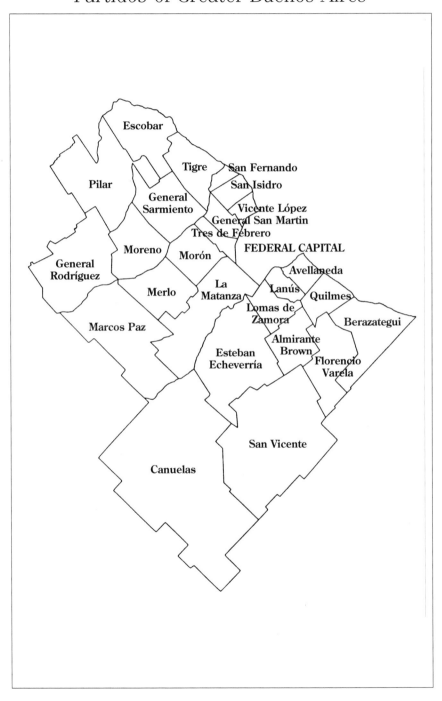

One

The Plague of Poverty

Children born in 1981 entered the work force in the 1990s. In most of the developing world, they were born during an economic crisis that capped a period of disappointing growth and little improvement in living standards for the poor. The economies of the 1990s are marked by high, even unprecedented, rates of unemployment and cutbacks in social services. How well prepared are the children born in the 1980s to work in the economy of the 1990s and the next century?

The medical association of the industrial city of Rosario, Argentina, monitored the development of all infants born there in 1981. It found that not one of the children from families in extreme poverty was able to satisfy age-appropriate norms for psychomotor development. Those norms include the expected ages at which an infant will lift or turn the head (one month); hold the head erect, or follow objects with the eyes (four months); sit, or attempt to grab an object and bring it to the mouth (six months); walk with help, or say *mamá*, *papá*, or any other word, or clap or wave (twelve and a half months) (Enria 1991, 66).

For a healthy child, those norms are not stringent, yet none of the very poor children (30 percent of all children in the study) had the motor and mental capacity to meet them. The Rosario study also found that at one year of age, 51 percent of the children of extreme poverty were below the twenty-fifth percentile for both weight and height, and 60 percent had a head circumference below the twenty-fifth percentile in national standards (Enria 1991, 66, 68).

One-third of the children born in Argentina in 1981 have not finished primary school, and fewer than one-third will finish secondary school. Some are already parents. Nearly 4 percent of children born in 1981 have died. What contribution will the surviving children make in the newly privatized economy of Argentina, touted by some as the "new tiger" of South America? The progress of Argentina and other developing countries will depend in large measure on the quality of their resources, including labor which is abundant and easily enhanced. The conditions in which the laborers of the new economy are born, grow up, learn, and work influence the economy for decades to come.

Most of Argentina's children are born in delivery rooms that are not inspected and that would not pass inspection, even by today's lax standards.

Thirteen percent are born weighing less than three pounds and with 40 percent fewer brain cells than a full-term adequate-weight baby.

Seven percent grow up in houses made of rags and flattened soda cans or other discarded materials, and another 30 percent live in other kinds of substandard housing.

Almost half drink water from contaminated wells, and many scavenge for food in dumps.

These children living in poverty have episodes of diarrhea and acute respiratory infection that follow in quick succession, so the children are sick most of the time.

If there is a health center to go to, children and expectant mothers stand in a cold, muddy waiting room and receive less-than-adequate, sometimes indifferent attention from overworked, underpaid, and sometimes badly trained doctors and nurses.

If the children go to the hospital, they are already weakened by malnutrition and catch new infections from the hospital staff or from other patients because the wards have no hand-washing facilities for nurses and doctors.

While they are in the hospital, no one asks if they have been vaccinated for measles, tetanus, pertussis, or tuberculosis.

If they are given medicine, it might be counterfeit—just contaminated water in a medicine vial.

Recurrent illnesses cause poor children to miss fifty days of school each year. They become discouraged at school and are needed at home to care for their siblings, so they leave school at age eleven or twelve.

This is how many of Argentina's workers have grown up. Their physical growth is stunted and their mental development thwarted, and now they enter the work force to build the new Argentina. What can any country build with workers who are tired, burdened with parasites, and of retarded mental capacity because of physical and emotional injury?

Poverty in the work force perpetuates national underdevelopment through the links between living conditions and health and between health and school or work performance. People get sick when they eat from garbage dumps, live in cardboard shacks, and are unvaccinated. When they are sick, they learn and work badly. There are countries in which 30, 40, even 70 percent of the work force is sick, and so national development is retarded. In more than 100 countries, the majority of people live in poverty. Globally, more than three billion people live in inadequate housing, drink contaminated water, or have little access to medical care.

From an ethical perspective, the definition of economic progress should be an increase in the well-being of the people. Even from a purely pragmatic viewpoint, the health and mental development of the work force is of paramount importance. People whose lives are stunted and limited because they have been deprived of the necessary inputs of food, shelter, education, and preventive health care are an obstacle to economic development. People are the tools as well as the proper beneficiaries of national development. Economists tend to analyze underdevelopment in the realm of models and numbers, tax rates, exchange rates, and investment ratios. We also need to know how people live and what their lives are like to know if our models can work.

Professionals in other fields also need to consider the living conditions of the poor: how they get sick, how poverty affects their lives, and why they do not escape its trap. Epidemiologists, for example, benefit from understanding the human ecology of diseases that affect the poor. When Ebola virus broke out in a hospital in Kikwit, Zaire, in 1995, patients fled to their homes in the surrounding villages. An international team of epidemiologists from the World Health Organization based their prediction of the spread of the disease on the assumption that each hospital patient lived in a house with only one to two persons per room. When researchers actually went to look for possible Ebola carriers, they had to revise their estimates upward because they found the people living five to ten to a room (Altman 1995*a*, C3). Without an understanding of how people live, epidemiology cannot adequately explain the spread of disease. The severity of an epidemic, even the mode of transmission, can be misunderstood if researchers are unaware of the conditions of housing, water supply, and other services.

It is difficult for economic planners, epidemiologists, and students in those fields who have lived healthy lives in comfortable homes to adapt their expectations to the reality of everyday life for the poor. For both epidemiologists and economists, the details of everyday life can help them understand why strategies that seem sound have so little benefit. It is pointless to try to understand models of economic development without first understanding the obstacles to development. Some widely used textbooks for courses in economic development contain only a line or two about health. Even more fruitless are the attempts of governments to follow complicated economic plans, fretting over tax rates and exchange rates, if they ignore one of the biggest obstacles to future growth, a sick work force.

This book describes the living conditions of the poor: their houses, their neighborhoods, their water supply, the safety of their food, drugs, and worksites. It also examines what medical services are available to the poor for the prevention and treatment of disease. Finally, it considers the effects of poor living conditions and inadequate health care on child survival, growth, and development, on school and work performance of adolescents and adults, and on prospects for national development. Practical solutions are offered in the final chapter.

An essential premise of the work is that health is primarily an economic, not a medical, problem. Health outcomes for the poor and the rich are conditioned more by their position in the economy than by any other factor. The good health that the affluent can enjoy and the ill health that afflicts the poor have more to do with living standards than with medicine. The same was true in the now-industrialized countries. Improvement in living standards, housing, sanitation, and nutrition, not medical advances, produced the dramatic declines in infectious diseases up to the middle of the twentieth century. Most of the worst microbial diseases, such as leprosy, plague, typhus, and malaria, had subsided in Europe long before people understood the etiology of those diseases (Neri 1982, 16, 21).

For the most part, the diseases that affect the poor are the result of the poverty of their environment. The rich generally do not contract cholera, summer diarrhea, tuberculosis, lice, worms, or leprosy. They do not suffer from burns caused by inadequate home heating or cooking facilities or electrocution from do-it-yourself wiring. Poverty also determines the availability and effectiveness of the medical response, which also plays an important role in health. Poor people do not get medical care for their poverty-induced conditions either because the country is poor or because they are poor in a country in which the market rations medical care only to the rich.

Shared Poverty, Shared Policies

The Third World includes three-fourths of the world's population (UNDP 1995, 14). The 126 countries in the developing world are of very different income levels. The poorest countries in sub-Saharan Africa have per capita annual incomes of only a few hundred dollars. In Latin America and East Asia, there are countries with average incomes of several thousand dollars, high enough to rank them as middle-income countries. There are great differences between the lives of the better-off in beautiful neighborhoods of Río de Janeiro and Buenos Aires and the comparatively modest luxuries of the elite in Dar es Salaam. When it comes to the lives of the poorer half of a population, however, there is much less difference between a country with an average income of $600 and one whose per capita income is $9,000. The rural poor live in mud-and-stick houses in both Argentina and Tanzania. Cardboard shanties are about the same whether they are on the outskirts of Caracas or of Nairobi. For those who eat from garbage dumps, it matters little that they are eating "middle-income" garbage. Infectious and parasitic diseases and a greater risk of accidental injury afflict the poor in all countries of the developing world. Prospects for national development are dimmed everywhere because of the ill health of the poor.

Not only are the living conditions of the very poor similar in most developing countries, so too are the economic development policies being pursued in Third World countries of all income levels and in the transition economies of former socialist countries. In the 1950s and 1960s, most countries attempted to foster economic growth through government intervention, using large subsidies to private firms and government ownership of public enterprises. Governments erected high tariff barriers to protect infant industries producing for the domestic market. By the 1980s, developing countries of all income levels, with a few notable exceptions, found their economies stagnating, burdened by unproductive state enterprises, with the private sector devoted more to rent seeking than to productive investment.

Since the mid-1980s, the trend in most of the developing world and even in most of the former socialist countries has been to move in the direction of liberal economic policies, including freer markets, privatization of state enterprises, fewer subsidies, reduction of tariff walls, and huge cuts in government spending. The need for many of those reforms is widely, although not universally, accepted among economists, just as the necessity of government intervention was widely recognized in the collapsing capitalist world of the 1920s and 1930s.

The debt crisis of the 1980s and the liberal economic medicine of the 1990s have produced a political climate in which budgets for health and education have been slashed in much of the developing world. The privatization and liberalization of those economies, however, did not necessitate such draconian cuts in social services. The governments could have achieved adequate budget cuts by reducing wasteful subsidies, unproductive bureaucracies, military spending, and payoffs to well-placed officials. Health and education were never the culprits in government fiscal deficits. In times of macroadjustment, when privatization and downsizing inevitably would lead to higher unemployment, social service budgets should have been increased. The health of the majority of the population in the developing world, of tomorrow's work force, is at risk or already compromised. When the burden of macroadjustment falls on populations already malnourished, ill housed, and unprotected from infectious disease, it worsens the countries' chances for success. Mean-spirited macroadjustment sows its own destruction, as is already being seen in some of the countries that have carried out structural adjustment at the expense of the poor. In the short run and the long run, the costs of that meanness will be borne by the whole economy.

Global Distribution of Health

The epidemiology of poverty is not absolute. Just as not every person who smokes dies of lung cancer, not every poor baby dies of the common cold turned to pneumonia, nor does every person who drinks contaminated water succumb to cholera. There is, however, enough of an association to justify the notion of causation between poverty and poor health (Hill 1992). Poverty and the living conditions it produces expose most of the poor to risks from infectious and parasitic disease to which the rich are not exposed. Cholera, typhus, leprosy, and many other diseases affect almost exclusively the marginalized population. Certain injuries afflict the poor to a far greater extent than the rich, including exposure to toxic substances, bus accidents, and birth trauma. The result of that greater risk is that poor people have a lower life expectancy. Moreover, poor countries generally have a lower life expectancy than rich countries.

There is a general correspondence in the rankings of countries by gross domestic product (GDP) per capita and life expectancy. Richer countries, in general, have better living conditions, sanitation systems, and health care facilities, all of which improve morbidity and mortality outcomes. Nevertheless, many countries do not conform to the correlation of GDP with life expectancy. Some countries have invested heavily in sanitary infrastructure or are making a concerted effort to distribute available food supplies. Some countries emphasize education, particularly female education, which significantly affects child survival and wellness. Finally, some countries spend more on medical services or focus their health care spending more effectively. Consequently, those countries have healthier populations than their GDP per capita alone would lead one to expect. China, Kerala State and parts of Maharashtra State in India, Sri Lanka, Costa Rica, Chile, and Cuba all have life expectancies that rank them above other countries or regions with higher GDP per capita. All the former socialist countries have life expectancies above what would be projected based on their present GDPs alone because of past investments in medical infrastructure, emphases on basic food distribution, and relatively more equal income distributions.

There also are countries whose failure in health is exceptional. The United States has the highest average living standard in the world but ranks eighteenth in infant survival. The United States has the most unequal distribution of income of any of the industrialized countries and is the only advanced industrial country without a system of national health coverage. The importance of factors other than per capita GDP is illustrated in life expectancy outcomes. In 1992, life expectancy at birth in Costa Rica, Cuba, and the United States was essentially the same. However, Costa Rica's GDP per capita was $5,480; Cuba's was $3,412; and in the United States, it was $23,760 (UNDP 1995, 155, 156).

Increase in GDP per capita can mean improvements in health, or it can be followed by increase in mortality rates if the distribution of income worsens. In the early 1970s, for example, GDP in Brazil increased at a rate of about 10 percent per year, but distribution of income worsened, and the military *junta* during those years did not invest in public health and disease prevention. From 1968 to 1976, infant mortality increased from 84 per thousand to 100 per thousand and to more than 130 per thousand in the impoverished northeast (Oya-Sawyer et al. 1987, 90). The effects persist. Brazil, with GDP per capita almost equal to that of Costa Rica, still has a life expectancy ten years less (UNDP 1995, 155).

The range of diseases and conditions is broader in poor countries than in industrialized countries. The illnesses that afflict the poor include infectious and parasitic diseases that result primarily from the physical environment. The injuries and poisonings that the poor suffer result from their countries' under-developed institutional environment. Because of exposure to environmental contaminants, low-quality foods, and lack of access to preventive health care, poor people also are more vulnerable to chronic diseases.

Epidemiologic transition describes the pattern of countries that have passed from a predominance of infectious diseases to a greater weight of chronic or degenerative disease, such as cancer or heart disease. Although rich people are less vulnerable to infectious diseases, it is not the case that poor people do not suffer from chronic diseases. In fact, poor people in both developing and developed countries have higher rates of noncommunicable diseases than the well-to-do (Phillips et al. 1992, 285). Poor countries have made some progress in reducing infant mortality and other deaths from infectious disease. People are living longer and so face the chronic diseases that generally have later onset. The same lack of access to good food, safe environment, or preventive medical care that puts poor people at greater risk of infectious and parasitic diseases makes them vulnerable to chronic, degenerative diseases. Poor women cannot easily get Pap smears or mammograms. Poor people do not get dietary counseling for diabetes or medication for hypertension. The notion of epidemiologic transition suggests that when heart disease, diabetes, cancer, stroke, and violence become the leading killers, a country has left behind the ancient scourges. On the contrary, there is more of an epidemiologic accumulation in which infectious and parasitic diseases remain along with chronic, degenerative diseases (Franco Agudelo 1988, 316).

In sum, poor health is encouraged by poverty and is aggravated by the lack of access to health services that the poor suffer. Improvements can be made by addressing income or health care or both. Specifically, health can be improved by increasing income, improving the distribution of income, expanding the sanitary infrastructure, and raising the quality and quantity of health service delivery. Significant improvements can be made in health, even in a poor country, as long as the resources are well directed. In the absence of economic improvement or as a short-run policy, preventive health programs work best. In the long run, improvements in living standards will have the greater impact on health outcomes (Terris 1991, 375).

Argentina as a Case Study

A doctor in a Buenos Aires slum asked me why I had not chosen Bolivia as the site for this study. After all, Bolivia has the lowest life expectancy in South America and is the second poorest country on the continent. It is true that in Bolivia I could demonstrate that poverty breeds disease and underdevelopment. Argentina, however, provides an even clearer example of the effects of poverty and underdevelopment on health. Even though Argentina has much higher average income and is much better endowed with medical infrastructure, the poor suffer as the poor do in Bolivia. In this environment of relative affluence, the poor still live in shacks, drink contaminated water, and lack medical care that is available to those who are better off. In Argentina, because of its relative affluence, we can isolate health as an economic, more than a medical, problem.

Argentina has more doctors per dollar of GDP than any other country in the world and more doctors per inhabitant than any other country except Israel. Buenos Aires has the very latest medical technology six months after it is available in the United States. Teams of surgeons in Buenos Aires can replace and repair severed limbs and conduct multiple-organ transplants. Two Argentines have received the Nobel Prize for medicine, and one for chemistry.

Almost everything a modern city should have, Buenos Aires has. In spite of its fine medical infrastructure, Argentina also has many things it should not. There are 25,000 lepers and, every year, 800 new cases of leprosy in Argentina. Twenty thousand child deaths a year are from avoidable causes, such as summer diarrhea—nothing exotic, not cholera, just summer diarrhea.

Argentina cultivates the image of a First World country inexplicably fallen on hard times. It is an Argentine obsession to appear to be First World. A Buenos Aires newspaper ran a banner headline because a minor visiting dignitary from Britain remarked, "Argentina is already in the First World." But Argentina is a Third World country in most respects, and its poverty and related health problems are representative of those of its neighbors in Latin America and, although different in degree, those of Africa and Asia as well. It is not unkindness on my part to want to deny Argentines the dubious honor of being in the First World. There are many countries like Argentina, with a veneer of modernity in their capital cities, whose development is held back by the poverty of the majority. The solutions to underdevelopment require unmasking the true condition of the population. Throughout this book, I describe conditions that are clearly Third World. The revelations may embarrass and infuriate many Argentines. Let us hope they also will stimulate change.

The economic crisis since 1980 has shown the fragility of Argentina's social infrastructure and the vulnerability of its middle and working classes. Infant mortality rates, generally considered an indicator of development, have been falling steadily around the world because of a few simple medical interventions advocated by the World Health Organization and UNICEF, including vaccinations, oral rehydration therapy, breastfeeding education, and prenatal checkups. In Argentina in the 1980s, however, infant mortality rates not only slowed their descent but actually began to climb. The deterioration of Argentina's health care system began twenty years earlier. Life expectancy already was falling in the 1960s. From 1960 to 1970, it fell 0.78 year, or 0.08 year per year. In the rankings in Latin America, Argentina had the highest life expectancy in 1940 and 1960. By 1970, Argentina had fallen behind Cuba, Costa Rica, and Panama (Accinelli and Müller 1978, 6, 8).

In countless ways, Argentina is representative of Third World conditions. One-third of the population live in housing with serious deficiencies. Access to clean water is worse for the poor in Argentina than in many African countries. Argentina, like most Third World countries, allocates its medical resources to a curative, urban, hospital-based system that does not adequately address the problems endemic to poverty. The regional distribution of health resources in Argentina is similar to that in most other Third World countries (but also to certain parts of the United States). While the ratio of doctors per person for the country as a whole (1:420) is one of the highest in the world, the distribution of doctors among the provinces and within provinces and between rural and urban areas is uneven. The city of La Plata, the capital of Buenos Aires Province and the seat of the University of La Plata medical school, has 1 doctor for every 150 inhabitants. The county of Moreno, part of the impoverished suburban sprawl of Greater Buenos Aires, has 1 doctor for every 2,000 residents (Katz and Muñoz 1988, 23), the same as Guatemala (OPS 1988, 30). In the Argentine interior provinces of Chaco and Salta, in indigenous communities and other marginalized populations, the ratio is 5,000 or more persons per doctor (Katz and Muñoz 1988, 24). In the Americas, only Haiti and Guyana have worse coverage (OPS 1988, 32, 34).

Highlighted in Argentina is the economic problem of choice: how a society uses its limited resources. Argentina has the resources, even in the midst of crisis, to provide sanitation and preventive health care to everyone, but it chooses not to allocate resources to public health. There are affordable solutions to health concerns. The ailments affecting the majority of the population can be identified, and practical solutions found. Basic health protection is not a scientific problem. It is a political and economic problem of how to make the benefits of scientific and technical advances reach all of the population (Neri 1987, 178). Argentina has doctors, hospitals, and equipment, but they are not available to the poor. Chile, Costa Rica, Panama, and Venezuela all spend ten times as much per capita on health as Argentina (OPS 1988, 211). All four countries have lower GDPs and lower GDP per capita than Argentina.

Spending for medical care is only part of the solution. Every day, public health facilities are inundated with waves of poor people with avoidable diseases and injuries. Their homes, their water systems, their jobs, the government's indifference, and, fundamentally, their poverty rob them of their potential and short-change the economy.

Part of the problem in identifying health problems is that information about health is highly political. Mortality rates, outbreaks of infectious disease, vaccination coverage, and other health data reflect on the success or failure of government policies as well as on the achievement of the coveted First World status. The data also have an economic impact if they suggest a level of economic well-being that would invite foreign investment. Consequently, governments provide false information to the public, to the press, and to international organizations. The data in the major annual reports of the World Bank, the United Nations Development Program (UNDP), and UNICEF have an aura of official validity, which then gives the fictitious data a life of their own.

The UNDP has devised an index of human development intended to counteract the false impression given by ranking countries solely by GDP per capita when their distribution of income, treatment of women and minorities, or other social factors create a living hell for the majority of the people. The new index, however, is subject to the weakness of data collected from national agencies. Argentina is ranked in the high category for human development, but the data behind that ranking in the same *Human Development Reports* are known to be incorrect. The international organizations are constrained to a certain extent in the degree to which they can differ with or criticize host countries. Their goals within a country cannot be met if they alienate the host. Officials of both UNICEF and the Pan American Health Organization told me that they were unable to accomplish anything in Argentina because they were blocked by the Argentine government. The United Nations' *Human Development Report 1995* reports measles vaccination coverage for Argentina for the period 1990 to 1993 to have been 95 percent of one-year-olds. That is impossible, and everybody working in public health in Argentina knows it. In 1990, Argentina did not buy any vaccines. It was the only country in the world not to buy vaccines, despite the efforts of UNICEF to explain the epidemic cycle of measles to Argentine health officials. Not surprisingly, Argentina had a serious measles epidemic in 1991. Numerous reports from doctors in the field tell of disease outbreaks that were covered up by the government, including a diphtheria outbreak in Misiones Province, whooping cough deaths in the Federal Capital, neonatal tetanus deaths, and the inability to obtain vaccines in the provinces for periods of many months (Rodríguez 1990, 750). Official data serve the short-term goals of the administration but not the interests of public health.

The Extent of Poverty in Argentina Today

It is important to recognize the extent and the severity of poverty in Argentina, both to assess Argentina's own possibilities for development and to judge the usefulness of Argentina as a case study of poverty in the Third World. Successfully packaged by top-flight public relations firms, Argentina receives good press in European and North American newspapers and magazines. Business economists see the possibility of fortunes to be made there. Like the speculators who have dominated the Argentine economy for decades, they have a limited perspective on economic prospects. In the short run, emerging capital markets can ignore the crushing poverty around them. Ultimately, the rosy forecasts for the "new tiger" of South America will cross paths with the more than ten million people whose hunger and disease make them unable to enter the labor force in a productive capacity.

Poverty is not new in Argentina. There are millions of people whose families have always been poor because they are part of the underdeveloped side of the Argentine economy. The census refers to those people as the "structurally poor." In addition, as poverty increases in Argentina, there now are many "newly impoverished," as they are called in census data. They used to belong to Argentina's middle class, white-collar workers in the public and private sectors and unionized industrial workers.[1]

Per capita income fell steadily from 1970 to 1990. According to World Bank figures, poverty doubled between 1980 and 1989 (*Buenos Aires Herald*, November 16, 1993, p. 11). Not only did the incidence of poverty double in the 1980s, but the proportion of people living in "extreme" poverty multiplied eightfold, and the percentage of "openly unemployed" increased fourfold (*Clarín*, November 21, 1993, p. 6).

Census figures for 1988 indicate four million people in Greater Buenos Aires, or 50.3 percent of the population of the nineteen counties surrounding the Federal Capital, living in poverty (INDEC 1989, 24–25). The situation continued to deteriorate for the poor after Carlos Menem assumed the presidency in 1989. In 1993, the bottom 29 percent of the income distribution earned 4 percent of income, compared with the 7 percent they earned in 1986 (Soltys 1994*a*, 3).

Real wages have fallen absolutely and as a share of national income. Wages and salaries were 47 percent of national income in 1975 but by 1981 were only 33 percent (Torrado 1986, 15) and by 1995 just 22 percent (Medina 1992*b*, 20). The spectacular rise in rents in 1991 and 1992 aggravated the already menacing pauperization of the middle class (*Buenos Aires Herald*, March 25, 1992, p. 10). Teachers and civil servants are joining the millions who never have known anything but poverty.

Unemployment is the chief cause of increasing poverty in the 1990s. The two periods of hyperinflation in mid-1989 and early 1990 caused unemployment to increase sharply. Surveys in Greater Buenos Aires (GBA) show what the hyperinflation meant at the neighborhood level. In four areas of GBA, among people living in "extreme poverty," unemployment increased from the usual 38 percent to 58 percent and 60 percent during the first and second hyperinflations. The structure of employment also changed with the crisis. Of persons working after the second hyperinflation, 72 percent were in the informal sector, compared to 47 percent before hyperinflation. Of those employed, 10 percent were in skilled jobs, compared to 20 percent before. People working *changas* (getting odd jobs in a shape-up) increased from 20 percent to 32 percent of the employed. People working in *cirujeo* (picking over garbage) increased from 3 percent to 8 percent of the work force, the largest percentage increase of any job category (Aguirre 1991, 18–19).

The official unemployment rates for 1995 showed 20 percent unemployment and 11 percent underemployment nationally, with significant variation among the regions. Unemployment dipped slightly in early 1996 but then rose again sharply. The government attempted to withhold the true unemployment figures until after the May 1996 midterm elections, but the actual condition of the poor came to the surface when the bishop of Rosario reported the growing number of people in his diocese whose diet consists of rats, grubs, slugs, and garbage.

It is extremely difficult for the poor to enter the formal economy. They live in squatter slums and remain isolated from the mainstream of Argentine society. Budget cutbacks have gutted an educational system that already had failed to integrate many of the poor. Primary school is a half-day program that goes through seventh grade. Nationally, more than one-half of the adult population have not finished primary school. That is not merely a reflection of an aged population who did not attend school in the early part of the century. Looking at children nationwide who entered school in 1971, more than 50 percent never finished primary school. In four provinces, over 70 percent of that age group never finished primary school. Only Buenos Aires Province, the most prosperous, had a much lower proportion (about one-third) who never finished primary (Manzanal and Rofman 1989, 60).

A government survey in 1985 found one-third of the adult population was either absolutely or functionally illiterate. The Menem government chooses not to count functionally illiterate adults. They report only 5 percent of the population as illiterate, a figure that does not include the 1.5 million adults who never went to school, another half million whose school attendance was unknown in the last census, and five million who abandoned school after just a few years. The Menem administration trumpets the fact that Argentina was ranked highly by UNESCO for literacy. UNESCO's ranking, however, relied on the erroneous data supplied by the Menem government (*Clarín*, December 12, 1993, Educación, pp. 2–3).

The majority of children in Argentina today are poor, and the majority of the poor are children. In Greater Buenos Aires, more than 60 percent of the children live in poverty. In a country of thirty-three million people, there are four million poor between the ages of six and eighteen. UNICEF and the International Labor Organization reported in 1993 that about 200,000 children between the ages of ten and fourteen, 6 percent of the population that age, were working on the streets and on farms. That is not high compared to countries such as Brazil, where 19 percent of adolescents are estimated to be street children, but it still amounts to an enormous waste of the country's resources (*Buenos Aires Herald*, November 19, 1993, p. 10). Argentina will not be able to compete in a modern world market with children who have spent their early teenage years in the streets and out of school. The backwardness of the economy pushes those children into the streets. Organized criminals live off the children's begging and prostitution, which bring in thirty or so pesos each per day (*Clarín*, December 10, 1993, p. 47).

Wage and salary workers also are hard hit by this economic crisis because of the persistent inflation that has raised the cost of living well above the average wage. In June 1992, the minimum expenses for a family of four in extreme poverty, eating one meal a day, were 881 pesos a month ($881 at the overvalued exchange rate). Average pay for the same month was 340 pesos for an unskilled industrial worker, 610 pesos for a skilled machine operator, and 622 pesos for a bilingual secretary (*Clarín*, June 7, 1992, Suplemento Económico, p. 10). Store clerks earned 450 pesos and bank clerks 600 pesos (*Clarín*, May 10, 1992, Suplemento Económico, p. 7). Pay scales for blue-collar government workers were even worse. Skilled forklift operators in the port of Buenos Aires were making 150 pesos a month for full-time work (María Teresa de Bravo, personal communication, March 1992).

The structurally poor in rural areas have no land. Some work as sharecroppers or seasonal farm workers. In urban and suburban areas, the last twenty years of economic crisis and the adjustment policies have marginalized both the structurally poor and the former lower middle class. They work at *changas* or as *cuentapropistas* (working for themselves), but that can mean selling tissue packs and pencils on street corners. The men also work as unskilled laborers in construction and the women as domestics. In border towns, importers pay no duty on goods carried across the border. So the *changa* there for men, women, and children is to carry loads through customs of as much as eighty pounds of goods on their heads for twenty-five cents a trip (Pazos 1992, 32). For decades, people have tried to get by in the informal sector, but the informal economy is saturated. There have been numerous closings of kiosks (tiny cigarette and candy stands, often run from the window of a house), many small-business failures, and the displacement of small food stores by large chains.

The vulnerability of the poor is seen in the proportion who, with or without work, have no social insurance coverage. That means no unemployment compensation, workers' compensation, health coverage, or pensions. In the Greater Buenos Aires area, at least 40 percent of the population have no coverage. In five other provinces, more than 50 percent of the population are not covered. In Formosa, a part of the undeveloped north, more than 70 percent of the population have no coverage. Even those figures overstate the population covered, because some people are double-counted when families have two working members.

Poverty continues to hold back Argentina's development. Roughly 40 percent of the population of Argentina live in poverty. Their work is unstable, their homes are precarious, their water supply is contaminated, and they have no health insurance. Argentines are searching for a way out of the stagnation that has plagued their economy for decades. The economy will remain mired in backwardness as long as its human resources are squandered. Chapter 2 examines the history of Argentina, in particular the missed opportunities for developing human resources.

A Note on Cultural Criticism

It has become unpopular to refer to countries or cultures as backward, and with good reason. Scholars from the industrial countries wrote much of the earlier literature on backwardness, the development economics of the 1950s, literature that was often arrogant, racist, and self-congratulatory. Dependency theory in the 1960s moved the debate forward by emphasizing the relationship between rich and poor and the role of imperialism in distorting peripheral economies. The weakness of dependency theory is that it puts all of the blame for poverty on external forces and fails to recognize the internal structure of poor societies as an impediment to development. A corollary feature of the 1960s was the emergence of liberation movements that were important in raising the issue of the dignity of people of color, women, and other groups. But a product of the wedding of the dependency and liberation movements was that scholarship was overwhelmed by cultural relativism.

Scholars of all kinds—anthropologists, economists, sociologists—should be careful in judging other societies by their own cultural standards. That is not the same as surrendering all judgment. Scholars (and other citizens) should judge societies, their own and others, by a standard of whether those societies advance or retard the dignity and well-being of their people. Cultures that throw young girls into volcanoes are not as fulfilling for humans as ones that do not practice human sacrifice, of this or a modern variety. Societies that practice genital mutilation or make women and girls wear metal masks so no man can see their faces, with the implicit notion of women's untrustworthiness, degrade both women and men. Cultures that make women feel so bad about their shapes that they starve themselves or allow doctors to implant dangerous substances into their bodies are not fully dignifying cultures. Countries so riddled with corruption that even medicine for child cancer patients is fair game for counterfeiting should be criticized. The criticism does not imply that the society in question is all bad nor that the critic's society is all good. The United States is a country of enormous resources and accomplishments, yet it throws some children on the garbage heap, both literally and figuratively.

In examining its history and some of the cultural aspects that impinge on the health of the poor, I am very critical of Argentina. This should not be interpreted as a lack of respect or affection for the people. The Argentines have enormous capacity. If I were not critical of the failures of their institutions, I would be guilty of patronizing a people I consider capable of solving their own problems. My choice of Argentina as a case study also does not imply that it is, by any means, the worst case. That is the tragedy in this story: there are scores of countries in which conditions are much worse than those in Argentina.

Two

Argentine History
and Society

At the beginning of the twentieth century, Argentina was one of the twelve richest countries in the world. Argentina's economy was growing rapidly, and members of its wealthy class were very, very rich. The twentieth century appeared to promise high living standards and sustained growth; the subsequent decline of Argentina has been a paradox to historians and economists.

An ongoing debate over what went wrong in Argentina has not answered why an apparently promising economy, with a relatively well educated population, the most even distribution of income in Latin America, and the largest middle class, became the economic and political clown of stop-go policies and military musical chairs. After a half century of decline, Argentina is a veritable theme park for macroeconomists, because everything that can go wrong there already has. Hyperinflation, massive unemployment, irresponsible expansion of the money supply (in fact, coexistence of several money supplies), huge federal deficits, and now, draconian structural adjustment policies—Argentina has it all.

Virtually all those engaged in the debate over Argentina's collapse have begun from the premise that the country is richly endowed in natural resources. Many have argued that it was bad policy that doomed Argentina (in particular, beginning in the era of Perón), or that it was the imperialist machinations of England and the United States that undermined a sound development strategy. Alternative explanations expand the debate but still adhere to the notion of a rich country fallen on hard times. Those analyses perpetuate several fallacies, including Argentina's presumed wealth of resources and the assumption that its institutional base in 1900 could have supported continuing growth and development. The reasons for Argentina's failure to thrive are complex and stem from many factors, including a narrow resource base, its Iberian cultural and political legacy, bad policies, and external obstacles. The result is an economy with many features of modernity whose growth is blocked by underdeveloped institutions and the poverty of half of the population.

Argentines have nurtured the belief in Argentina as a First World country, but that belief has interfered with understanding the nature of the development problem the country faces. The economic and political crises of the 1970s and 1980s were not anomalies. They were symptoms of the chronic backwardness of a country that is First World only on a few boulevards of Buenos Aires.

The Land and Its Resources

Argentina is the eighth-largest country in the world and extends from the tropics to subarctic Tierra del Fuego.[1] Buenos Aires, the federal capital, is a city of three million people in a metropolitan area of eleven million, situated on the Río de la Plata (the River Plate), an estuary of the Atlantic Ocean. There are four distinct geographic zones in Argentina: the pampa, the riverine northeast, the arid northwest and west, and the Patagonian desert of the south. (See map of Argentina.)

The pampa is a flat grassland with adequate rainfall and rich soil, excellent for growing grain and pasturing cattle. The pampa covers 30 percent of the territory of Argentina and has almost 70 percent of the population. The humid pampa extends in an arc for about 400 miles around Buenos Aires. Beyond that, to the west and the south, the land becomes drier and ultimately desert.

The Northeast is an extremely poor and undeveloped subtropical area. The province of Misiones (named after the Jesuit missions of the eighteenth century) extends fingerlike between Paraguay and Brazil and produces lumber, yerba, tea, tung, and subsistence food crops. The province of Corrientes, low lying along two rivers, is subject to flooding. Its main products are rice, cattle, and sheep. Formosa and Chaco, the poorest provinces, lie to the west of the Paraguay River. Impenetrable scrub brush covers one-third of the Gran Chaco geographical region (a part of which is even called El Impenetrable). The more hospitable riverine areas of Formosa and Chaco produce cattle and soybeans. Cotton is grown in the middle one-third of the region. Drier areas have been cleared and overgrazed, resulting in an ecological imbalance that has serious health effects. (See Chapter 4, "Chagas' Disease.")

The entire western border of Argentina is formed by the high Andes Mountains, which produce a rain shadow effect, blocking moisture for the length of the country. The Northwest stretches from the *altiplano*, or high plateau of the Andes, to lowlands bordered by the Gran Chaco and the dry pampa. Almost the entire region, consisting of the provinces of Jujuy, Salta, Catamarca, La Rioja, Santiago del Estero, and Tucumán, is arid, underdeveloped and chronically poor.

The central western zone, called Cuyo, consists of Mendoza, San Juan, and San Luis. Irrigation has played a critical role in developing Cuyan agriculture. Without irrigation, the land in Cuyo is useful only for grazing goats and cattle. Mendoza stands out in the interior as a relatively prosperous province due to its irrigated vineyards for wine production.

Patagonia is a cold desert that has been overexploited for sheepherding. It now has some oil production and fruit cultivation in the northern river valleys. The provinces of Santa Cruz, Tierra del Fuego, Chubut, Neuquén, and Río Negro make up Patagonia, which comprises 28 percent of the land of Argentina but has only 4.5 percent of the population (INDEC 1991a, 19, 22).[2]

The reality is that Argentina is not well endowed in resources. The fertile pampa produces goods (corn, wheat, beef, oilseeds) that made Argentine landowners wealthy at the turn of the century but that no longer command high prices on world markets. The rest of the country is quite unproductive, or would be without expensive and ecologically harmful clearing, irrigation, and soil degradation. Most of the agriculture of the interior was promoted by tariff protection, which now is being eliminated. Argentina has some oil but few other mineral resources.[3]

The myth of Argentine resource wealth plays a perverse dual role in the national psyche. Argentines are proud of the country's supposed natural wealth, based on what they see on the pampa. The fact that the country has not developed economically engenders a sense of failure and inferiority when Argentines compare themselves with countries that are presumed to have a similar resource base, such as Canada and Australia. A joke Argentines tell on themselves evokes this duality: When God was allocating resources to the various countries, the angels complained that Argentina was getting too much. God replied, "Wait 'til you see the people I'm going to put there." This self-image as fractious, argumentative squanderers of a rich resource base prevents Argentines from recognizing the poverty of the country or appreciating Argentina's real achievements.

Ambitious subsidy programs to develop the interior have not taken into account the poverty of resources, the political and economic backwardness of the interior, and the limits on development they both imply. That backwardness is evident in the sketch of Argentine history given in the next section. Argentina has more in common with its South American neighbors than with First World countries. There are some notable differences, including the flourishing of the Argentine medical infrastructure in the 1890s and the late 1940s. The existence of that medical infrastructure only strengthens the argument of this book, that the health of the poor is an economic problem, not a technical problem. The Argentine poor are menaced by leprosy, tuberculosis, cholera, and other diseases of poverty, as are their counterparts in the rest of the developing world.

History of the Argentine Political Economy

The brief history of Argentina given here focuses on the characteristics of the Argentine economy that contribute to its poverty. It also surveys the development of health care services in the context of other economic events. Argentina became a politically unified country only in the 1860s, and a national economy emerged in the decades that followed. From 1890 to 1914, exports of wool, beef, and grain gave Argentina the world's highest rate of economic growth. The country attempted to maintain the momentum by exploiting the land and by inward-oriented development behind a high tariff wall. External factors, including two world wars, the Great Depression, and stagnant postwar demand for its traditional exports, limited Argentina's options. Policy mistakes compounded the weaknesses of an economy that was modern only in the coastal pampa. Urban industrial workers and rural peasants supported the populist movement of Juan Perón in the mid-twentieth century. A small increase in the share of national income going to workers and recognition for union representation led to a half-century of conflict among competing interests. The expectation that the resources of the country should provide an easy living led Argentines to fight among themselves over the redivision of the national product rather than looking outward to a world economy that was fast outpacing an isolated and stagnant Argentina. Each new regime tried to lay claim to wealth that no longer was being produced. Special privileges, in the form of tariff protection, subsidies, government favors to business friends, or, in the case of trade union leaders, lucrative pension plans to pillage, were surrogates for real investment or expansion of output. As the economy worsened, the struggle became more brutal, descending finally into a bloody, secret war with tens of thousands of casualties. The debt crisis of the 1980s was another phase in Argentina's struggle to redivide a shrinking output. The structural adjustment program implemented in Argentina does not address some of the historical weaknesses of the economy—a speculative propensity, corruption, rent seeking, and a narrow base for purchasing power. The national government has failed to promote the long-term interests of the country.

Colonial Days and Caudillos, 1536 to 1860

Argentina was thinly populated when the Spanish first settled the area. The goal of early Spanish colonization in the Americas was the extraction of precious metals. Consequently, what is now Argentina was unimportant in the early years and only provided mules from Salta for the silver mines of Potosí (Bolivia). Argentina was part of the Upper Peru viceroyalty of the Spanish Empire. Buenos Aires was first established in the sixteenth century, but only in the late eighteenth century did it emerge as an important port, as a conduit for smuggling European goods behind imperial tariff barriers. Spain created a new viceroyalty of the River Plate in 1776, with Buenos Aires as its capital, to control the illicit trade.

The Spanish imperial system was based on tribute, which encouraged extractive industries, such as mining, over those that developed the land. Labor practices in much of the Spanish colonial world were precapitalist, including several forms of forced labor for indigenous peoples. Even manufacturing in early Buenos Aires used nonwage labor in coercive arrangements (Rock 1985, xxv–xxvi). Although slavery was officially abolished with Independence, the practice of forced labor continued in the interior until the days of Perón in the 1940s.

Argentine independence was declared in 1810 but not secured until 1817. Independence was not equivalent to the establishment of a nation-state as a coherent economic and political entity. It would take forty-five years of fighting and some fortuitous external events to provide that cohesion. Even then, the country would be wracked by continuing revolts until the end of the nineteenth century.

The years 1816 to 1853 were dominated by violence and rule by local *caudillos* (strongmen). The economy was based on hunting cattle that had run wild from the early settlements. They were used for hides and later for salted beef. Most of the interior, including much of the pampa, had not been wrested from the indigenous population. The various leaders of the port of Buenos Aires and its hinterland, whether *caudillo*, governor, or triumvirate, were not really national leaders, and neither the economy nor the political structure conformed to a modern nation-state.

By 1861, Argentina was far behind the industrializing world, and its distance from Europe and the United States made Argentina peripheral to the growing world economy. In the 1860s, when U.S. mills had already turned out 10,000 miles of railroad track and the United States had hundreds of textile factories, the Argentine economy essentially was based on hunting cattle and sheepherding.

In spite of the liberal ideas embedded in the constitution (modeled in part on that of the United States), the cult of personalism pervaded Argentine political culture. Reliance on the *caudillo* frustrated both democracy and economic development. Argentina remained an outsider to the economic and political transformation of Europe and North America. The failure of civic maturation rendered the Argentine mood pessimistic, except when rallied by xenophobia and nationalism (Calvert and Calvert 1989, 47).

Formation of a Nation-State, 1861 to 1890

It was not until 1861 that a nation-state began to emerge. In that year, the blockade of the South in the United States during the Civil War led to a skyrocketing price of fibers, making Argentine wool a valuable export. War with

Paraguay produced another boom in 1865 and helped to consolidate government control over northwest Argentina. The wool boom and the war, combined with the pacification of the pampa in the late 1870s in the Campaign of the Desert, formed the basis for a national economy. By 1876, the railroad reached beyond the pampa to Tucumán, and grain exports from the pampa soared. Refrigerated ships made frozen and chilled beef a significant export by the 1890s.

Land Ownership and Exploitation. Argentine political philosophers, influenced by European liberal ideas dating back to the 1780s, had argued for the settlement of the country by yeoman farmers. Instead, the pampa and parts of the interior were settled through the granting of huge estates to generals who had served in the Campaign of the Desert. Equally important was the sale of federal land in the interior in huge blocks, the largest of which was the size of Massachusetts, Connecticut, and Rhode Island combined. Those large land grants and sales to people already well connected and well off are considered the original sin, the missed opportunity in Argentine history (Halperín 1986, 43).

Besides concentrated land ownership, the way the pampa developed gives an insight into the later structure of the Argentine economy. In the last quarter of the nineteenth century, the large landowners rented their land to immigrant sharecroppers in four- to seven-year leases. The sharecropper would break the sod, grow grain, and, when the lease was up, sow alfalfa and move on. The landowners got alfalfa pastures with no investment on their part. Even the plowing and harvesting were contracted out, so the landlords did not invest in equipment. Most landlords were purely rentiers. Their tenants had very low fixed investment, as one would expect; consequently, their productivity was very low (Tulchin 1986, 34). Short-term profit maximization by the tenants led to farming methods that hastened the destruction of the soil. Government agricultural research and rural education were lacking. Natural resource exploitation rather than development and a reliance on windfall profits from nature rather than investment characterized the actions of owners, tenants, and government alike (Solberg 1987, 58, 65, 229).

The concentration of land ownership and its manner of exploitation reflected and reinforced the importance of connections rather than effort or productive investment. Status is accorded in Argentina to persons of "important last names," deriving from the great landed estates. Being a member of the landed rich or one of their descendants is what matters. *Ser,* to be in Spanish, is what counts. *Hacer,* to do, is not important. Breaking the sod, building the infrastructure, and developing agriculture were not tasks to engender prestige (Fillol 1961, 14–16).

The lack of investment in corollary industries negated the advantages of flexibility and low fixed costs of the pampean system. For example, the port of Buenos Aires was not mechanized when port cities of other nations modernized their loading systems. Consequently, port charges at the time were 6.5 times as much in Buenos Aires as in Montreal, a chief competitor. Grain had to be loaded in jute bags, which added 4 percent to the price of wheat (Solberg 1987, 125, 141). The lack of investment in the land, the absence of an agricultural extension service, and the failure to mechanize the port reflected the notion that land wealth was enough. The Argentines did not see land wealth as an advantage to be developed through corollary investment. An overdeveloped sense of destiny and expectation of ease is the legacy that still afflicts Argentine development.

Fate. The structure of the Argentine economy encouraged the view that human beings are passive recipients of nature's bounty or nature's curse, that effort is pointless, and waiting for good fortune is rational. When the fates control your life, you are subjugated by nature and must accept the inevitable. Argentines can feel blessed by nature in the fertility of the pampa and, at the same time, cheated of the wealth that was supposed to flow effortlessly from that fertility. The stifling effect of this fatalism on human productivity is strengthened by the importance of *ser* over *hacer.* People are judged by what they have inherited, by their lot in life. Consequently, professional work is not esteemed and lacks a sense of purpose. The process of education is depreciated. Helping one's friends at university (connections) is more important than the effort of study. A corollary of the role of fate and of *ser* is that getting caught in misdeeds is a matter of bad luck, not justice (Fillol 1961, 9, 16, 20). Indeed, disgraced officials keep resurfacing in other positions of public trust.[4]

The "Other." Perhaps the most important implication of being at the mercy of fate and a supernatural environment is the view it contains of other human actors. When the fates control your life, the elements of your environment are hostile. Argentines view their neighbors as potentially dangerous and assume that other people envy their prosperity and wish them harm. Suspicion is thought to be a reasonable attitude toward nonintimates (Fillol 1961, 9). Since only the inner circle can be trusted, it is a group that needs to be cultivated and protected. Because no one on the outside matters, everyone is an enemy in a sense. Consequently, the level of civility among strangers in stores, on the street, or in traffic is low.

In the political realm, hostility toward the "other" has inhibited the development of a national consciousness, of a citizenry, and of a constructive political dialogue. Calls for unity based on nationalism stress the Argentine versus the outsider (the Chilean, British, Paraguayan, or Brazilian threat or U.S. imperialism) rather than the Argentine as citizen. Even the appeal of solidarity is not a national clarion. It is a class-based rallying cry, generally restricted to the unionized sector of the working class. The absence of a notion of citizenship facilitated the rationale for violence from both the right and the left in the chaos years of the 1970s and the military regime of 1976 to 1983. That same lack of civic identity allows the sacrifice of the lower third to half of the income pyramid in the economic adjustment schemes of the 1990s. The perceived hostile environment fostered by superstition made Argentina a cauldron, rather than a melting pot.

Increase in Immigration. The growth of the Argentine economy encouraged a flood of European, especially Italian, immigration in the second half of the nineteenth century. The ratio of immigrants to receiving population was the highest ever recorded for any country in the modern era, much higher than in the United States. Most of the immigrants were men. Buenos Aires became the most important destination for the white slave traffic from about 1880 to 1920, raising alarm in Europe. In France and in eastern Europe, the "road to Buenos Aires" meant sale into prostitution for poor women and girls in the late 1800s (Londres 1928).

The population of Buenos Aires increased more than sevenfold between 1855 and 1895 and doubled again by 1910, to 1.3 million. Housing, the sanitary infrastructure, and hospital facilities were inadequate for the waves of European immigrants the city absorbed in those decades. Until the 1870s, when the first trams were built, construction was confined to a small area of the city. One-fifth of the population lived in *conventillos*, or tenements, whole families to a room with several families sharing a kitchen. The paving of city streets became a priority because most had been cobbled over garbage fill. The putrefaction of animal and vegetable matter released noxious gases and contributed to higher rates of epidemic outbreaks in those neighborhoods where garbage had been used to fill the streets (Escudé 1989, 61–62).

The low level of sanitation and the high rate of influx of immigrants contributed to recurrent epidemics from 1850 to 1900, including smallpox (1852), yellow fever (1852, 1857, 1858, and 1871), cholera (1867, 1868, 1886, 1887, and 1890), typhus (1862–1864 and 1868–1871), measles (four outbreaks), dysentery (seven outbreaks), scarlet fever, diphtheria, and plague. In 1871, nearly 12 percent of the city's population died, a large proportion from yellow fever (Escudé 1989, 62).

By the 1880s, it was clear that the meager resources applied to public health were insufficient, and high death rates from infectious diseases threatened to discourage immigration. In 1861, the death rate per thousand in Buenos Aires (27.8) was slightly better than in New York (28.4). Over the next decade, New York's death rate rose to 33 per thousand in 1872, but in Buenos Aires, the rate climbed dramatically until 1871, when it reached almost 118 per thousand. From

1855 to 1869, life expectancy in Buenos Aires fell from thirty-two years to twenty-six years and still had not returned to the 1855 level by 1887 (Escudé 1989, 62, 67).

Up until 1880, the city had only three hospital beds per thousand inhabitants in public and private medical establishments. In colonial times, the viceroyalty and the Church maintained dispensaries for the isolation of those with infectious diseases. In the mid-nineteenth century, nationality-based fraternal organizations in Buenos Aires established health centers that evolved into hospitals. The first of those were the British Hospital in 1844 and the French Hospital in 1845. The Italian, Spanish, German, and Israelite Hospitals followed. A Physicians' Court judged the qualifications of physicians and surgeons practicing in the city and established norms of medical procedure. The court also initiated preventive measures against smallpox, leprosy, and tuberculosis (*Buenos Aires Herald*, July 3, 1994, Supplement, p. 4).

The immigrant flow and the epidemics of the late nineteenth century necessitated a large expansion of hospital facilities. From 1880 to 1909, the number of beds increased to over eight per thousand, with the state providing 81 percent of the funds for the hospitals. Services were free to the "solemnly" poor and inexpensive for the less poor. Nationally funded hospitals in the interior were initiated only after 1906 (Escudé 1989, 63, 64).

Several of the important hospitals in use in the 1990s date from the construction boom of the last century. In 1882, the Municipal Isolation Home opened in Buenos Aires. It was renamed the Muñiz Hospital for Infectious Diseases and is today charged with the care of AIDS patients. In 1883, the Hospital of Buenos Aires took the place of the old Hospital for Men. It became the Hospital de Clínicas General San Martín, today the main teaching hospital of the University of Buenos Aires. Other hospitals from that era still operating are the Ramos Mejía, the Rivadavia, the Argerich Military Hospital, the Ricardo Gutiérrez Children's Hospital, and the Pirovano (*Buenos Aires Herald*, July 3, 1994, Supplement, p. 3). In Mendoza, the Emilio Civit Children's Hospital, in use until 1993, dated from that era.

The other critical public health measure undertaken in the 1890s was the construction of water and sanitation systems. Street paving, hospital construction, and water and sewer systems contributed to improved health for the population. By the first decade of the twentieth century, the death rate in Buenos Aires again was lower than in New York, Philadelphia, or Montreal. Some of that advantage, however, reflected a younger population on average in Buenos Aires than in the North American cities (Escudé 1989, 67). In Buenos Aires, the improvements at the turn of the century gave the city essentially the health infrastructure it would have for the next fifty years. In the interior, sanitary infrastructure developed much later.

The Golden Age to the First Military Revolt, 1890 to 1930

The export-led growth of 1895 to 1914 financed the construction of opulent palaces, the opera house, broad avenues, and monuments, giving the heart of Buenos Aires an air of Paris of the same era. The French expression of the time to connote vast wealth was "as rich as an Argentine." The urban middle class was growing. Pressure to broaden the franchise led to a Radical Party victory in 1916, unseating the conservative forces of the landed oligarchy that had controlled the government up to that time. It appeared that Argentina could follow a modernizing path. But the golden age of Buenos Aires had much in common with the rubber boom in Manaus or the gold rush in the Klondike. Extraction of rent, rather than investment or broad-based development, characterized the golden age.

World War I and England's recession in the 1920s slowed the rate of growth of Argentine exports. The structure of Argentina's agricultural growth also stifled the economy. Land leases required the tenants to sell their crop to wholesalers, who were also credit providers. These *acopiadores* drove the farmers into debt peonage. Violent rent strikes ended in failure (Solberg 1987, 141). While North America developed an independent yeomanry that provided a market for domestic industry and a base for democratic institutions, Argentina crushed its peasantry with landlord privilege.

Profits in Argentina came from land rent and from oligopolistic quasi-rents that were the result of collusive practices and tariffs, quotas, and special permits. Much of the investment, for example, in railroads, was financed by foreign capital. Growth based on rent and foreign capital encouraged a nonproductive attitude and a speculative approach to economic activity. Industry was developed with a strategy that was collusive rather than innovation intensive, which would have required a different attitude toward organization and risk taking (di Tella 1986, 120–124).

From 1916 to 1930, the Radical Party maintained its support among the urban middle class through patronage and machine politics. To take up the slack in labor markets caused by the mechanization of agriculture, the closing of the frontier, and the lack of industry, the government employed 28 percent of the labor force by 1930 (di Tella 1986, 125). The collapse of world trade and tariff revenues in that year made it impossible to balance the budget and also maintain the patronage system and led to the nation's first successful military coup.

From 1890 to 1930, pampean cities and pampean agriculture prospered. In retrospect, however, the weaknesses are apparent: a narrow base in agriculture, concentrated land ownership, speculative and collusive investment strategies, and urban employment heavily dependent on patronage. Even so, income distribution in Buenos Aires was the most equal of Latin America, and some potential for growth was there, if as yet unexploited.

The Argentine interior was another world. *Estancieros*, who owned estates the size of Connecticut, kept peons in virtual slavery. The interior, from the beginning, was developed only by special exemption from the supposedly liberal policies of the federal government. To gain the political support of the provincial *caudillos* and to secure the border areas, the federal government sought to develop agroindustries in the interior by awarding subsidies and imposing tariffs and other trade restrictions on a number of agricultural products. From a long-run efficiency perspective, those were bad policies. But how else the interior could have developed, even to the extent it did, is another question.

The interior remained backward politically and left the construction of an infrastructure to the federal government. In spite of repeated epidemics of cholera, bubonic plague, smallpox, and dysentery, the city of Salta failed to construct a water system. Servants collected rainwater in cisterns for the well-to-do, but the rest of the population scooped their water out of drainage ditches that accumulated human and animal waste, dead animals, garbage, factory waste, and stagnant water. Butchers washed their meat in the ditches and bakers got their water there (Scobie 1988, 91, 98). That was Argentina's golden age. Indeed, they were golden years, but the gold did not extend far inland from Buenos Aires, nor did it trickle down very far in the *porteño* (Buenos Aires) population.

Presidential Musical Chairs, 1930 to 1955

A civilian regime took over from the military in 1932. With the market for its exports gone, Argentina lacked the foreign exchange for imports. The government quietly supported import substitution industrialization (ISI), a policy of promoting domestic industries to produce goods that previously were imported. ISI requires tariff protection for the infant industries and sometimes subsidies from the government budget. An overvalued currency makes imported component parts cheaper and serves as one of many subsidies to domestic industry. Supporters of ISI argue that it requires a domestic market, which implies broad purchasing power. In practice, it has meant privilege for a small urban industrial work force at the expense of rural and informal sector workers. It subsidizes protected industry at the expense of exporters, who cannot export at overvalued exchange rates. It increases, rather than decreases, the import bill because all components have to be imported. The products of ISI, sheltered from international competition, are shoddy and overpriced. Government subsidies lead to budget deficits and recurrent inflation. The large import bill and the collapse of export revenues lead to foreign exchange crises that, in concert with high inflation, make the economy unstable.

The weaknesses of ISI took some years to show up in Argentina, especially since the world economy of the 1930s offered so little competition. As a result, there was moderate growth in industry in the 1930s, and Argentina maintained its status as a middle-income country with a sizable middle class. Because the economy grew in the years of isolation and faltered in later years, some economists reasoned that it must have been imperialism that stymied Argentina's ongoing development. That argument ignored the changing international economic climate, as well as the internal obstacles to development. There is more reason to believe that precapitalist conditions in the interior, the speculative bias of domestic investors, and the political grip of the oligarchy provided sterile ground for Argentine growth. Because that growth was premised on tariff-protected industries and furthered with state enterprises that were grossly inefficient, there is no need to look for villains outside Argentina, common though they may have been.

Economic conditions in the interior by mid-century suggest some of the internal obstacles. Life had changed very little from the nineteenth century. Investigations into social conditions in Jujuy and Salta in 1942 found forced labor and inhuman conditions. One-third of the economically active population of Catamarca worked as seasonal migrants, 60 percent of whom returned home penniless, indebted to the labor contractor's company store (Rutledge 1975, 99, 106).

The isolation of the depression was alleviated somewhat with the sale of beef to Britain during World War II. But the war played a critical role in Argentina's economic future. Argentina's neutrality until March 1945 protected Britain's supplies of beef from attack by the Axis, but neutrality also suited the ideological inclination of the Argentine military. Trained by Prussian and Italian troops, the army was sympathetic to the fascists. Nevertheless, Argentina sold its most valuable asset to England in exchange for blocked (nonconvertible) sterling balances.

In spite of the concrete support to England that Argentine neutrality had afforded, the fascist sympathies of the Argentine military were not forgiven by the United States, which enforced a strict boycott of Argentina after the war. The only chink in the blockade was the continued sale of beef to Britain for blocked sterling in the years 1946 to 1948 and trade with fascist Spain. Depression, war, and then blockade isolated the economy and reinforced Argentine nationalism and chauvinism.

Juan Domingo Perón came to power in October 1945 (he was elected president in 1946), after two years in the wings. He intensified the policies of import substitution industrialization, in part because it suited the nationalism and interventionist leanings of the military, but also because Argentina was cut off from the developed world. ISI also favored urban and industrial interests at the expense of the *estancieros*. The populist rhetoric of the Perón regime necessitated some shift in the relative shares of labor, land, and capital, and the assertion of Peronist power required breaking the political grip of the old landed class.

During the Perón years (1945 to 1955), there was an increase in labor's share of national income, unions gained strength under government protection, women got the right to vote, and social programs, hospitals, and retirement protection were expanded. The populist regime of Juan Domingo Perón effected an expansion of health services under Health Minister Ramón Carrillo and the María Eva Duarte de Perón Foundation. In the Perón years, the number of hospital beds doubled and the number of health workers on government payrolls tripled. Between 1946 and 1951, the health budget increased fourfold, and the infant mortality rate decreased from eighty-four per thousand to sixty per thousand (Escudero 1987, 526). Under Carrillo's health administration, the most successful programs were those that attacked endemic diseases, including goiter, Chagas' disease, and malaria (Neri 1982, 101). The coup of 1955 that ousted Perón interrupted the Carrillo-Perón expansion of health facilities and programs.

An ironic twist in the development of public health in Argentina is that Perón both expanded public (government) health facilities and initiated a process that would undermine the public system. He empowered the unions, which later administrations made the agents and beneficiaries of a system of compulsory social security that included union-owned health plans (discussed in Chapter 7).

The real gains in public health and social services during the Perón years were not institutionalized sufficiently to be sustained by subsequent regimes with different visions of health care. The Pan American Health Organization conducted an assessment of the public health sector after Perón and concluded that it was characterized by general disorder, an oversized and bureaucratic national ministry, uncoordinated duplication of services, and corruption (Neri 1982, 103).

The Perón years were an important epoch in the formation of modern Argentina. The intense feeling for and against Perón and his wife, Eva, has barely subsided in the half century since they attempted to redirect the course of Argentina. They are detested by conservative forces because of the Peronist assault on the privilege of the landed oligarchy and their export-fed wealth. After Eva's death, Perón also incurred the wrath of the Catholic Church because Peronist mobs destroyed churches in a show of defiance against the bishops. Revisionist history recasts Perón as a defender of conservative interests because he diverted labor's strength from communist unions in the critical postwar years. Nevertheless, his populist rhetoric obscured such a role at the time.

The costs of the Perón years were class antagonisms brought to the surface in Argentine politics, bankruptcy of the state treasury and foreign reserves, a larger state apparatus, and a continuation of the political manipulation of the economy. Recessions in 1949 and 1952 caused Perón to ease up on his statist manipulation of the economy and return to more liberal economic policies. To enhance his control of the government, Perón neutralized traditional power centers (Portantiero 1989, 26). He ruined the *estancieros* by lowering commodity prices and checkmated industry by building the labor movement. The persistence of his popularity to the present day, in spite of the suffering he caused in later years, can only be attributed to the intensity of the oppression felt by the workers up to that time. With their populist rhetoric, he and Eva struck a responsive chord, even if Perón's policies were only somewhat prolabor. Their movement elevated work and the working person. That such appreciation took a factional and divisive tone is understandable in the antagonistic context in which it emerged.

Descent into Chaos, 1955 to 1976

Throughout Argentina's history, misfortune played a role in thwarting economic development, but the failure to seize opportunities may be the defining feature of Argentina's frustrated development. Among the opportunities missed was one in the year 1955, when the military deposed Perón. Ten years of Peronism had tilted the income distribution toward salaries and wages, widening the market for domestic industry. The improvement of the infrastructure (particularly in the social sector), combined with higher wages, produced an increasingly educated population that could utilize the technological advances of the postwar era. By the mid-1950s, Perón was out, the U.S. boycott was over, and Argentina could link up with the developed world's technology through freer trade.

The winners in the 1955 coup, however, took a very short sighted view of correcting what they saw as the errors of Peronism. Instead of using the progress of the Perón years as stepping stones to a modern economy, the Liberating Revolution sought revenge, by turning back the increase in workers' share of national income. Second, instead of seeing Argentina's further progress as built on investment (including investment in human capital), they continued to base the economy on skimming quasi-rents from the land and from collusive practices, including tariffs.

Reversing Wage Gains. In 1945, the share of wages in national income was 40.1 percent; by 1949, it was 49 percent. Personal consumption increased 7.5 percent per year. Between 1950 and 1955, recession and the changes in policy it forced caused wage income to fall from the 1949 high to an average 41.8 percent of gross national product (GNP). From 1956 to 1958, it averaged 39.6 percent. For the period 1959 to 1961, labor's share fell to 35.8 percent (ECLA 1969, 122, 136). That 26-percent decrease in ten years was imposed on a work force that had been empowered and politicized under Perón. The outcome was labor resentment and unrest, as well as a smaller market for domestic industry. Short-term profit taking at the expense of the working class took precedence over expansion of the domestic market and political stability, both of which would have contributed to long-term economic health. The outcome of the redivision of the national pie was eleven governments in eighteen years, including six military revolts.

De facto governments after 1955 tried to reduce the role of the state in health services that had been affirmed in the Perón years. The Pan American Health Organization suggested decentralization of the federal infrastructure to the provinces, but the attempt had to be reversed because of the lack of technical and financial capacity in the interior (Neri 1982, 104).

Although the federal government had begun to abandon the public health system in 1955, the medical infrastructure survived into the 1970s, and the quality of care and research maintained some momentum through that time. Several renowned research institutes were founded in the early 1900s, and others were established by Carrillo in the late 1940s. Those institutes supported research, publishing, conferences, and medical attention, which they were unable to maintain when federal funds were withdrawn. Among the casualties were the National Institute of Endocrinology, founded in 1947 and closed in 1966, and the Model Institute of Clinical Medicine, founded in 1914 and closed in 1978 (Pasqualini 1988, 107–108).

The most important health care innovation of the post-Perón era was the emphasis on the social security system, the *obras sociales*, that had its origins in the mutual systems of railroad workers. After 1955, the social security system gradually was extended to those unions that were recognized during the Perón years. The *obras sociales* constituted a fundamental ideological shift from the concept of health as a right of citizens (or at least as a begrudging duty of the government to curtail epidemics) to health care as a component of the wage package. In addition to the ability to buy food, clothing, and shelter, labor's incentives (in the formal sector) now included medical care. In 1970, membership in the *obras sociales* became compulsory for those employed in the formal sector (Isuani and Mercer 1986, 18).

That approach to medical care contributed in another way to social stability, anticipated or not by its creators. A stratified social security system impedes social action around health care issues. Under such a system, the means of acquiring medical care is an individual action—getting the right job—rather than political action for broad coverage. In other words, "the blame is perceived to rest with the individual for not having the right job, not with the state for failing to provide a universal service" (Ward 1986, 128).

Expanding Protectionism. The other missed opportunity in 1955 was in not dismantling the expensive, inefficient system of subsidizing and protecting both industry and agriculture. The military, from 1955 to 1958, and the civilian administration, from 1958 to 1961, continued and even strengthened ISI, relying on high tariffs and subsidies for private industry, and maintained state ownership of much industry. By the 1960s, Argentina had one of the most protected economies in the world.

Low productivity in key industries stifled the rest of the economy. Well into the

1990s, Argentina was attempting to compete in world markets in the telecommunications age with a phone system that was available to only a small percentage of the population and that was pathetically unreliable.[5] Run by political cronies, state industries kept no balance sheets nor any record of how much they were spending. They just spent it, and the government printed the money they needed (José Martínez de Hoz, November 23, 1989). Private industry was not much better. High tariff walls protected goods that were shoddy and out of date. Exports stagnated because few other countries wanted Argentina's overpriced goods.

The government tried to resolve the competing demands of industry and labor by running a deficit and printing more money. The mounting subsidies and wage increases led to a cycle of budget deficits, annual inflation of 15 to 20 percent, balance of payments crises, and devaluations that made the economy unstable and unattractive for productive investment. In periodic attempts at monetary discipline, the government would institute an austerity plan, and the economy would come to a screeching halt. Stop-go policies followed each other in monotonous succession.

The competing interests might have been pacified with a growing pie, but instability discouraged investment, and the economy was not growing. Beyond the problems of inefficiency and instability, the economy had no particular logic; Argentina had no niche. The beef and grain that fueled Argentina's growth from 1880 to 1930 faced shrinking world markets. The United States and Canada competed with Argentina as exporters; by the 1960s, Europe could feed itself and soon would begin exporting food. Lacking significant amounts of coal, iron, and waterpower and situated 5,000 miles from any significant markets, Argentina is not a great place for manufacturing. Other late industrializing countries, such as Japan, invented their own niche, but Argentina's economic and social culture did not foster such innovation.

The lack of investment led to the progressive deindustrialization of Argentina. The workers expelled from industry joined the ranks of the self-employed (*cuentapropista* in Spanish, "on their own account").[6] Urban self-employment is the category of the work force that has shown the highest relative expansion since the days of the first Perón administration. In 1947, 355,000 persons were in that category; in 1970, there were 1,141,000. In the next decade, the number of urban self-employed increased to over 1.6 million, or 16 percent of the economically active population. That represented 11 percent of those working in industry, 30 percent of those in commerce, and 34 percent of those in construction (Palomino 1987, 150).

The political environment of the late 1960s was more volatile than the economic scene. After an uprising in Córdoba in 1969, the country descended into political chaos, with terror from both the left and the right. The Peronist movement split into two camps, reflecting the contradictions of its ideology. Perón encouraged both the right and the left wings of the movement, met with both while he was in exile, and directed the violence perpetrated by the extremes of both wings, often against each other. Perón calculated accurately that the unrest he sowed would force the military to call him back from exile.

Perón returned in 1973 to chaos. He died after nine months in office, and his wife and vice president, Isabelita, a former nightclub dancer whom he had met while in exile in Panama, took over. The power behind Isabelita was her Rasputinish advisor, José López Rega. They ran the country into such utter disaster, politically and economically, that most Argentines welcomed the military takeover in 1976.

The Proceso, 1976 to 1983

The Process of National Reorganization (the *Proceso*), as the military called its regime, is most remembered outside Argentina as the years of the Dirty War, when many thousands of persons disappeared and were killed by the military and police. Government reports name 9,000 of those killed, but credible estimates of the number of dead range from 20,000 to 30,000 persons (Graham-Yooll 1995, 13). Argentines also remember the *Proceso* as years of disastrous economic policy.

Spending Spree. Economy Minister José Martínez de Hoz, whose family owned the fifth-largest estate in the province of Buenos Aires (Solberg 1987, 63), attempted the liberal experiment that already had been introduced in Chile and Uruguay. The program would have entailed privatization, deregulation, elimination of the federal budget deficit through cuts in spending, tariff reduction, and maintaining a realistic exchange rate. It was unsuccessful because the military did not exercise any more self-control in economic matters than they did in the political realm. The government failed to correct the budget deficit because the generals spent billions on themselves and on their military hardware. Despite gaping deficits, they refused to cut subsidies to a wide range of unproductive industries they considered militarily strategic. When the military took power in 1976, the government owned 10 percent of the economy. When the military left in 1983, it owned 40 percent of the economy. With the private economy in collapse, public spending in Argentina was the highest in relation to GDP of all the nonsocialist world. From less than half of GDP in 1976, government spending amounted to 80 percent of GDP after 1979. That increased the budget deficit, made all the worse by inflation, which reached hundreds of percent annually. What little tax revenue was collected was paid late, when its real value had fallen to a fraction of the amount levied. The currency was repeatedly devalued.

Worldwide Recession and Debt Crisis. The spending spree continued, fed by recycled petrodollars loaned at low or negative real interest rates. A new oil crisis and worldwide recession and inflation precipitated a debt crisis for all those Third World countries, including Argentina, that had been borrowing petrodollars. By 1981, the peso was greatly overvalued and capital flight enormous. Anyone with assets sought safe haven in banks abroad, in Miami or Zurich. What the military had to show for the public portion of the debt were a few roads and bridges in border regions considered strategic. The bulk of the debt was private.

Industrial employment dropped from 38 percent of the work force in 1974 to 26 percent of the work force in 1982 (Palomino 1987, 48). In another economy, those data might be interpreted as reflecting increasing capitalization of industry, releasing labor to the tertiary (services) sector. But in Argentina, it is clear that the decrease in industrial employment represented the closing of factories, not their modernization. In the 1980s, the United States spent 2.8 percent of GNP on research and development, compared to Argentina's 0.4 percent of a much smaller GNP. Argentina's spending on research and development as a share of GNP was half that of Kenya (*Clarín*, September 22, 1991, p. 24). The decrease in industrial employment also had the effect of ultimately breaking the power of the labor movement.

Until about 1975, the self-employed in Argentina were part of the formal economy, stable and integrated into the industrial system. They had a fixed workplace, and two-thirds had been in their work for more than five years. One-third had been self-employed for more than ten years. They were middle class and had higher average incomes than salaried workers. Essentially, the self-employed in Argentina were like those in the United States. Since 1975, the self-employed increasingly are not middle class but part of the informal economy and have no fixed workplace (Palomino 1987, 161). They are marginal, selling packs of gum while walking between lanes of traffic, demonstrating ten kitchen knives with both hands while standing in a lurching, crowded bus or passing out holy cards and sentimental bookmarks for whatever passengers offer in return.

Changes in the Health Sector. Falling real wages, growing rates of unemployment and underemployment, and a large reduction in the population of wage and salary workers added to the demands placed on the public health system. As former industrial workers became *cuentapropistas*, they lost their affiliation with employment-based health plans. In 1975, it was estimated that 80 percent of the population had health coverage. By 1983, only 65 percent were covered. The rest now had to go to public hospitals. Health plans faced financial crisis because of mismanagement and shrinking membership. To cover their shortfalls, the health plans instituted copayments for services. Consequently, even people with health coverage started to go to public hospitals because they could not afford the copayments (Belmartino 1991, 24).

At the same time that the public sector faced increasing demand, the financing of public health was slashed. In 1978, the *Proceso* handed national hospitals

over to the provinces but did not provide the funds to support the decentralization (Isuani and Mercer 1986, 19). The portion of the federal budget going to
health was reduced from 6 percent in 1975 to 2.5 percent in 1983 (Belmartino
1991, 23). That led to a further deterioration of public-sector services and infrastructure. The military regime cut back on social spending more than debt service constraints required. Social services in general and health and education in
particular bore the brunt of the military government's rising debt-service problems (Looney 1987, 25–32). Another change introduced by the military was the
charging of fees in the public hospitals. The *aranceles*, as they were called, could
be waived in cases of demonstrated need, but they represented a bureaucratic
hurdle that was enormous for some of the very poor.

Among the casualties of provincialization and lower health care spending
were the campaigns against endemic diseases. Malaria, which had been eliminated in the subtropical and tropical north, and Chagas' disease, which was controlled through house-spraying programs, both saw a resurgence. Prior to
decentralization, 5,000 sprayings annually were carried out in Santiago del Estero
for control of Chagas' disease. In 1989, there were only 150 (De Genaro 1989,
240).

The economic policies of the *Proceso* gave a permanent technological advantage to the private sector. The overvalued peso enabled the private hospitals to
import the latest in medical technology. Imports of medical equipment were duty
free in exchange for a certain number of uses granted to public hospital patients.
The national price schedule instituted in 1977 *(Nomenclador Nacional)* benefitted the kind of services offered in the private sector, which are specialized, technologically advanced, and hospital based. The *Nomenclador* also priced doctors'
services lower than the use of technologically advanced equipment (Arce 1988,
105).

Burdening the Nation with Debt and War. When the presidency changed
hands in 1981, Domingo Cavallo became economy minister (1981–1982). Arguing that the debt had quintupled in value in peso terms, Cavallo nationalized the
private debt. The entire nation became responsible for private debt that had been
contracted between private firms and private banks and that had made some people so rich. (The private accounts in Miami and elsewhere of those wealthy
Argentines exceed the national debt.)

The structural adjustment policies now deemed necessary are the prescription for a disease with distant antecedents, seriously aggravated by the spending
of the military regime and even further by the whitewashing of the debt under
the stewardship of Cavallo. All the countries facing debt crises instituted some
form of structural adjustment program to reduce government deficits and provide funds for debt service through export promotion. The International Mone-

tary Fund (IMF) recommended halting wasteful government spending on bloated, unproductive state enterprises and using the government budget for things the market cannot adequately do, such as mass education and public health. The Argentine interpretation of structural adjustment has meant no pay increases for a decade for lower-ranking public employees and slashed spending on education and health. Even the IMF criticized such draconian measures.[7]

Faced with public opposition to the wretched state of the economy and increasing discomfort due to the disappearances, the military resorted to rallying support through nationalism. In 1982, it attacked the British-held Islas Malvinas (Falkland Islands). The military adventure was as much of a disaster as its handling of the economy. Hundreds of Argentine lives were lost, and the military finally called a truce after three months. Added to the loss of life and humiliation of defeat was the shameful revelation that officers had abandoned their untrained conscripts in the field of battle and returned to Buenos Aires, having embezzled funds intended to supply the troops. Defeat in the Falklands War finally roused the population, and the military announced it would allow elections and hand over control to civilians.

Democratic Chaos and Thuggish Stability, 1983 to the Present

The primary task of the new Radical government of Raúl Alfonsín (1983–1989) was the restoration of democracy in a country scarred by more than a decade of violence. The top military officials were tried and imprisoned for their role in the Dirty War, but a series of military mutinies, with a menacing show of force, pressured Alfonsín to halt the judicial process. Those convicted later were pardoned by President Carlos Menem, who took power in 1989.

The Radicals inherited a huge external debt, which they could not pay when world commodity prices fell after 1985. Per capita GDP fell 1 percent per year through the 1980s. The Radicals again relied on patronage and subsidies to the interior to maintain political support. Excess federal spending was magnified by the dual or even multiple money supplies. Provincial payrolls were paid with provincial bonds that circulated as currency within the province. Since half the employed persons in some provinces worked for the provincial government, that was a significant amount of money.

What good policies the Radicals did propose, the Peronists in Congress blocked at every turn. The Peronist union leadership undermined the government by calling repeated strikes, including several general strikes, and kept the economy in turmoil. Perhaps the biggest obstacle to progress was that fortunes large and small were to be made in currency speculation, where success depended on the failure of the government's plan. Real private investment was almost nonexistent.

While investment subsidies grew from 0.3 percent of GDP in 1980 to 2 percent of GDP in 1986, investment as a share of GDP fell from 24 percent in the 1970s to 15 percent in the 1980s. The subsidies were pocketed, not invested. Argentina's decline in investment as a share of GDP was twice what it was in other highly indebted countries. From 1980 to 1984, export subsidies amounted to $1.5 billion. The average export subsidy was 22 percent. During the same period, promoted exports declined in value from $1.5 billion to $1.1 billion (Nogues 1989, 49).

Although both the share of national income going to workers and the share going to government fell in the 1980s, capital's increasing share was not invested. The share of wages and salaries in national income fell from 43 percent in 1970–1975 to an average of 30 percent in 1976–1989, a loss to wage and salary workers of approximately $80 billion. Subtracting from that $80 billion the $35 billion transferred to creditors abroad during the same period, there still remained some $45 billion available for investment with the transfer of incomes from labor to capital. Instead, average net investment fell from almost 16 percent for the earlier period to 4 percent for the period 1976–1991, with net investment in the last three years being negative. The difference was not taken by the government in profits tax. On the contrary, the proportion of taxes paid by wage and salary workers increased from 32 percent in the period 1970–1975 to over 50 percent in 1981–1988. At the same time, the Central Bank calculated that for the period 1980–1990 it had lost $105 billion to corporations and private banks in the form of subsidies, overpricing by suppliers, nationalization of the debt, and manipulation of exchange rate changes in billing (Medina 1992b, 20).

The paralysis of the Alfonsín government in contending with speculative fever, Peronist obstructionism, and its own deficit spending ensured Peronist victory in the 1989 presidential elections, a frightening prospect for asset holders. Carlos Menem, the Peronist candidate, campaigned as a populist, provoking capital flight and the hyperinflation of July 1989. The tripling of prices in the first week of July sparked rioting, widespread looting of grocery stores, and a wave of unemployment. The loss of confidence forced Alfonsín to turn over power to Menem six months early, an ironic outcome since it was the fear of Menem that, in part, had triggered the capital flight and hyperinflation. The handover of power in 1989 was the first transition from an elected president to another elected president since 1928.

Menem and the La Rioja Bandits. Carlos Menem had been governor of the underdeveloped province of La Rioja. It was easy for the poor, illiterate voters to recognize him in campaign posters because he wore bushy, full-face sideburns, just like the nineteenth-century La Rioja *caudillo* Facundo Quiroga, whose picture appeared on the provincial money. For Menem, every bank note was a campaign flyer.

The Menem administration talked a liberal economic policy but, faced with a second bout of hyperinflation in December 1989, resorted to the confiscation of private bank accounts. The only unifying principle of the regime seemed to be unbridled corruption. Every La Riojan that Menem brought with him eventually was indicted. His appointments secretary was found to have secured the contract for providing milk to the maternal-child nutrition program and then to have fulfilled that public trust by supplying spoiled, worm-ridden dry milk that had been rejected for public consumption. The spoiled milk kept turning up like a bad penny; each inspector who confiscated it would resell it instead of having it destroyed. The president's sister-in-law was indicted in Spain for laundering drug money. Menem's disregard for the dignity of office seemed clear in his appointment of the son of his tarot card reader, a fugitive from justice, to a judgeship (Cooper 1994, 14). Like the spoiled milk, bad officials kept resurfacing. Being disgraced in one job just meant moving to some other lucrative position. Matilde Menéndez had to resign as minister of health due to a scandal over the starvation deaths of inmates of the psychiatric hospital under her stewardship. Menem then appointed her to be director of the largest health insurance program in the country, the social security system's program for the retired (PAMI—Programa de Atención Médica Integral). Although accused of presiding over a multimillion-dollar kickback scheme at PAMI (*New York Times*, April 14, 1994, p. A5), she did not resign until the scandal cost the Peronists the Federal Capital election in 1994 (*Buenos Aires Herald*, April 17, 1994, p. 4). An Argentine journalist compiled a list of all the Menem officials under indictment and the crimes of which they were accused, a list that filled nine pages of small print (Horacio Verbitsky, *Robo para la corona*, 1993).

Plan Cavallo. Besides being preoccupied with the pillage of the treasury, the Menem government was slowed down by the deaths of two economy ministers in the first two years. In 1991, Domingo Cavallo joined the Menem government as economy minister. What Cavallo was able to accomplish was in many respects remarkable, although not the miracle that the foreign press credited to him. He managed to keep the peso at one dollar, even though prices kept climbing for a year after the peso's value was fixed. That produced a much overvalued currency, which penalized exports. He used the revenues from the privatized government enterprises to shore up the peso. The government claimed that inflation was checked without resort to price controls. But the single most important price in the Argentine economy is the exchange rate, which was fixed. It now takes an act of Congress to devalue the currency. It was an important step to stop the inflationary cycle, which was suppressed but not cured.

   The official statistics showed impressive growth, but much of that growth was in the overvaluation of the peso. Capital inflow financed the deficit on current account, but that was short-term capital, which is volatile and influenced by factors beyond Argentina's control, such as United States interest rates and Mexican uprisings and presidential scandals.

Successes in Argentina have been achieved by edict, not in a free economy under normal political conditions. In the first five months of *Plan Cavallo*, Menem issued thirty presidential decrees, more than had been announced in the previous 130 years since the constitution was enacted. From 1991 to 1993, there were 300 decrees, with 100 cosigned by Cavallo (who held no elective office). In the past, presidential decrees had to be ratified by Congress. But Menem expanded and packed the Supreme Court, which then decided that decrees stand unless overruled by Congress. The administration threatens and bullies the press and the opposition.

The changes in the health sector begun under the *Proceso* were reinforced in the 1980s and 1990s. After the restoration of democracy in 1983, public spending on health continued to fall. The Radical plan for a national health service was blocked by the unions. Throughout the inflationary period, the *obras sociales* and the public hospitals suffered because employers paid their contributions to the health plans late and the health plans paid the public hospitals late, if they paid at all. The crisis in the economy, aggravated by the hyperinflation of 1989, further thinned the ranks of unions and filled the public hospitals and health centers with patients who had no coverage or poor coverage. By the mid-1990s, unemployment reached 20 percent and underemployment another 11 percent of the labor force. The segment of the population covered by health plans dipped as low as 50 percent (Goñi 1993*b*, 2).

The paralysis of the private economy, the massive unemployment that is the continuing legacy of the period of hyperinflation, and the job losses due to the government's adjustment policies have been disastrous for workers. Sixteen months after the convertibility plan took effect (fixing the value of the peso at one dollar), the share of national income going to wages and salaries was calculated to be between 22 and 25 percent (Medina 1992*b*, 20). Economy Minister Cavallo claimed that pushing labor's share to historic lows would result in renewed investment. Previous attempts at supply-side stimulus were unsuccessful. Subsidies during the *Proceso* and the Alfonsín years failed to generate growth. Redistribution of income from labor to capital in the 1980s also failed to confirm the supply-side approach. The investment so far in Argentina consists mostly of short-term capital inflows on the *Bolsa* (stock exchange). For economic resurgence, it would be more useful to attack the maze of regulations, taxes, and licenses that businesses face and that stifle innovation and harbor corruption (Goñi 1993*b*, 2). The billions wasted on employee and employer contributions to useless medical plans also raise Argentine cost unnecessarily. (See Chapter 7 on the social security health sector.) There are ways to encourage investment that do not compromise the long-term health of the economy by crushing workers. Labor is a resource as well as a cost.

As far as the government budget goes, while spending on health and education has been cut to the bone, it is business as usual for government officials. When Menem went on a ten-day European swing in 1992, he found it necessary to take along eighty-four people, including three hairdressers for himself. It was not clear what the purpose of the trip was (*Buenos Aires Herald*, October 13, 1992, p. 10). In 1995, Menem had a golf course built at his presidential estate at public expense and a new jet delivered at a cost of $66 million (Sims 1995*b*, A16). Meanwhile, the city of Buenos Aires announced it would no longer provide a glass of milk each day to 150,000 schoolchildren because of the expense. The city had been paying forty cents per serving per day for the milk, although it could have obtained the milk at six cents per serving by contracting directly with producers (*Buenos Aires Herald*, March 27, 1994, p. 4).

In 1992 and 1993, the government finally started to dismantle the subsidies and tariff protection for agriculture in the interior but so quickly that the provinces of the interior rose in revolt. Sugar production fell 49 percent and cotton production 50 percent. Cutting the subsidies to the uncompetitive provincial industries and ending the dole to provincial governments that act as alternatives to local economies were steps that had to be taken. The way those measures were carried out, however, led to unemployment of up to 35 percent in the provinces and violent reactions in most of the interior's capitals. Rioters destroyed the state house in more than one provincial capital, and several deaths and numerous injuries resulted. Santiago del Estero erupted in violence in December 1993, when the provincial government announced it would not pay the monthly wages of $350 to public employees who had gone unpaid since August, although it would continue to pay senior officials their $16,000-a-month salaries (*Buenos Aires Herald*, January 9, 1994, p. 20).

Liberal economic policy is the strategy that many would agree is necessary in Argentina in the 1990s. But liberal economics in Argentina is associated with the military *Proceso* of 1976 to 1983. The regime that killed infants and displayed their preserved bodies in military museums as part of its antiguerrilla campaign used liberal economic policy as revenge. During the first Perón administration in the 1940s, the share of wages in national income had tipped slightly in favor of workers. Since 1955, each administration has struggled to push back labor's share. The Liberating Revolution, the *Proceso*, and then Menem identified labor cost as the prime obstacle to Argentine development. Consequently, structural adjustment is defined as breaking labor, while numerous other areas of economic and institutional backwardness are neglected. Corruption and government waste could provide fertile ground for adjustment projects. Corruption continues to foster a climate of insecure property rights and is an important obstacle to efficiency and genuine growth. When Cavallo finally spoke out about corruption in the government, he was fired in mid-1996.

The long-run impact of impoverishing the working class and failing to tackle corruption will be the continuation of underdevelopment. Structural adjustment plans and liberal economic policies cannot be separated from the political and historical setting in which they are executed. What the administration wants to do is what Argentine profit seekers have always done, reap where they have not sown. Their rent seeking consists of expecting quality work out of a labor force in which nothing has been invested. It is biological rent seeking from human capital. The long-term effects will be a broken working class, which is the aim, but they will be broken physically and mentally as well as organizationally. Growing in the information age with a destroyed school system, competing in the global economy with workers who are retarded by malnutrition and repeated illness are not realistic goals.

The result of this history of conflict and missed opportunities is a divided economy. A few people, mostly those with "important last names," live extremely well. The middle class, which used to make up much of the Federal Capital's population, is going hungry. The government eliminated jobs, but industry has not taken up the slack. A large proportion of the industrial working class has slipped into the informal economy, without health coverage or pensions.

Millions of Argentines live and die in poverty. Part II describes how the poor live, heirs of Argentina's failure to develop a self-sustaining economy. The condition of the poor in Argentina is replicated in more than one hundred countries around the world. More than one billion people live on less than one dollar a day. One dollar in Africa or five dollars in Argentina buys squalor, dirty water, danger on the job, and little medical attention. It provides a weak foundation for sustainable human development.

Part II

How Poor People Get Sick

Three

Housing and Health

W here people live has a significant influence on their physical and mental health and on their ability to integrate into society. The home is more than just the structure in which a person sleeps, eats, works, and plays, although the structure itself is important. The human habitat includes the neighborhood in which a person lives and the facilities or lack of facilities in the area. Habitat plays such an important role in defining quality of life that three of the five indicators used by the census to define poverty in Argentina concern housing: crowding, type of house, and sanitary services (INDEC 1990, 321).

The inadequacy of housing for the poor affects their health and safety in many ways. Constructed of flimsy material, shanties offer little protection from the elements and often are located in areas that are unprotected from natural hazards, such as flooding. City tenements are badly designed or maintained, with hazardous stairs, windows, heating and cooling systems, and fire escapes. Lack of housing codes or weak enforcement allows the use of unsafe building materials, such as lead-based paints and asbestos. People uneducated about environmental hazards may use discarded materials that are unsafe for dwellings, such as creosote-soaked lumber or synthetic materials that emit noxious fumes. Insufficient kitchen space and faulty wiring or gas connections can lead to fires and other accidents. In houses without gas and electricity, people use open fires with poor ventilation, which produces indoor air pollution and increases the risk of burns. Crowding and multifamily households allow little privacy. In city slums and periurban shantytowns, safe play space is rare, and traffic accidents and environmental hazards are a threat to children (WHO 1991b, 20).

This chapter discusses a number of aspects of housing and health, including the reasons for Argentina's housing deficit, the distribution of substandard housing in the country, types of construction of substandard housing, equipment and location of poor housing, and the health effects of inadequate housing on the poor.

We begin with housing because the home is where the vast majority of illness and disability occur for the poor. The home is meant to shelter, comfort, and protect. For the poor, however, home is the place of transmission of infectious disease because of crowding, the place where minor infections become life threatening because of exposure to the elements, the site of accidents and contact with toxic chemicals. Housing, more than anything else, distinguishes the lives of the poor from those of the rich. The housing inadequacies described here, in one form or another, affect more than ten million Argentines and more than two billion people around the world.

The Home Environment for the Poor

The home environment plays a larger role in health for the poor than it does for the more affluent because, for many, it is their only environment. The world of the poor may be very restricted. They cannot afford to travel. Busy with work and family and short of cash, they do not go downtown for a night out or to the beach on holiday. Their lives are confined to the urban slum or suburban shantytown. Small shops in the neighborhood sell groceries, and vendors come through the neighborhoods hawking goods. What social life and relaxation they have are with their neighbors.

Women

The majority of women in poor neighborhoods in Argentina do not work outside the home. For the country as a whole, the proportion of women fourteen years of age and over in the work force was 23 percent in 1960 and 27 percent in 1970 and 1980 (INDEC n.d., 153). Labor force participation of poor women is much lower than of nonpoor women, and unemployment for poor women is much greater than for nonpoor women (INDEC 1990, 72, 74).

Preschoolers

In poor neighborhoods, children up to the age of six generally are home all day. Rates of kindergarten attendance are markedly different among economic strata. Fewer than one-third of poor children who are four years old attend preschool, compared to over 80 percent of nonpoor four-year-olds. Of poor children five years old, about two-thirds attend kindergarten, compared to over 90 percent of the nonpoor. Most public and private preschools are in urban areas, inaccessible to the majority of poor children, who live in periurban slums (UNICEF 1990a, 107, 112). Young children at home, in the care of a parent or grandparent, are spared exposure to the myriad infectious diseases found among children in child care centers and preschools. They are exposed twenty-four hours a day, however, to all the health and safety hazards of the substandard home and the unhealthy environment of the shantytown or urban slum. Worse yet, if they are at home and cared for by an older child or are unattended, those hazards are substantially greater.

School-Age Children

Children in primary school—up to seventh grade in Argentina—have only a half-day of school, usually in the neighborhood. Free, compulsory education is officially available to all children age six and over, but fewer than 80 percent of chronically poor children are enrolled, compared to 100 percent of the nonpoor. Starting school late is common among children in shantytowns and tenements. School abandonment begins early among the poor, as well, and at every age is more severe for the chronically poor than for the nonpoor. Approximately one out of every twelve poor children ages eight to eleven is not in school. For almost every age group, school enrollment is lower for girls, in particular for those age twelve and older (UNICEF 1990*a*, 109, 112).

From about age twelve on, many girls are kept home to take care of the house and younger children. In 1980, 25,000 fourteen-year-old girls in Argentina were out of school and keeping house. Of girls fifteen to nineteen years old, over 270,000 were out of school and keeping house (INDEC 1985, 75–76). After a few years of school, which takes up only part of the year and a few hours a day, the girls are back full-time in their homes and neighborhoods.

Self-Employed Workers

Even the poor who are employed might not leave the neighborhood because they are self-employed, working in the home or nearby. As the crisis of the Argentine economy deepens, the informal economy employs an ever greater proportion of the work force, particularly of the poor. More than 20 percent of the work force is self-employed, and often the whole family participates.

There are positive aspects to families spending so much time at or near home together. Some neighborhoods are very peaceful, and I found them a pleasant refuge with warm, welcoming people just a few blocks from noisy, busy downtown Buenos Aires. The fancy apartments and towering hotels are in sight, the traffic noise is distant, and the chickens peck around at your feet. But to be there all the time in any weather and in the houses that they have, makes people sick. When winter comes, they may never set foot in a warm, dry place. They may never use a bathroom with running water. Even the hospital they go to when their children are sick may be missing exterior walls and have no heat or running water. Because the poor have no place else to go, the cold, wet filth of their neighborhood is their constant environment.

Housing Deficit in Argentina

The ongoing crisis and the speculative nature of the Argentine economy have had a serious impact on the housing market nationwide in both quantity and quality of housing units. In absolute terms, it is the Greater Buenos Aires area that has the greatest housing deficit. Greater Buenos Aires is significant in Argentina, both demographically and economically. The area contains one-third of the population of the country and the greatest concentration of the poor.

Population growth in Greater Buenos Aires has exacerbated the housing deficit there. From 1960 to 1980, immigration from the provinces, bordering countries, and the Federal Capital swelled the population of the suburbs of Buenos Aires by over 80 percent. From 1976 to 1981, the military government prohibited those who were "unworthy" from living in the capital. The poor were forced out at gunpoint, and their homes were bulldozed. From 1975 to 1980, 400,000 people left the Federal Capital, 75 percent of them for the nearby areas of the Province of Buenos Aires (Abba et al. 1986, 68). The construction of housing space has not kept up with population growth, nor have real wages kept up with soaring construction costs and rents. Because of chaos and speculation in capital markets, investment in housing is lacking.

Housing Costs and Shortages

In the Federal Capital from 1970 to 1982, more than 22 million square meters of dwelling space were built, but 75 percent of the construction was in the most affluent neighborhoods (Belgrano, Palermo, Barrio Norte, Núñez, Villa Crespo, Caballito, and Flores), which make up 30 percent of the city's area (Abba et al. 1986, 62, 70). The increase in housing space was essentially an increase in the number of units for more affluent families and in the amount of space for those families.

Purchasing power for floor space has fallen to about half what it was in 1970. The apartment that the average worker could have bought with 7 years' wages in 1970–1974 would have taken 12.5 years by 1977–1984 (Abba et al. 1986, 64, 68). The crisis has deepened since then, in particular with the hyperinflation of 1989.

Because of the falling incomes of lower- and middle-income people and the rising costs of construction, the construction industry has just stopped building for those sectors, leaving a huge housing deficit for low- and moderate-income people. After 1991, because the peso was held fixed in dollar terms but prices kept rising, the usual hedge against inflation in currency speculation was closed. People sought security in real estate, pushing up prices still further in both purchase and rental markets.

Another factor contributing to the shortage of housing space is the fact that much space is unused. In a normal market, perhaps 5 to 10 percent of units are unoccupied. In 1980, 16 percent of units in Buenos Aires were unoccupied. In

1983, due to fears that the civilian government would reinstate rent controls, another 40,000 to 60,000 units were withdrawn from the market, increasing the units unoccupied to 22 percent of the city's housing stock (Abba et al. 1986, 62).

The very poor have dropped out of the rental market entirely. By 1980, roughly 100,000 families, or about 300,000 people, faced a serious housing deficit in the Federal Capital (Abba et al. 1986, 59, 74). In Greater Buenos Aires, the deficit now affects 500,000 families, of which 200,000 families face a housing emergency. That means they are technically homeless and live in shanties they have pieced together from trash (*Clarín*, September 22, 1991, second section, p. 4).

Due to the lack of housing space, high rents, and the policy of the military government, new migrants to Buenos Aires have located in the nineteen suburban counties *(partidos)* that make up Greater Buenos Aires. Since 1970, the greatest growth has been in six outlying counties that are now included in some studies in the new Greater Buenos Aires area. In 1980, the population of the outer six counties (Cañuelas, Escobar, Pilar, General Rodríguez, Marcos Paz, and San Vicente) was 299,000; in 1991, it was 442,000 (INDEC 1991*a*, 52). (See map of Greater Buenos Aires.)

Squatters

Between 1960 and 1980, the number of illegal tenancies in Greater Buenos Aires quadrupled, from 46,000 to 200,000 (Lumi 1990, 190). In Buenos Aires, squatter status used to be temporary. As long as there was some industrial growth and because of the redistributive effects of the first Perón administration, people moved out of slums. When even modest economic growth ceased, the *villas miseria*, as shantytowns are called in Argentina, became permanent. Thirteen percent of all dwellings and 62 percent of those that are precarious are occupied by squatters, who illegally occupy either the houses or the land. Lack of legal rights to houses or land is closely associated with precariousness because of the disincentive to invest in improvements in the dwellings. Since 1980, the number of squatters in Greater Buenos Aires, Greater Rosario, and other urban areas has continued to grow rapidly. Census data tend to understate squatter populations because people respond to a question about their status as they see it. They answer, *"dueño"* ("owner") because they own the houses they have erected, although they do not own or rent the land on which the houses stand, which is the meaning intended by the census (Dr. Mario Rípoli, November 27, 1991).

Before the military *Proceso*, there had been many thousands of shanties in the Federal Capital. One squatter area, the *villa* of Saldías, in the railyards of Retiro station, had over 30,000 people (Dr. Pablo Muntaabski, June 26, 1992). In 1974, during the government of Isabel Perón, the parish priest of Saldías, Padre Mugica, was murdered. Later, the military regime bulldozed the *villa* and destroyed its health center. After the expulsion, only forty-seven families re-mained in Saldías, hiding in the freight containers.

The *villa* population began to increase again after the return of civilian gov-ernment, in 1983. In Saldías, the forty-seven families that remained were joined by 8,000 people who inhabited the new *villa* of Retiro. The community flourished for ten years, almost in the shadow of the Sheraton Hotel but unseen, until the construction of a new highway. The economy ministry decided that valuable downtown space was being wasted and decided to evict the squatters once again to allow the construction of malls and hotels along with the highway. The *villa* of Retiro grew to 9,000 in the spring of 1992 (González Toro 1992, 6).[1] The relo-cation of the population, promised in 1992, still has not been resolved as of this writing.

Most of the new squatter communities in the Federal Capital are in the south-west part of the city, in Mataderos, Soldati, and Flores Sur. In 1980, 1 percent of the population of the Federal Capital (about 30,000 people) lived in shanties as squatters, in 6,677 dwellings. By 1984, it was estimated that 35,000 people lived in *villas* in the capital (Abba et al. 1986, 69). In the nine years after the military stepped down, the *villa* population of the Federal Capital grew to 50,000. That may be an underestimate, because by mid-1991, Villa 21 alone, the largest shan-tytown in the Federal Capital, had 35,000 residents, including 18,000 children (*Buenos Aires Herald*, May 12, 1991, p. 4).

There are shantytowns in every one of the nineteen *partidos* of Greater Buenos Aires, but they are not evenly distributed across the region. The greatest concentrations are to the south and the southwest of the capital. Table 3.1 lists the populations of *villas miseria* in Greater Buenos Aires according to a survey by the Province of Buenos Aires. While the province undercounted the number of people in shantytowns, the distribution of the *villero* (*villa* dweller) population among jurisdictions is fairly accurate.

The changes in the 1970s in the southern suburbs were dramatic. Between 1970 and 1981, the shantytown population of the county of Quilmes increased by more than 10,000 people, or 43 percent. By 1981, the *villero* population was 8 per-cent of the total population of Quilmes and 9.7 percent in Lanús (Cuenya 1985, 97–98).

It is not only *villeros* who live in precarious, substandard housing. Shanty-towns, *villas miseria*, or squatter camps are only one aspect of inadequate hous-ing. In Quilmes, for example, while 8 percent of the county population live in *villas*, 29 percent of its population live in homes with unsatisfied basic needs, which are the census categories used for estimating poverty. Of children in the county under five years of age, over 40 percent live in such homes. There is no piped water in 50 percent of those homes, and over 60 percent are not connected to the sewer system. In squatter neighborhoods, the proportions are even higher (Cuenya 1985, 97).

_____ *Table 3.1* _____
Population in Shantytowns in Greater Buenos Aires (GBA), 1981

County *(Partido)*	Number of Shanty Dwellings	Population in *Villas*	*Villeros* as Percentage of GBA	*Villeros* as Percentage of County Population
Lanús	11,223	45,209	15.5	9.7
La Matanza	8,405	36,238	12.5	3.8
Quilmes	8,709	35,727	12.3	8.0
Lomas de Zamora	6,647	28,198	9.7	5.5
General San Martín	6,367	26,070	9.0	6.8
Avellaneda	6,010	23,796	8.2	7.1
General Sarmiento	4,111	15,902	5.5	3.2
San Isidro	3,467	15,742	5.4	5.4
Tres de Febrero	2,615	10,874	3.7	3.1
Vicente López	2,513	10,550	3.6	3.6
Tigre	2,078	9,131	3.1	4.4
San Fernando	1,861	8,206	2.8	6.1
Morón	1,750	7,899	2.7	1.3
Merlo	1,117	4,743	1.6	1.6
Esteban Echeverría	693	3,006	1.0	1.6
Berazategui	606	2,940	1.0	1.5
Moreno	617	2,690	0.9	1.4
Florencio Varela	511	2,083	0.7	1.2
Almirante Brown	453	1,916	0.7	0.6
Total GBA	69,753	290,920	100.0	4.3

Source: Cuenya 1985, 99, and my own calculations based on 1980 population data from Rofman and Marqués 1988, 36.

In addition to *villas*, there is another category of settlement on illegally occupied land, called organized neighborhoods, in which the residents organize into neighborhood councils. The physical environment is essentially the same as a *villa*, but the political status is somewhat different, at least since the return of democracy. In one such settlement, Quilmes West, 91 percent of the population live in homes with unsatisfied basic needs (Cuenya 1985, 151). As of 1991, there were 101 registered settlements in Greater Buenos Aires, with 36,400 families, or 173,000 people (*Clarín*, September 22, 1991, second section, p. 1).

The Homeless

Among people living on the street are many abandoned children, some delinquents, and many girls twelve and thirteen years of age who have left home because they were being sexually abused by relatives or neighbors, according to provincial delegate Marta Modernel (Vidal 1992, 6). Among the older homeless are people who are out of work and out of funds for whom living on the street is temporary. As soon as they secure employment, they move into boarding houses. Some people become homeless due to illness. While they are in the hospital, their one-room houses and the contents are stolen, so they have nothing to return to (Dr. Lucía Saracco, August 21, 1992). In addition, there are permanent street residents who are, according to city officials, mentally ill and number about 1,000. All the homeless share the problems of a lack of hygiene, contaminated food taken from garbage cans, water from runoff, and infestation with lice, crabs, and other parasites (Pazos and van der Horst 1993, 44).

Housing Conditions in Argentina

One out of every three families in Argentina is ill-housed. Over ten million Argentines live in shanties or tenements, in houses without sanitary facilities, in mud houses, lean-tos, or caves, or crowded three or more to a room. The 1980 census indicated deficiencies in 2.4 million housing units. By 1986, that number had climbed to 2.8 million units, of a total housing stock of 7.1 million units (Lumi 1990, 184). The census considers five types of housing substandard:

- precarious dwellings, those made of discarded materials
- *ranchos*, which are typical of rural areas and rusticly built, with materials of local origin, walls of mud or cane, straw roofs, and dirt floors
- tenements, dwellings with four or more households sharing a kitchen and a bath
- type B houses, which have dirt floors or lack piped water and flush toilets
- others, which includes certain kinds of trailers, lean-tos, and caves (Lumi 1990, 219)

More than two million housing units fit into those five categories. There is an undercounting of inadequate housing because other categories of deficiencies are not considered. Single-family apartments and single-family houses are assumed to be adequate, regardless of location, noise levels, age of the structure, or other factors that reduce comfort and safety, such as lack of heating.

Table 3.2 shows the number of housing units in each substandard category. Over one-half million houses in Argentina in 1980 were made of discarded materials patched together with great effort but meager results. Over one-quarter million rural houses were made of mud and sticks or cane walls with straw roofs and dirt floors. Over a million more houses lacked water and toilets or had dirt floors. Of all those substandard houses, about 30 percent could be rehabilitated. For the rest, it would cost less to start over than to bring them up to standards (Lumi 1990, 186).

The distribution of poor housing nationwide is uneven. In absolute numbers, the housing deficit is an urban and suburban problem, but 36 percent of poor housing is in rural areas, although only 17 percent of the total population is rural.

_____ *Table 3.2* _____

Substandard Houses by Type, 1980

Type of Dwelling	Urban	Rural	Total
Precarious houses	425,217	110,047	535,264
Ranchos	79,691	209,350	289,041
Tenement units	61,644	2,719	64,363
Type B houses	741,419	402,247	1,143,666
Others	9,327	7,168	16,495
Total	1,317,298	731,531	2,048,829

Source: Lumi 1990, 210. Reprinted with permission of UNICEF.

Almost half of the country's substandard housing is in the provinces of Buenos Aires, Córdoba, and Santa Fe, but the proportion of poor housing is greatest in the Northeast and the Northwest. In the Northeast (Entre Ríos, Corrientes, Misiones, Chaco, and Formosa), 62 percent of all dwellings are substandard. In the Northwest (Catamarca, Santiago del Estero, Tucumán, Salta, Jujuy, and La Rioja), 57 percent of the regional total housing stock is substandard. Table 3.3 shows the distribution of inadequate housing among the regions and also the percentage of dwellings in each region that are precarious. While Cuyo (San Luis, San Juan, and Mendoza) and Patagonia (La Pampa, Río Negro, Neuquén, Chubut, Santa Cruz, and Tierra del Fuego) make up a small percentage of the national total, the proportion of substandard housing for each area is high (30 percent and 38 percent, respectively).

_____ *Table 3.3* _____

Regional Distribution of Substandard Housing, 1980

Region	Substandard Units	Percentage of Total Nationally	Percentage of Units in Region
Greater Buenos Aires	464,729	22.7	17.4
Pampas	553,522	27.0	23.8
Northeast	435,435	21.3	62.1
Northwest	354,409	17.3	57.0
Cuyo	128,315	6.3	30.2
Patagonia	112,419	5.4	37.8
Total	2,048,829	100.0	28.8

Source: Lumi 1990, 210. Reprinted with permission of UNICEF.

An analysis of the regional disparities conducted by CEPAL (United Nations Economic Commission on Latin America) and using data from the 1980 census illustrates the modest standard of living in many of the interior provinces. In seven of the Northeast and Northwest provinces, more than three-fourths of rural houses and more than one-third of urban houses have dirt floors. In three provinces (Chaco, Formosa, and Misiones), fewer than half of urban dwellings are electrified. Only in bitter cold Santa Cruz and Tierra del Fuego are more than one-third of rural homes electrified. In most of the country, well below one-third (an average of 19 percent) of homes are electrified. In five provinces, 5 percent or fewer rural homes have electricity (Gatto c1982, n.p.).

In the Greater Buenos Aires area, as well, the distribution of substandard housing is uneven. The *partido* of Florencio Varela has the highest proportion (58 percent) of inadequate housing. General Sarmiento is the *partido* with the smallest percentage of houses with running water and sewer connections (5.4 percent) (*Buenos Aires Herald*, August 23, 1993, pp. 1, 7).

Types of Construction of Substandard Housing

What substandard houses actually are like depends on the area. *Ranchos* generally are found in rural areas, but they also are common in towns and even provincial capitals of the Northwest. In big cities, especially Buenos Aires and Rosario, tenements are the predominant form of slum housing. In periurban areas, shanties, often on illegally occupied land, are the main form of housing for the poor. Type B houses (without sanitary facilities and with dirt floors) are found in all regions, in provincial capitals, in suburban areas of large and small cities, and in rural areas. This section describes the characteristics of the first three classes of substandard housing: shanties, *ranchos*, and tenements. (Type B houses are of various forms of construction and so are not detailed further.)

Ranchos

In rural areas, the poor house typically is the *rancho*, built of local materials. It has two, perhaps even three, rooms, including the kitchen. The walls are of cane, mud, or mud pressed over a frame of sticks, similar to the wattle and daub construction common in Africa. Roofs are of straw or sometimes sheet metal. This type of house is common in the Northwest and Pampean regions. The floor generally is dirt. In parts of the Northeast of Argentina, some *ranchos* are made of wood, due to its greater availability in the region.

A *rancho* generally does not have water or sanitary facilities inside the house. If there is a latrine, it is located in an outhouse. The water may come from a hand pump on the property, but not every rural house has its own well.

Another category of rural housing is that of migrant farm workers. In Río Negro and Neuquén (Patagonia), the housing provided by employers typically has a corrugated metal roof, a cement floor, potable water, and an indoor toilet, but only 14 percent have electricity. Only one-third of the workers have beds. The rest sleep on crates or blankets or directly on the floor.

In the Northeast, forestry workers live in company housing in precarious dwellings in the remote forests without water, sanitary facilities, or electricity. In the Northwest, sugar cane harvesters live in the cane fields in groups of 300 to 1,000, without water, sanitary facilities, or electricity. As many as three families live in a room four meters square. In Tucumán, the cane workers build their own dwellings of mud walls with cane or burlap roof (Neffa 1986, 99).

Tenements

A large proportion of the urban poor live in tenements, dilapidated, walk-up buildings in congested city areas. The buildings are poorly constructed. Although some tenements in La Boca and other areas of the Federal Capital have exterior walls made of corrugated metal, many are of wood. Often the tenement buildings are not connected to essential services, such as gas and electricity, and the residents have to improvise cooking and heating facilities. Tenement apartments, called *conventillos* or *inquilinatos*, consist of one room for a family, with five or more families sharing a kitchen and a bathroom.

In the city of Buenos Aires in 1980, 28,000 housing units classified as tenements housed 3 percent of the city's population. The actual number of people living in such accommodations is understated in the 1980 census because hotels and boarding houses are not included. Many tenements are called hotels to avoid legal restrictions regarding rents and tenants' rights. Because such camouflaged slums are not subject to inspection, fire and other hazards persist (*Clarín*, December 10, 1993, p. 18). Although people live in these quasi-hotels on a permanent basis, they are grouped in the census with collective homes such as convents, prisons, barracks, and hospitals (Abba et al. 1986, 65). Like tenements, they are crowded, both in persons per room and in families per sanitary unit or kitchen. They also often lack essential services or are precarious or dilapidated (Lumi 1990, 220). Counting recognized tenements as well as substandard hotels and boarding houses with permanent residents, 4.3 percent of the city population live in dilapidated one-room apartments sharing baths and kitchens, with an average of fifteen persons per house. The total population residing in such accommodations was estimated to be 125,000 persons (Abba et al. 1986, 66).

In Buenos Aires, the tenements are concentrated in the older sections, to the southeast, in La Boca, and to a lesser extent in Congreso and Barracas. La Boca has both a large percentage of the tenements (one-fourth) and a large proportion of its inhabitants (23 percent) living in such accommodations (Abba et al. 1986, 68). In the stretch of La Boca along the Riachuelo River, 80 percent of the people live in homes with unsatisfied basic needs. One hundred percent of the children under two years of age in this area live in such homes. In Barracas, 81 percent of the people living in the area along the Riachuelo live in homes with unsatisfied basic needs (Rofman 1992, 20).

Villas Miseria

The *villa* dwelling, like the rural house, uses locally acquired materials and usually has a dirt floor. But local materials in urban and periurban settings provide even less adequate protection than in rural areas. The result sometimes is little better than people pulling newspapers over themselves on park benches. *Villa* dwellings are diverse in the materials used, the state of completion, and amenities. In Retiro, some of the people who have resided in Barrio Güemes the longest have constructed their houses of concrete. The president of Barrio Comunicaciones even has a concrete yard, where meetings can be held and nurses can set up temporary health stations. But some houses are extraordinarily modest. Other people in Comunicaciones live in wood houses that sit directly on the dirt. One house in that neighborhood is a cargo container of the kind tractor trailers pull.

The worst houses in Retiro are in the Autopista neighborhood. Some are made entirely of blankets, others of scraps of plastic sheeting. Still others are made of plastic bags, like those used to package fruits and vegetables in a supermarket, taped and tacked together, or of flattened soda cans or cardboard. Some houses are made of corrugated or sheet metal, not in whole wall-sized strips but patches the size of license plates or dinner dishes. The houses have one, sometimes two, small, dark rooms. The more precarious houses have one room, with one bed for a family of four. A wooden house, such as in Comunicaciones, might have two rooms for six people.

It is better to visit Retiro after plenty of rain. Then the streets are full of water and what is underneath is unseen and unsmelled. The flooding hides the permanent muck. When the water recedes, the pools of standing water are wretched, and the ruts that run with wastewater from each house lie exposed. The piles of garbage, as well as the random garbage strewn about by people and scavenging animals, are more visible. Even on a chilly winter day, the smell of garbage and human waste is noticeable. Children with no shoes frolic in the muck, and toddlers sit in the dirt with nothing to play with but dirt and chips of brick (visits to Retiro, June–September 1992).

In Quilmes West, the first houses were made from branches, trunks, sheets of metal, cardboard, and nylon. Even two and a half years later, when a thorough survey of the housing was carried out, many of the homes were still the same. Lack of security in the land had kept people from improving their houses (Cuenya 1985, 114).

Almost 80 percent of the dwellings in Quilmes West use light materials for exterior walls and interior partitions. Wall lining, when it is used, is cardboard or plastic, contributing to the shabby look of the houses and providing shelter for disease-carrying insects. In 50 percent of the houses, the floors are dirt, which makes it impossible to keep out rain, rodents, and insects (Cuenya 1985, 121).

Almost all the houses have one or two rooms about three meters square. If the bedroom is a separate room, it has no window or other opening to sunlight or ventilation. That is done to keep the room as warm as possible in the winter, but it prevents the airing and sunning of the rooms. The latrine and sometimes a shower are located outside. Many household and family activities, like playing, eating, and clothes washing, take place outside (Cuenya 1985, 115, 116, 125).

The construction of the houses is varied and ingenious. One-room houses for a family of four are of wood, sheet metal, or cardboard and have no water in the house and no latrine on the lot. Some houses of more than one room are made entirely of cardboard and have electricity and water inside. Another house of more than one room, made of wood with a roof of metal and cardboard, might have a cement floor, electricity, and water (but no toilet) inside (Cuenya 1985, 117–119).

There is a *villa* in the area of the meatpacking plants in the Federal Capital that is called Ciudad Oculta (Hidden City). Some of the residents object to the name, which refers to the wall built by the military government to hide the slum it was unable to bulldoze completely in time for the 1978 World Cup Soccer championships. There are 8,000 residents in the *villa*, 40 percent of whom are under fourteen years of age (Dr. Mario Rípoli, November 27, 1991). The houses in Ciudad Oculta generally are one room, two meters by three meters and barely high enough to stand in. Eight to nine people live in each house (Dr. Graciela Spatz, December 6, 1991). There is no space between the houses, only passageways running along the blocks of houses (visit, November 27, 1991).

Most of Greater Buenos Aires is flat, so in built-up areas one can see only what is nearby. There is a place in La Matanza near La Tablada (where the armed uprising in 1991 occurred) where the road comes to a rise and it is possible to see a great distance. All around, in every direction, stretch miles and miles of shanties.

Crowding

One characteristic shared by *ranchos*, *villa* houses, and tenements is crowding. According to the census, housing is crowded if there are more than two persons per room. Of the substandard housing already counted in the preceding section, 880,000 units are also crowded. Of houses of adequate construction, 435,000 are crowded. The more than two million substandard houses and the crowded but otherwise adequate houses yield a total of almost 2.5 million deficient units for 1980. Crowding without precariousness is mainly an urban problem; 92 percent of those units are in urban areas. Greater Buenos

Aires alone has 40 percent of the country's crowded, nonprecarious houses (Lumi 1990, 211).

Table 3.4 shows the degree of crowding for five urban areas. In all five cities, one-fourth or more of the population live in crowded conditions. In rural areas, too, people live in crowded homes. The availability of open space does not outweigh the high price of building materials nor the disincentive to build when tenancy is uncertain.

In all five areas, between 36 percent and 46 percent of the structurally poor are crowded more than three persons to a room. And in all areas, two-thirds or more of the structurally poor live in dwellings with more than two persons per room. In all the areas, about one-third of the impoverished and 10 percent of the nonpoor live more than two to a room.

There is a high degree of crowding in shantytowns. Often a family of four shares one small room. In a survey of Quilmes West, 39 percent of the homes

_____ Table 3.4 _____

Number of Persons per Room, by Poverty Group, 1990

Number of Persons per Room	Percentage of Homes			
	Total	*Structurally Poor*	*Impoverished*	*Nonpoor*
Greater Buenos Aires				
• Fewer than 2	77.1	28.5	67.0	90.0
• 2 to 3	17.5	25.1	33.0	10.0
• More than 3	5.4	46.5	0.0	0.0
General Roca				
• Fewer than 2	75.1	32.5	67.1	92.4
• 2 to 3	18.6	24.2	32.9	7.6
• More than 3	6.2	43.3	0.0	0.0
Neuquén				
• Fewer than 2	71.6	35.2	64.7	90.2
• 2 to 3	22.5	26.5	35.3	9.8
• More than 3	5.9	38.2	0.0	0.0
Posadas				
• Fewer than 2	68.4	32.6	68.5	89.2
• 2 to 3	22.4	30.7	31.5	10.8
• More than 3	9.2	36.7	0.0	0.0
Santiago del Estero				
• Fewer than 2	71.5	34.3	67.8	91.2
• 2 to 3	20.8	29.7	32.2	8.8
• More than 3	7.7	36.0	0.0	0.0

Source: INDEC 1990, 344.

_____ *Table 3.5* _____

Provinces with Extreme Crowding, 1980

Province	Percentage of Population in Homes of Eight or More Persons	Persons per Room
Catamarca	27.6	2.9
Corrientes	24.3	3.2
Chaco	23.3	3.8
Formosa	25.6	3.8
Jujuy	25.4	3.0
Misiones	22.1	3.2
Santiago del Estero	24.0	3.5
Tucumán	24.5	3.2

Source: Derived from 1980 census, INDEC n.d., 263–266.

had between two and four persons per room; 36 percent had four or more persons per room (Cuenya 1985, 127).

In Argentina as a whole, 13 percent of the population live in private homes with eight or more occupants. The ratio of persons per room in these houses is greater than three. An additional 9 percent of the population live in homes with seven occupants. The person-per-room ratio for those homes is greater than two.

The distribution of crowded homes corresponds to the distribution of poverty in the country. In the eight provinces with the most severe crowding, about one-fourth of the population live in homes with more than eight occupants and with three or more persons per room. Table 3.5 gives the percentages of persons living in such homes and the degree of crowding for the eight provinces.

In the counties *(partidos)* of Greater Buenos Aires, 10.4 percent of the population live in homes of eight or more persons, averaging 3.2 persons per room. In all those regions, additional crowding with seven persons per room accounts for another 10 to 15 percent of the population (INDEC n.d., 263–266).[2]

Promiscuity

Another measure of crowding called promiscuity indicates the number of persons per place in a bed. The term in this context does not mean sexual promiscuity, but it is well chosen because of the consequences of such bed crowding. Promiscuity with extended families and multiple families and in social conditions that lead to marginalization and poor mental health results in high levels of child sexual abuse, as well as precocious sexual activity, teen pregnancies, and associated health problems.

Table 3.6 demonstrates the high degree of promiscuity, especially among the

_____ Table 3.6 _____

Homes with More Than One Person per Single-Bed Place, 1990

		Percentage of Homes		
City	Total	*Structurally Poor*	*Impoverished*	*Nonpoor*
Greater Buenos Aires	10.2	44.9	13.9	2.4
General Roca	15.4	41.9	23.4	2.7
Neuquén	14.4	42.0	18.7	1.2
Posadas	21.1	46.5	26.1	2.6
Santiago del Estero	19.4	49.4	24.1	2.3

Source: INDEC 1990, 345.

structurally poor. In every urban area, 40 to 50 percent of the homes in this economic group have more than one person per bed place. In many *villa* houses, there is only one bed for a family of four. One-room tenements, sheltering an entire family, also have one bed for the entire family.

Family Crowding

Family crowding is the sharing of housing units by more than one family. Government surveys in 1978 indicated a rate of family crowding ranging from 2.8 percent of households in Patagonia to 5.9 percent in Cuyo, with a national average of 4.5 percent (Lumi 1990, 212). Family crowding does not include extended or multigenerational families. This category is for unrelated families sharing homes and facilities. The 1980 census counted one-person homes, nuclear families, extended families, and "composite" homes *(hogar compuesto)* and found family crowding even greater than in the 1978 survey. In 1980, of the 27.5 million persons living in private homes, 2.7 million, or 9.9 percent, lived in multifamily homes. Over half a million of the 7.1 million private homes were multifamily (INDEC n.d., 117). Since that represents 7.4 percent of private homes but 9.9 percent of the population, it is clear that family crowding and crowding per dwelling go together. It also should be noted that it is unusual for Argentine young people to live with other single people in apartments, as is common in the United States; generally they live at home until marriage. Therefore, composite homes are not groups of students or young workers.

Equipment

Besides being poorly constructed, precarious, insubstantial, and crowded, the houses of the poor lack equipment for and connections to heating

_____ *Table 3.7* _____

Lack of Residential Heating or Cooling, by Poverty Group, 1990

	Percentage of Homes without Heating or Cooling			
City	Total	Structurally Poor	Impoverished	Nonpoor
Greater Buenos Aires	17.3	32.0	19.8	13.6
General Roca	1.5	3.5	0.5	1.7
Neuquén	6.3	9.7	8.0	3.7
Posadas	22.2	51.8	24.4	3.3
Santiago del Estero	16.9	52.2	13.9	2.7

Source: INDEC 1990, 353.

and lighting services. They also lack space for food preparation and food and water storage. All those deficiencies present additional health and safety hazards.

Heating

Rural houses, squatter shanties, and often even city tenements are not connected to gas and electricity services. Inhabitants have to use kerosene lanterns and heaters, which are especially dangerous in combination with the highly combustible construction materials that are typical in these types of dwellings (Abba et al. 1986, 75). Another type of heater commonly used in poor homes is a charcoal burner, similar to a hibachi or small barbecue grill, on legs about twenty to thirty centimeters high. The open fire is placed in the middle of the living room/bedroom floor, directly in the path of toddlers and careening baby-bouncers. Besides the danger of contact burns, house fires, and noxious fumes, charcoal and kerosene heaters also do not distribute heat very well. The drafty, patched-together shacks and poorly constructed tenements are cold and damp.

Table 3.7 lists for five urban areas the percentages of homes that lack heating or cooling. In Greater Buenos Aires in the four winter months, the temperature can dip below freezing; it is common in July and August to have weeks of rainy weather with temperatures not far above freezing. Greater Buenos Aires has an average of seventy days of frost per year and a significant amount of rainfall every month. Temperatures reaching 100 degrees are possible in the four summer months. One-third of the structurally poor and one-fifth of the impoverished in Buenos Aires have no heat.

Neuquén and General Roca have an average of 186 days of frost per year. In Neuquén, 10 percent of the homes of the structurally poor and 8 percent of those of the impoverished have no heat. In Posadas and Santiago, the numbers given in

Table 3.7 shows the proportion of homes without means of cooling or ventilating. In Posadas, temperatures climb over 86 degrees every month of the year and, for four months, day and night temperatures average eighty degrees (INDEC n.d., 60, 62, 65). In Santiago and Posadas, more than half the homes of the structurally poor have no ventilating or cooling.

Cooking

The lack of gas or electrical connections also means that cooking is done over open charcoal grills or with bottled gas. In addition to the danger of fire, the use of such grills and gas stoves exposes families to noxious fumes, especially in poorly ventilated tenements and rural houses. Table 3.8 shows the type of cooking fuel used by each economic group in the five urban areas.

In General Roca, wood is the cooking fuel most used by those who lack gas stoves. In Posadas, more than one-fourth of the structurally poor use wood or charcoal for fuel. In Santiago del Estero, almost half of the poor burn wood or charcoal for cooking.

Food Preparation and Storage

A serious problem for poor households is the lack of food-preparation space. In cramped shanties or *ranchos*, where one room may serve as both kitchen and bedroom/living room, or in tenement kitchens shared by several families, there is no place to put anything down. In addition, it is difficult to keep a house clean that has a dirt floor and a leaky roof and that is easily accessible to insects and rodents. In *ranchos* and *villas,* chickens, pigs, dogs, and cats are, if not in the house, in close proximity. Feces and parasites of those animals are carried, especially by children, into the house. The food inevitably is contaminated because of the lack of clean preparation space.

Food storage is another problem. Table 3.9 shows the proportion of homes without refrigeration, by economic group, for the five urban areas. Summer temperatures climb well into the eighties and nineties in Buenos Aires, where over one-fourth of the structurally poor have no refrigerators. In Santiago, almost half of the structurally poor lack refrigeration. In Posadas, where the temperature reaches 100 degrees four months out of the year, over half the homes of the structurally poor and over one-fifth of the homes of the impoverished have no refrigerators. In such temperatures, food spoils rapidly. Foods usually are stored in fruit crates standing on the dirt floor or hung on the wall, where they are accessible to rats, cockroaches, and other pests (Cuenya 1985, 126).

Because most of the houses of the poor do not have piped water inside, water storage is also a health problem. Even where water is obtained from a supposedly potable source, it has to be carried and stored in the house. The containers become contaminated from dirt in the house and from hand contact.

_____ Table 3.8 _____
Type of Cooking Fuel Used, by Poverty Group, 1990

		Percentage of Homes		
		Structurally		
Fuel	Total	Poor	Impoverished	Nonpoor
Greater Buenos Aires				
• Gas connection	59.2	16.8	43.0	73.3
• Tank gas	39.7	78.6	55.3	26.4
• Kerosene or charcoal	0.8	2.9	1.2	0.2
• Wood or other	0.3	1.7	0.4	0.0
General Roca				
• Gas connection	74.8	33.9	71.2	88.4
• Tank gas	21.8	54.1	25.2	10.7
• Kerosene or charcoal	0.6	1.1	0.6	0.5
• Wood or other	2.8	10.9	2.9	0.5
Neuquén				
• Gas connection	71.9	38.5	63.7	90.6
• Tank gas	26.9	56.6	35.7	9.1
• Kerosene or charcoal	0.3	1.7	0.0	0.0
• Wood or other	0.9	3.3	0.6	0.3
Posadas				
• Gas connection	8.1	0.5	6.0	14.1
• Tank gas	80.7	71.4	83.9	83.7
• Kerosene or charcoal	3.2	10.0	1.4	0.6
• Wood or other	8.0	18.1	8.7	1.6
Santiago del Estero				
• Gas connection	41.3	10.6	26.5	65.7
• Tank gas	46.1	46.5	63.7	33.7
• Kerosene or charcoal	9.8	32.9	7.7	0.5
• Wood or other	2.8	10.0	2.1	0.0

Source: INDEC 1990, 352.

_____ Table 3.9 _____
Homes without Refrigerator, by Poverty Group, 1990

		Percentage of Homes		
		Structurally		
City	Total	Poor	Impoverished	Nonpoor
Greater Buenos Aires	6.7	25.2	8.8	2.5
General Roca	13.7	39.6	17.3	4.1
Neuquén	16.0	36.2	17.5	7.8
Posadas	21.7	55.3	20.7	3.0
Santiago del Estero	14.5	44.5	13.5	1.4

Source: INDEC 1990, 350.

Other Appliances

The appliances considered essential for cleanliness, comfort, and food preparation in middle- and upper-class homes simply do not exist in the houses of the poor. Vacuum cleaners, washing machines, toasters, microwave ovens, blenders—none of those is found. Clothes are washed by hand in a basin or in a stream.

The telephone, which in the United States is considered a vital organ, is a luxury of the upper and upper-middle classes in Argentina. Certainly none of the houses described here would have a phone. Many middle-class people, including doctors, cannot afford telephones in Argentina. The rural *rancho* is already isolated. Without a phone, help in an emergency is always a ride on horseback away. In studies of childhood mortality in the Argentine interior, it was found that the death rate among children in isolated areas was much greater than in urban areas. The rural zones of San Juan Province had child mortality rates twice that of the provincial capital (Burke 1979, 29).

Electricity

Most of the urban and suburban poor in Argentina have electricity. Even in the shantytowns, many of the houses are connected to electric lines. In Retiro, the older houses have electricity, but the shanties of Autopista do not. The electrical connections to a shantytown, however, are likely to be clandestine. Consequently, the wiring is not always done correctly. In the houses, too, the wiring as well as the connections to the main line are do-it-yourself and very likely not in conformance with appropriate safety standards.

Screens

Many areas in Argentina are low lying and damp, with frequent precipitation. The entire littoral (which is what Argentines call the provinces along the great Paraná and Uruguay rivers), Greater Buenos Aires, and most of the Northeast fit that description for at least half the year. Such a climate fosters the spread of mosquitoes. For a reasonably well-built house, screens would be useful in protecting inhabitants from mosquitoes and the diseases they carry. Unfortunately, in most of the houses described here, screens would be of little use because the houses sit on dirt. Walls do not meet the dirt for the entire perimeter, and the doors, if there are any, do not fit their openings.

Location

For many of the poor, it is the location of their miserable homes as much as the construction that is injurious to their health. Rural *ranchos* are isolated, remote from schools, recreational and cultural facilities, and health centers.

According to UNICEF, only 21 percent of the rural population of Argentina has access to health services (UNICEF 1991, 107).

City housing markets ensure that tenements are not well located. In Buenos Aires, most of the tenements are located in the neighborhoods of La Boca and Barracas, settled in the early years of the city near the port and the pestilential Riachuelo creek. After the yellow fever and cholera epidemics of the late 1800s, the wealthier residents abandoned these areas for the more healthy sites in Barrio Norte. The class division in location remains. Because of its low elevation—La Boca lies below the high-tide line—there is frequent flooding of sewers, storm drains, and underground electrical wires.

The location of the *villas miseria* produces the greatest number of problems. Essentially, squatters occupy no-rent land, land that has so little worth that no one bothers to have or enforce property rights to it. The worst squatter shanty-towns are those built on or around garbage dumps (see Chapter 5, "Water, Waste, and Garbage").

Only marginally better off are people who live on former garbage dumps. In some cases, these landfills are former toxic dumps for industry, filled-in lakes, or built-over cemeteries. Villa Soldati, a neighborhood in the Federal Capital, and the nearby public housing project of Ramón Carrillo were built over a former lake, a toxic dump, *and* a cemetery and in a flood zone. The basin of the Cildáñez drains into Soldati Lake, which is highly contaminated because 3,000 industries dump liquids and sewer effluents into the Cildáñez. Studies by the University of Buenos Aires have found mercury in the soil. In 1991, the subsecretary of health for the city of Buenos Aires, Alberto Morán, said the city has no idea with what the land is filled, but he assured the population that there was no danger of chemical or other environmental contamination (*Clarín*, September 22, 1991, pp. 38–39).

Shantytowns commonly are located in flood zones, which can be creek flood zones, low areas that collect rainwater, or coastal flood areas. Greater Buenos Aires has all three. The Riachuelo-Matanza, Resistencia, and Luján rivers all have shantytowns located in their flood plains. In fact, a favored place to erect a shanty is under the protection of bridges over those rivers. Because all the rivers and streams in Greater Buenos Aires are dead from industrial, chemical, domestic, and sewer system dumping, the flooding is extremely unhealthy for those inhabitants.

Greater Buenos Aires is very flat, very close to sea level, and poorly drained. Consequently, every rain of any magnitude leads to rainwater flooding throughout the region. Rains accompanied by southeast winds lead to flooding of all low-lying coastal areas from La Boca to Tigre in the delta of the Paraná. Thousands of squatters live in this estuarine area. Southeasters bring not only flooding but also untreated sewage that has been dumped into the Río de la Plata. All these areas that are vulnerable to flooding also are perennially damp.

Another locational disadvantage is that the poor live where others cannot stand to, downwind from the meatpacking plants. The stench in the neighborhoods of Mataderos and the so-called Ciudad Oculta is nauseating. (The hazards of parasite infection from living near abattoirs are discussed in Chapter 5.)

Safety

Shantytowns in Buenos Aires and in the surrounding metropolitan area have different personalities, depending on the composition of the resident population. Some, such as Villa Fátima (near Villa Soldati) in the Federal Capital, are composed of honest, hard-working families. In these *villas mansas* (tame slums), there is considerable solidarity. The people look out for each other, there are few criminals and drug addicts, the people organize day care centers and soup kitchens, and it is safe to walk around (visit, September 24, 1991).

At the other extreme are the *villas bravas* (tough slums), which are populated largely by criminals and drug addicts. They have their own *cacique*, or chief, and the police do not enter the area. In the fancy suburban county of San Isidro is one of the worst *villas bravas*, called *La Cava*. Another tough slum is in the garbage dumps of San Fernando on the fashionable north side (visits, 1991, 1992, 1993).

The Retiro *villa* is peaceful during the day, and doctors and nurses feel safe making rounds. At night, however, people stay in their houses (numerous interviews and visits, June–September 1992, September 1993). Ciudad Oculta, downwind from the meatpacking plants, is a tough area populated with many criminal types. The medical center staff do not go into the community, day or night, because they are afraid. Residents interviewed in Ciudad Oculta reported spending the whole weekend, every weekend, with an entire family of eight inside their one-room house to protect the children from drug pushers. Because of the drugs and delinquency, families tend to be young in Ciudad Oculta. Parents try to move out before their children become adolescents (visit, November 27, 1991). A new *changa*, or job, has been invented in the *villas bravas*, that of people guarding the houses of those who go to work and women walking children to school so others do not have to leave their houses unattended. The neighborhood of Villa Corina has 40,000 people, but its streets and paths are deserted at night (Alvarez and Alvarez 1992, 6). In Buenos Aires, it should be noted, deserted streets are a rarity, even at night. Until very recently, people were quite safe at all hours of the day and night all over Buenos Aires.

Public Services and Amenities in Shantytowns

The housing of the poor almost always is in areas poorly served by public facilities. Even in cities in which services exist, they generally serve higher-income neighborhoods and commercial districts. Periurban areas, especially illegally occupied land, lack even basic municipal services.

Homes in Neighborhoods without Various Facilities, 1990

| | Percentage of Homes | | | |
Facilities	Total	Structurally Poor	Impoverished	Nonpoor
Greater Buenos Aires				
• Street lighting	6.1	17.0	8.1	3.3
• Storm sewers	15.0	27.2	17.7	11.7
• Paved streets	24.9	50.8	33.3	16.8
• Sidewalks	13.4	32.8	17.4	8.2
General Roca				
• Street lighting	7.4	18.4	9.3	3.1
• Storm sewers	n.a.	n.a.	n.a.	n.a.
• Paved streets	46.9	71.4	58.6	32.3
• Sidewalks	36.9	66.3	43.5	24.3
Neuquén				
• Street lighting	3.9	12.0	3.9	1.2
• Storm sewers	n.a.	n.a.	n.a.	n.a.
• Paved streets	4.6	75.8	67.3	36.2
• Sidewalks	28.8	57.2	34.0	14.4
Posadas				
• Street lighting	16.5	34.4	16.2	6.3
• Storm sewers	22.0	38.6	16.9	16.1
• Paved streets	64.2	88.1	68.0	47.5
• Sidewalks	44.8	75.9	48.2	24.1
Santiago del Estero				
• Street lighting	1.5	6.8	0.0	0.0
• Storm sewers	36.0	62.6	39.8	21.0
• Paved streets	23.2	54.0	24.7	8.0
• Sidewalks	10.2	32.2	8.5	1.2

Source: INDEC 1990, 326, 327, 330, 331.

These areas almost never have garbage collection. Sometimes people bury garbage or burn it, but generally it is left in piles in the streets. There are no storm drains or sewers, so rainwater and household wastewater run in open ditches in the dirt streets. The stagnant and putrefying pools, which are breeding grounds for vectors (carriers) of gastrointestinal and parasitic diseases, are also play areas for the children.

Table 3.10 gives the proportion of homes, by poverty group, that lack various public services. In some neighborhoods, usually affluent residential areas or commercial zones, certain facilities are available for an entire neighborhood. In other areas, some facilities may be available on some blocks of a neighborhood, which makes living more convenient even for those on unserved blocks because they pass through the served areas. Table 3.10 lists for each urban area studied the percentage of households in neighborhoods in which *none* of the streets had a particular service.

In item after item, the lack of facilities means another way in which quality of life, safety, physical and mental health, and vitality are undermined for the poor. Unlighted mud streets, flooded by rains and filled with garbage, are the constant environment of the poor.

In all five urban areas, the most critical deficit in poor neighborhoods is paved streets. Over half the structurally poor in all five cities live in neighborhoods in which no streets are paved. In three cities, the proportion is over 70 percent. For the impoverished, as well, the proportion living in neighborhoods without any paved streets is high: one-fourth of the impoverished in Santiago, one-third of those in Buenos Aires, and well over half in the other three urban areas. These five cities are not country towns; they include the national capital and three provincial capitals.

Table 3.10 does not evaluate storm sewers in General Roca and Neuquén, because of the arid climate. In Santiago, few areas have storm sewers, but because of the dry climate that is not a critical factor. In Buenos Aires and Posadas, where there is significant rainfall throughout the year, the lack of storm drains, combined with dirt streets, means roads are impassable for long stretches of time. In Buenos Aires, 27 percent of the structurally poor and 18 percent of the impoverished live in neighborhoods in which no streets have storm drains. In Posadas, nearly 40 percent of the structurally poor live in neighborhoods in which there is no storm drainage.

Living at the fringes of a city and on the fringes of society cuts poor people off from educational, cultural, and social activities. Table 3.11 lists, for five urban areas, the percentage of homes located more than ten blocks from primary and nursery schools and from child care centers.

In Buenos Aires, the location of 8 percent of the structurally poor more than ten blocks from a primary school helps to explain the late starting age that is common for poor children. The distance from a nursery school is greatest for this group. For all economic groups, more than 60 percent of homes are located more than ten blocks from a child care center. The isolating effect, however, is greatest for the structurally poor, because it compounds the other forms of separation from society.

In General Roca and Neuquén, the proportion of homes of the structurally poor that are distant from nursery schools and child care centers is significantly greater than for the nonpoor. In Santiago and Posadas, a high percentage of homes in all economic groups are distant from child care centers, but the proportion is higher for both poor groups.

_____ *Table 3.11* _____

Homes More Than Ten Blocks from Schools, 1990

Type of School	Total	Structurally Poor	Impoverished	Nonpoor
Greater Buenos Aires				
• Primary school	5.3	8.2	6.7	4.3
• Nursery school	14.3	20.0	16.0	12.6
• Child care center	63.2	65.2	63.7	62.6
General Roca				
• Primary school	5.8	7.5	6.9	4.6
• Nursery school	14.2	26.7	18.7	7.9
• Child care center	38.7	48.9	49.9	28.5
Neuquén				
• Primary school	0.8	4.2	0.0	0.3
• Nursery school	15.6	31.5	17.4	8.6
• Child care center	37.5	57.9	39.5	28.8
Posadas				
• Primary school	8.0	14.4	8.2	4.2
• Nursery school	10.5	20.0	8.9	6.1
• Child care center	55.2	72.5	63.2	39.2
Santiago del Estero				
• Primary school	1.5	5.3	0.9	0.2
• Nursery school	3.7	7.7	3.1	2.2
• Child care center	80.8	91.6	89.1	70.2

The "Percentage of Homes" header spans the Total, Structurally Poor, Impoverished, and Nonpoor columns.

Source: INDEC 1990, 333, 334, 335.

Table 3.12 gives the percentage of homes for each economic group located more than ten blocks from a public telephone. Considering that there are no phones in private homes or businesses in poor neighborhoods, the isolation of the poor is stark. For every urban area, more than one-third of the poor live more than ten blocks from a public telephone. For example, the neighborhood of Ramón Carrillo was built by the city of Buenos Aires to relocate squatters who had taken over a building elsewhere in the city. By 1991, there were 2,000 adults and 1,800 children in the neighborhood and not a single telephone.

Firehouses

The county of La Matanza has over one million residents but only four volunteer firehouses. Although each house has a total of twenty-five men on whom it can call, the house is staffed by about four firefighters at a time. Thus, sixteen men protect one million people in shacks, apartments, individual houses,

Homes More Than Ten Blocks from a Public Phone, 1990

| | | Percentage of Homes | | |
| | | Structurally | | |
City	Total	Poor	Impoverished	Nonpoor
Greater Buenos Aires	18.1	35.9	23.2	12.9
General Roca	17.6	36.1	18.9	11.6
Neuquén	23.4	34.8	27.5	15.9
Posadas	30.1	54.2	32.1	14.5
Santiago del Estero	23.2	36.3	24.1	16.6

Source: INDEC 1990, 337.

factories, schools, and offices in an area of 125 square miles. The force is entirely volunteer, and all their resources are financed by donations from the residents. They have enough support from the residents that they are able to protect the force with equipment that is up to U.S. standards (visit, Gregorio La Ferrere firehouse, November 6, 1992). I found no information in any of the INDEC sources or elsewhere about firehouses in the rest of Greater Buenos Aires or in provincial cities.

Impact of Inadequate Housing on Health

The effect of all these deficiencies on the health of the poor is devastating. The extent of the effect generally is underestimated because so many of the poor are illegal occupants and do not appear in official figures. Neither the numerator of the problem (mortality, morbidity, fertility) nor the denominator (size of the population, distribution) is properly estimated. When asked for the infant mortality rate in Ciudad Oculta, the director of the health center there could not really say because the actual population or the number of births was not known. His best estimate was that the infant mortality rate was well over 100 per thousand (Dr. Mario Rípoli, November 27, 1991).

This section outlines some of the health effects of bad housing. Poor people also suffer the effects of bad water, bad food, and other factors discussed in subsequent chapters, all of which contribute to the respiratory, skin, and gastrointestinal diseases, mental illnesses, and injuries discussed here.

Respiratory Illnesses and Common Infectious Diseases

The combined effect of poor housing construction and a cold damp environment is the increased severity of colds and other infectious diseases.

Crowding encourages the transmission of diseases such as flu and meningitis. The incidence of respiratory infections is similar in developed and developing countries and among children from different socioeconomic strata—four to eight episodes a year (PAHO 1990*a*, 78)—but the outcomes are worse for the poor. A leaky roof, a drafty wall made from a blanket, a dirt floor turned to mud in every rain, no heat—none is conducive to quick recovery from the usual childhood illnesses. In fact, the most common cause of death in children in precarious urban, periurban, and rural housing is the common cold. The cold worsens to pneumonia, and, already malnourished from poor diet and repeated gastrointestinal and respiratory infections, the child dies.

Argentina's rate of mortality from acute respiratory infections is ten times that of Canada (PAHO 1990*a*, 75). The mortality rate among children in Third World countries in general is thirty times that of industrialized countries (Leowski 1986, 138). The third leading cause of death in children under one year of age and from one to four years of age is pneumonia and influenza, which claimed over 1,000 Argentine children under the age of five in 1986 (PAHO 1990*a*, 430, 437). In Ciudad Oculta, infectious diseases, especially respiratory diseases, are still the leading cause of death in children (Dr. Graciela Spatz, December 6, 1991). In all ages, over 5,000 deaths nationally in 1986 were due to pneumonia and influenza (PAHO 1990*a*, 403). Including other forms of acute respiratory infections, the actual death toll was much higher. The census-recorded deaths among children under one year of age due to respiratory causes ranged from 1,500 to 2,100 for the years 1980 through 1983 (INDEC n.d., 136). The deaths included those from acute bronchitis, diphtheria, pertussis (whooping cough), and otitis media (middle-ear infection).

Open fires for heating and cooking and cigarette smoke contribute to indoor air pollution, which aggravates respiratory conditions. Doctors in Argentina are beginning to realize that much of the bronchial disease thought to have been viral is in fact due to particulate pollution. The number of children brought to the hospital with attacks is significantly higher on days when the particle count is high (Giménez 1991, 130). The World Health Organization reports that, in some large cities of the developing world, vehicular emissions of air pollutants are increasing by 5 to 10 percent per year (WHO 1991*b*, 12). Unfortunately, few doctors work in the area of environmental contamination, because they get little training in medical school and there would be few jobs for them if they did specialize in that field. In addition to damage to the respiratory system, indoor pollution is toxic because of the carbon monoxide from not only open charcoal burners but also gas heaters and cookers. Even when a child is removed from the toxic home environment, the effects, such as demyelinization (the destruction of the protective sheaths around nerve fibers, similar to the effect of multiple sclerosis), persist (Giménez 1991, 131, 139).

The Inter-American Investigation of Mortality in Childhood was carried out in fifteen locations in the Americas. Households with a child death were compared to a random sample of households to investigate the correlation between household circumstances and child deaths. Two of the sites were in Argentina: one included rural and urban areas of Chaco; the other included rural and suburban areas of San Juan. The study found a significant amount of crowding in both the sample and the death groups in San Juan and Chaco, but in all study sites, a larger percentage of households with a child death had more than three persons per room. In the city of Resistencia, Chaco, 30 percent of sample households had more than three persons per room, compared with 66 percent of households with a child death. In rural areas of Chaco, 53 percent of sample households and 75 percent of households with a child death had such severe crowding (Burke 1979, 34).

Location is also important in determining the severity of respiratory illnesses, such as in flood zones that are perennially damp. The children attended to in Health Center Number 6 who live in low-lying *villas* near the Riachuelo creek suffer from very high rates of asthma and other respiratory disorders (Dr. Aprigliano, September 24, 1991). There are 1,000 asthma deaths a year in Argentina, of which half occur in the Federal Capital and Buenos Aires Province (Mazzei et al. 1988, 714). It is probable that the prevalence of asthma is underreported because doctors are reluctant to label a child as chronically ill with an incurable disease (Roncoroni 1989, 544; Gené et al. 1989, 546).

Besides the little protection offered by precarious housing, it appears that crowding leads to increased infecting dosages of pathogens, aggravating the severity of acute respiratory infections. The combination of indoor pollutants with immunosuppression caused by malnutrition also might account for the severity of respiratory infections among the poor (Denny and Loda 1986, 1).

Another disease that is particularly dangerous for children already weakened by gastrointestinal, parasitic, or infectious diseases is measles. Measles is not life threatening for well-nourished and well-housed children, but in the circumstances of the poor, measles can lead to fatal respiratory infections. Worldwide an estimated 2.5 million deaths from measles occur each year (Styblo and Rouillon 1991, 391). Because the Menem government has neglected to maintain immunization programs, measles still poses a serious health problem for poor children.

In an investigation of the 1984 measles outbreak, in which there were 32,000 reported cases, it was found that among children under five years old there were three times as many cases of measles in poor areas than in nonpoor areas. The study found that 45 percent of the difference could be attributed to socioeconomic causes (Manterola et al. 1987, 49). In the 1991 outbreak, there were more than 95,000 cases. Argentina has the same rate of measles infection as the United

States did in 1924, many years before the vaccine was invented. In Argentina, the vaccine was introduced in 1971, but epidemics still occur on a predictable basis (Dr. Graciela Spatz, December 6, 1991). (The failure of the Argentine government to maintain an adequate immunization system is discussed in Chapter 8, "Primary Health Care.")

There are 600 to 700 deaths from meningitis every year in Argentina, about half of them in Greater Buenos Aires. Bacterial meningitis is transmitted through respiratory passages and is spread more easily in crowded conditions (Camps 1992*b*, 41).

Strep infections have a higher incidence in conditions of crowding and inadequate housing and in households that consist of a large number of persons. Noting that the incidence of strep tonsillitis varied greatly in different studies in Argentina, researchers compared its incidence among children of working-class homes and middle-class homes. They found that the greater incidence of strep tonsillitis among working class children was statistically significant and varied with the degree of household crowding (Roncoroni et al. 1987, 443).

Tuberculosis

Tuberculosis (TB) is the greatest cause of death from a single pathogen and perhaps the disease that has caused the most deaths in human history. In 1990, three million deaths worldwide were attributed to tuberculosis. The search for a cure for TB was protracted and difficult because of the resistance of the bacillus to chemotherapy. The bacillus dies in direct sunlight but can survive in dust for months. An estimated 1.7 billion persons in the world are infected (Ryan 1993, 6, 396, 397). Not all of them have active cases of TB, but the disease establishes a node of infection in the lungs or elsewhere and then can remain dormant, even for decades. The disease becomes active when the infected person's resistance is lowered. An extremely dangerous situation has developed since the emergence of AIDS worldwide; about 40 percent of AIDS sufferers develop TB. Tuberculosis and human immunodeficiency virus (HIV) have a synergistic relationship. Tuberculosis triggers AIDS in HIV-positive patients much earlier than in non-TB patients, and AIDS promotes devastating effects from TB.

In developing countries, there is rarely a better than 50-percent cure rate for TB because of the difficulties of case surveillance. Incomplete treatment creates a more dangerous public health situation than no treatment, because sufferers survive longer and expose a much larger number of people. Incomplete treatment also contributes to the development of drug-resistant strains of the bacillus (Styblo and Rouillon 1991, 391). Since 1992, drug resistance has developed in Argentine strains of TB.

In some African countries with very good surveillance, cure rates of 80 percent or more have been achieved, for example, in Tanzania. Wealthier countries have had less success, in part due to a lack of commitment on the part of public health authorities and in part due to the composition of the patient pool. Tuberculosis sufferers in developed and middle-income countries often are dysfunctional people, such as drug addicts, who cannot maintain a drug therapy program for the six months it takes to achieve a cure. Community-based programs have failed because people tend to stop coming for treatment when they feel better. When infected people remain in the community, they continue to spread the disease. Even a person who continues the medication remains contagious for as much as two months (Ryan 1993, 391).

Crowding and promiscuity, as well as poor quality of housing, create an environment conducive to the spread of tuberculosis. The likelihood of contracting TB is increased by the intensity of contact with infected persons, as well as by the virulence of the case. The overcrowded poor household is the ideal climate for TB. Argentina has a serious TB problem, with an average of 1,500 deaths per year (PAHO 1990a, 340–341). Official figures give 13,000 new cases per year, out of a population of 33 million (Sainz 1992a, 19). A doctor whose primary work is tuberculosis control in the *villa* of Ciudad Oculta asserts that the actual rate of new infections in Argentina is 18,000 per year (Dr. Graciela Spatz, December 6, 1991).[3]

As early as the 1930s, it was recognized that TB resulted from overcrowding in the tenements of Buenos Aires. Provincial governor Manuel Fresco promised better housing to combat tuberculosis, which was the infectious disease with the highest mortality rate in Argentina at that time. In 1938, when Fresco was governor, 15 percent of deaths in Buenos Aires were from infectious diseases, of which three-fourths were caused by TB (Dolkart 1969, 234). Almost sixty years later, people are living in the same tenements, and TB still causes about 20 percent of the deaths from infectious diseases. Eighty percent of infantile tuberculosis is among children from the *villas* (Noguero 1988, 497). In Córdoba, the second-richest province, 5 percent of TB cases are in teenagers. The disease is more dangerous in the young due to its tendency to cause progressive lesions (Valdés et al. 1986, 322).

The risk of transmission of TB depends on the number of cases. The risk of becoming ill depends on a person's immune status and environment. In 1988, Argentina reported a national rate of 19.6 contagious people per 100,000 population. The distribution in the country, however, was uneven, with 11.6 per 100,000 in the Federal Capital, 29 per 100,000 in Corrientes, and 74 per 100,000 in Jujuy (PAHO 1990a, 175, 176). More up-to-date data indicate a growing epidemic of TB in Argentina, which is not surprising given the worsening economic situation, with falling living standards and cuts in government spending on TB control, as well as the growing AIDS epidemic. As of June 1991, the national average was

52.3 TB cases per 100,000, with a range from 22 to 214 in different regions (de Kantor et al. 1991, 461).

Skin Diseases

The location of slum dwellings on former landfills, toxic waste dumps, and filled lakes and cemeteries leads to epidemic skin disease. The residents, especially the children, are in constant contact with contaminated soil. Acid soil always leads to skin problems. The University of Buenos Aires found high acidity and mercury in soil samples in the Flores area of Villa Fátima. Dr. Gabriel Muntaabski of Health Center Number 6, which serves the area, says that 10 percent of center visits are for skin problems, including mange, scabies, and infected lice infestation (*Clarín*, September 22, 1991, pp. 38–39).

In addition to location, the lack of facilities for bathing, the lack of water, or the absence of a habit of bathing and the marginalization that makes some people dysfunctional lead to inadequate use of water for bathing. The chronic lack of cleanliness is responsible for numerous skin diseases, such as mange and scabies (Dr. Aprigliano, September 24, 1991). Head lice is a problem of enormous proportions in Argentina. The endemia has established itself so firmly in the population that no school, including elite private schools, is spared.

Another skin disease that is the result of location and quality of housing is leprosy. A warm, moist climate, miserable living conditions, and prolonged proximity to infected persons encourage contagion. In the early 1980s, there were about 1,000 new cases a year. In the second half of the 1980s, 700 to 800 new cases of leprosy were reported each year. In 1987, there were 17,000 lepers in Argentina, with a prevalence of 5.4 per 10,000 population (PAHO 1990*a*, 165). The Pan American Health Organization considers prevalence of more than 1 per 10,000 population a significant problem. As of 1990, the Ministry of Health reported 20,000 to 26,000 lepers in Argentina.

Because leprosy is a disease of warm climate and of poverty, the national rate of 5.4, which in itself is quite serious, disguises a regional problem of much greater proportions. The areas of highest prevalence are also those of greatest poverty. Chaco has 36.9 lepers per 10,000 population; Corrientes, 35.7; Formosa, 30.4; Misiones, 15.6; and Santa Fe, 9.7 (*BEN* 1990*a*, 60). The areas of highest incidence are not remote regions. In Misiones, for example, the greatest number of cases are not in the hinterland but in the shadow of the health centers of Posadas, the provincial capital.

It is known that "there is no disease which is less readily transmitted from person to person than leprosy, or so easily controlled by simple methods of hygiene or by what we should today regard as normal standards of cleanliness" (Fiennes 1978, 26). In most of the world, leprosy has decreased substantially over the past decade. In the Americas, however, because of ineffective control programs new cases have continued to increase (Noordeen 1992, 300).[4]

Mosquito- and Fly-Borne Diseases

Several diseases endemic to Argentina are borne by mosquitoes. Both the location of a house and its construction contribute to the spread of those diseases. Siting near breeding areas, near pools or swamps, places people in close proximity to mosquito populations. People are exposed in poorly built houses with doors and windows that do not fit openings, with cracks in the walls and between the walls and the floor, and without screens.

Dengue fever is carried by the *Aedes aegypti* mosquito. Yellow fever is carried in the Brazil-Argentina border area by *Aedes albopictus*. Both diseases recently have extended their range in South America and in some countries have returned after being suppressed. In Argentina, both mosquitoes have returned. In a study to evaluate the risk to the population of northeast Argentina, it was found that only a small proportion of the people surveyed had antibodies to dengue because it had been absent for a long time. With the presence of the vector in the areas near Posadas, dengue fever now threatens an unprotected population (Alonso et al. 1987, 55).

One of the biggest killers of Third World children and adults and an important cause of lost work time and vitality is malaria. The incidence of malaria has been rising annually in the Americas since 1974. By 1988, there were four times as many cases as fourteen years earlier, and chloroquine-resistant strains now are found in many countries. Chloroquine is a relatively inexpensive and safe prophylaxis against malaria, but in resistant areas, prevention now requires more potent and more expensive drugs.

In Argentina, malaria is not a major disease nationally because the endemic zone is small for this generally tropical and subtropical disease. Malaria had been eliminated in all of Argentina, but it has returned. In 1986, there were 2,000 cases of malaria in Argentina. In 1987, 1,521 cases were reported; in 1988, there were 666 cases. By the early 1990s, however, malaria was a cause for increasing concern as living conditions worsened and government control programs were cut back. So far, the strain in Argentina is not the chloroquine-resistant type. The World Health Organization lists inadequate sanitation and precarious living conditions first among the difficulties encountered in malaria prevention and control (WHO 1990, 70, 74).

Leishmaniasis, a disfiguring disease carried by sandflies in forest zones, is endemic in Salta, Jujuy, Santiago del Estero, and Tucumán. The parasite causes large craters in the skin, particularly on the face but also on the legs and arms. It is incurable.

_____ *Table 3.13* _____

Working Mothers Leaving Children under Four Years of Age with Siblings

City	Total	Percentage of Working Mothers		
		Structurally Poor	Impoverished	Nonpoor
Greater Buenos Aires	7.2	18.5	12.2	3.1
General Roca	15.9	28.3	20.9	4.0
Neuquén	7.3	25.9	9.4	0.0
Posadas	11.3	18.1	14.3	0.0
Santiago del Estero	19.7	31.4	20.8	12.0

Source: INDEC 1990, 230.

Burns and Punctures

The majority of patients at the special hospital for serious burn victims in Buenos Aires are shanty dwellers. Numerous burn hazards exist in the poor household. The most obvious on entering a *villa* dwelling is the coal-burning heater, propped in the middle of the living room/bedroom floor. The open fire in the hibachi-like apparatus is just about at face and hand level for a crawling infant or toddler. It is a natural target for a baby in a wheeled walker, which some mothers use to keep babies out of the dirt. Any child running into the house is likely to knock into the heater and spill the fire into the bed coverings nearby.

Adequate habitat for children includes having a person of responsible age present. Unattended children have more accidents, burns, and poisonings (WHO 1991*b*, 23). In Table 3.13, the percentages of mothers who leave their small children in the care of another child is given by economic group for the five urban areas.

In all areas, the proportion of mothers leaving children under four years of age in the care of young siblings is highest for the structurally poor and is from one-fifth to one-third of working mothers for that group. Doctors in the *villas* confirm that children are left in the care of other children. Three thousand children in Ciudad Oculta are under the age of fourteen. The neighborhood has four day care centers, with a total capacity of about 150 children. Children as young as ten are left to care for younger siblings while parents work (visit, November 27, 1991). In a visit to Villa Fátima, the director of the health center and I were approached by a child of six who was caring for a younger sibling and needed help (September 24, 1991).

The inadequate kitchen space makes burns and scaldings more likely. Doctor Coruja, director of the burn hospital, reported a high number of mother and child burns and scaldings, particularly in shanties, where there usually is no stable surface on which to place a pot removed from the single burner.

The materials used in construction (wood, blankets, plastic sheets, cardboard) make the houses and the inhabitants particularly vulnerable to fire. The lack of adequate fire protection means that fires can spread easily and quickly among the closely crowded shacks.

The houses are made of scrap materials, whatever can be found. Doors are closed with rusty, twisted wire that juts out at eye level of the resident tots. Barbed wire is everywhere. Try to avoid the sewage and mud that fill most of the passageways, and the barbed wire on both sides of the road gets you. Dirt floors conceal sharp objects. Inadequate garbage disposal results in streets and yards full of trash. Lack of drainage causes mud streets to retain water, further concealing puncture hazards. Through all of this, children scamper barefoot and inevitably suffer numerous puncture wounds. Keeping wounds and burns clean in such an environment is next to impossible.

Wiring and Electrical Hazards

In the self-constructed houses, the wiring is precarious and provisional. Hookups to the power grid are do-it-yourself. In tenements, wiring and main grid connections are often unsafe. The hazards are multiplied during the frequent storms that lash Buenos Aires and the littoral. After every storm, the newspapers report the number of deaths caused by fallen wires. As of 1993, the power authorities have begun to cut off entire zones during storms because of the inevitability of downed wires.

Commuting and Street Hazards

The great distances people have to travel to work mean long rides on overcrowded buses, with people coughing in other riders' faces—the buses are so packed that passengers literally cannot raise their hands to cover their mouths. The bus rides are exhausting and frustrating. People line up in queues of sometimes one hundred or more, only to see bus after bus pass, too full even to close the doors. Several people hang from the handrails at the steps. Not surprisingly, one person per day is killed by a bus in Buenos Aires. The rest of the passengers emerge exhausted from a trip that may have lasted two hours, with little time left in the day for food shopping, food preparation, or relaxation. The shantytowns and tenements are located in areas of heavy road traffic with little play space. Consequently, being hit by cars is a serious hazard for children in those neighborhoods. In urban areas, 75 percent of traffic deaths are pedestrians, particularly old people and children (*BEN* 1990*b*, 36).

Mental Health

A pleasant environment, with clean open space and recreational facilities, contributes to good mental health. In some shantytowns, there is no open
space between the houses. In others, there is space but no facilities. The only
open space in the *villa* of Retiro was the soccer field. The impending expulsion of
the residents of the neighborhood of Autopista threatened to divide the *villa*,
since it was feared that those whose houses were bulldozed for the highway construction would rebuild on the holy ground of the soccer field.

Lacking any alternative activities and exposed to all the same influences of
children in big cities around the world, many of the slum children in Buenos
Aires use drugs, the cheapest and most popular being glue and alcohol. The
national health ministry lists teenage alcoholism as the country's second most
important endemic illness after Chagas' disease. The health secretary of the city
of Buenos Aires reports that 5 percent of children under twelve years of age
drink alcohol on a regular basis and that 5 percent of those under eighteen years
of age are chronic alcohol abusers. There are three million alcoholics in Argentina (*Buenos Aires Herald*, August 3, 1992, p. 7).

There are few pleasant public spaces in Buenos Aires (except the Botanical
Garden). Almost every public space is full of garbage and worn out. The water-
front parks, although far from most people's homes, could be pleasant areas for
free relaxation. Instead, they are covered with garbage and spoiled by human
waste. Among the plans for the use of the bulldozed Retiro *villa* is an enormous
green space, perhaps as much as 400 hectares (1,000 acres). The area, however,
probably will be used for malls and hotels.

Buenos Aires has 2.5 square meters of park space per person compared to
New York's 30 square meters per person and Brussels and Amsterdam, which
have nearly as much as New York. Based on World Health Organization recom-
mendations for green space per person, Buenos Aires, which has 865 hectares,
should have 3,865 hectares (Johnson 1995, 13).

Another factor that contributes to poor mental health is crowding and promiscuity (bed crowding). It is not surprising that a UNICEF study of the *villas* of
Greater Buenos Aires and Greater La Plata found that promiscuity was associated with a high degree of psychological backwardness among children
(UNICEF 1990*b*, 92).

Gastrointestinal Diseases and Parasites

The lack of proper storage and preparation space for food and the lack
of refrigeration contribute to gastrointestinal diseases and diarrhea. Dirt floors
add to the likelihood of parasite infestation. Lack of excreta disposal and the presence of numerous dogs and cats also spread parasitic diseases. Location in and

around garbage dumps presents hazards of disease, parasites, and poisonings. In rural and periurban households, the presence of chickens inside the houses and goats in the yard presents another source of oral-fecal contamination, particularly for young children. Many of the illnesses to which a child is exposed are not serious, but for children whose immune systems are already compromised by malnutrition, bacteria, viruses, and parasites pose serious threats. (Chapter 5, "Water, Waste, and Garbage," examines these diseases in greater depth.)

Desamparado

The word in Spanish for homeless is *desamparado*, meaning left without shelter, unprotected. To a greater or lesser extent, ten million Argentines are *desamparados*. They may have a roof over their heads, but their home does not protect them from the myriad hazards of infectious disease, accidents, parasites, toxic waste, and violence. The house itself, its size, its location, and its equipment—all should contribute to physical and mental well-being. People need to go home to a comforting place after a difficult day at school or a trying day at work. When going home is frustrating at best and life threatening at worst, vitality suffers. The whole country is impoverished when so many of its people live in shacks and tenements, when their opportunities for recreation are so limited, when they come to work and to school beaten down instead of renewed.

Chapter 4 examines in greater detail a specific disease that results from poor housing and that is the most widespread endemia in Argentina, Chagas' disease.

Four

Chagas' Disease

On an expedition to South America from 1831 to 1836 on HMS *Beagle*, Charles Darwin described in his diary a night spent in a village located at the present-day site of the state-owned oil refinery near Luján de Cuyo, Argentina.

> March 25th. . . . We slept in the village of Luxan, which is a small place surrounded by gardens, and forms the most southern cultivated district in the Province of Mendoza; it is five leagues south of the capital. At night I experienced an attack (for it deserves no less a name) of the *Benchuca*, a species of Reduvius, the great black bug of the Pampas. It is most disgusting to feel soft wingless insects, about an inch long, crawling over one's body. Before sucking they are quite thin, but afterwards they become round and bloated with blood, and in this state are easily crushed. (Darwin 1958, 284)

What Darwin recorded is the nightly experience of many millions of people in the Americas whose houses are infested with the *vinchuca*, a winged bedbug. He possibly also was recording his own infection with an incurable, degenerative disease known as Chagas' disease, caused by the parasite *Trypanosoma cruzi*, whose vector is the *vinchuca (Triatoma infestans)*. Later in life, Darwin suffered from debilitating physical disorders that his contemporaries considered psychosomatic. Chagas' is a disease of the Western Hemisphere, unknown in Darwin's England and at that time unidentified even in its endemic zone.

The Prevalence of Chagas' Disease in Latin America

Chagas' disease, also called American trypanosomiasis, is named for the Brazilian physician who first identified it, Carlos Chagas. The parasite that causes the disease, *T. cruzi*, exists from Maryland and California in the United States to southern Argentina and Chile. The endemic zones for Chagas' disease, however, are more restricted, with its highest concentrations in Central America and southern South America. The World Health Organization estimates that ninety million people are at risk of contracting the disease and that prevalence in the Americas is no fewer than sixteen million to eighteen million people (PAHO 1990a, 160–161). In the countries where Chagas' disease is endemic, it presents a major public health problem, even though the actual number of cases is unknown in many countries.

Estimates of the extent of the disease are based on local serological surveys in which prevalence ranges as high as 30 percent (Argentina, Bolivia, Colombia, and Honduras) and 83 percent (Paraguay). Sampling at blood banks has been another source of data. Seropositive cases in such surveys were found to be around 25 percent in Argentina and Brazil and 63 percent in Colombia (PAHO 1990a, 163). Mexico has perhaps as many as 3.8 million people infected with Chagas' disease, over 4 percent of the population (Rojas et al. 1989, 115).

In Bolivia, public health specialists estimate that as many as half the country's population of six million may be affected by the disease. Although Bolivian data on morbidity and mortality from Chagas' disease are incomplete, the Sucre Health Project investigating Chagas' found evidence of a much higher prevalence of the disease than had been anticipated reflected in the age structure of the population. In high-altitude communities, above the range of the Chagas' disease vectors, there are many old people. In valley communities, where Chagas' disease is prevalent, few people are over fifty years old. The team found much anecdotal evidence suggesting Chagas' pathology. There were many cases of young and middle-aged people dying of sudden heart failure, which likely would not have been entered in the death statistics as Chagas'-related, although Chagas' disease would be the probable cause (Renshaw and Rivas 1991, 244, 246).

A Brazilian specialist in Chagas' disease, João Carlos Pinto Dias, says that about five million people in Brazil (over 3 percent of the population) are infected and that over 4 percent of deaths in Brasilia are caused by the disease. The distribution of Chagas' disease throughout Brazil is uneven, but regardless of the region, the "prevalence is always higher among lower social classes and in regions where the socioeconomic indicators are poorest" (Dias 1987, 70, 72, 78).

Distribution of Chagas' Disease in Argentina

Chagas' disease is the most commonly reported parasitic disease in Argentina (PAHO 1990b, 16). Out of a population of 32 million, 2.5 million people, or 8 percent, are infected with this potentially fatal and incurable disease. In areas of greater endemicity, a much higher percentage of the population is infected. Table 4.1 shows the prevalence of Chagas' disease in army conscripts for the years 1981, 1982, and 1983 by province. The worst affected provinces at that time

_____ Table 4.1 _____
Prevalence of Chagas' Disease among Conscripts, by Province, 1981–1983

	Percentage of Conscripts		
Jurisdiction	*1981*	*1982*	*1983*
Federal Capital	2.3	0.8	1.6
Buenos Aires Province	2.5	2.5	2.3
Catamarca	24.3	14.3	11.3
Córdoba	4.4	3.9	3.5
Corrientes	2.1	2.8	2.6
Chaco	30.6	17.7	27.3
Chubut	6.0	0.7	1.8
Entre Ríos	2.6	1.9	2.0
Formosa	18.1	8.6	28.5
Jujuy	14.6	7.4	9.9
La Pampa	10.4	5.6	7.1
La Rioja	6.2	9.0	9.2
Mendoza	6.5	3.2	6.8
Misiones	4.3	2.3	2.1
Neuquén	3.0	1.6	2.2
Río Negro	4.4	1.4	2.0
Salta	11.9	7.7	14.6
San Juan	2.4	5.2	3.1
San Luis	17.3	15.4	13.0
Santa Cruz	2.3	2.8	0.6
Santa Fe	4.4	5.4	4.6
Santiago del Estero	23.7	23.7	15.6
Tucumán	7.8	6.2	6.9
Total	5.8	4.8	5.2

Source: INDEC 1985, 121.

were Catamarca, Chaco, Formosa, and Santiago del Estero, all with over one-fourth of the population infected. Also seriously affected were the provinces of Jujuy, Salta, and San Luis, in which more than 15 percent of conscripts were found to be infected.

Results of blood tests of conscripts after 1983 indicated that La Rioja and Córdoba had joined the provinces of high prevalence, with 18.25 percent of the conscripts infected (Goyoaga 1990, 10). Conservative estimates for the early 1990s are that more than 10 percent of the population of Santiago del Estero, Chaco, Salta, San Luis, and Formosa are infected (Del Rey and Basombrío 1992, 4).

Health Zone Number 4 of the province of Formosa comprises 31 percent of the province's territory (almost 23,000 square kilometers) but has no paved roads. Many of the inhabitants are Wichi and Toba Indians. A household survey of the zone found that 80 percent of the population are infected with Chagas' disease (Ferrero 1987, 169–172).

The highly endemic areas include the fourteen provinces of the Northeast, the Northwest, and the center of the country, in which six million people, almost 20 percent of the population, live. An additional seven provinces constitute an area of lower endemicity. Eighty-six percent of the territory of Argentina is affected. In fact, due to the territorial extension of the range of *T. cruzi*, only Tierra del Fuego and probably the province of Santa Cruz are so far free of the parasite. Although cases of the disease have been detected in those two provinces, infected persons probably migrated to the area (Becker 1985, 306).

Chagas' disease is not restricted to the rural areas. Besides being carried to the cities by new migrants, the disease also is transmitted in the hovels and shantytowns in the urban and periurban areas of large and small cities of Argentina, just as in Latin America generally. In Gregorio LaFerrere, a very poor neighborhood in La Matanza, a county adjacent to the Federal Capital, a child reported in at the morning clinic with a probable case of new Chagas' infection (Hospital Materno-Infantil Gregorio LaFerrere, November 3, 1992). The same conditions of precarious housing that make poor rural people susceptible to infection affect shantytown dwellers in urban and periurban areas.

Transmission of Chagas' Disease

The most common way that Chagas' disease is transmitted is by the bite of the *vinchuca*. The insect bites, usually in the vicinity of the eyes, sucks the blood, and then defecates in the wound. The parasite *T. cruzi* is carried in the feces of the insect and enters the bloodstream of the human or animal host at the site of the bite and defecation. Sometimes a red rash occurs in the area of the bite, but recent studies in Brazil indicate that no more than 5 percent of new cases present the rash, called Romaña's sign. In spite of eradication campaigns, there probably are still about 100,000 new cases of Chagas' disease each year in Brazil due to vectorial transmission (Dias 1987, 73, 74). With an average annual population growth of about half a million (derived from INDEC 1991*a*, 21–22), maintaining a rate of infection of 8 percent in the Argentine population would mean about 40,000 new cases a year.

Chagas' disease also is transmitted from infected mother to child during gestation (congenital Chagas'), from infected mother to child through lactation, through blood transfusions, and, less frequently, by the ingestion of insect waste in food.

The transmission of Chagas' disease through blood transfusions has increased the population at risk to those outside the endemic zone. Donated blood is generally, although not universally, screened for Chagas' disease. In 1987, Dias estimated that there still were about 20,000 new cases per year in Brazil due to transfusions, even though it has been known since the 1940s that the disease can be transmitted that way (Dias 1987, 73). According to the World Health Organization, "Only five countries of the region (Argentina, Brazil, Honduras, Uruguay and Venezuela) have adopted laws that make serological testing of blood donors for *T. cruzi* mandatory. However, even in countries where the legislation exists, a government may not have the political will or the power to enforce it. Financial constraints may also hinder the full implementation of the law" (WHO 1991*a*, 54).

Doctors in the United States are becoming concerned with Chagas' disease, because of its prevalence in areas of recent emigration to the United States. Roughly 25 percent of recipients of blood from infected persons contract the disease (Skolnick 1989). Since Chagas' disease almost never is seen in the United States or other affluent countries, infected blood recipients very well could remain undiagnosed, and their condition would be worsened by the failure to receive what corrective measures are available (Skolnick 1991). In a study of Central American immigrants in the Washington, D.C., area, 5 percent of those tested were found to be infected with *T. cruzi*, although they were asymptomatic (Kirchhoff et al. 1987, 915–920).

The Nature of Chagas' Disease

Chagas' disease presents itself in two phases, acute and chronic. The acute phase occurs shortly after transmission; the chronic phase may not exhibit pathological symptoms for twenty years. The pathology and the outcomes are very different in the two phases.

Acute Chagas' Disease

According to Dr. Roberto Castellucchio, a neurologist who works with the Argentine Foundation for the Fight against Chagas' Disease, the first acute stages often are not correctly diagnosed, and the mortality rate, especially among children, can be as high as 15 percent. Symptoms during the acute phase include meningitis and myocarditis (inflammation of the inner layer of the heart wall). A child who survives may suffer severe consequences, such as mental retardation (Goyoaga 1990, 10). That acute cases are more severe in young children appears to be verified by the high proportion of child deaths in Argentina that are due to heart disease. The Pan American Health Organization lists heart disease as the second leading cause of death in children one to four years old, apart from congenital anomalies, which rank fifth (PAHO 1990*a*, 70).

Mortality in young children often results from a combination of Chagas' disease with measles and pneumonia. Vulnerability to Chagas' infection appears to be associated with malnutrition and diseases of poverty, such as diarrheal infections, other parasites, and tuberculosis (Dias 1987, 59, 77). Studies in rats suggest an important link between zinc deficiency and resistance to infection by

T. cruzi, indicating a synergistic interaction with nutritional deficiency in attacking the immune system (Fraker et al. 1982, 1224–1229).

Chronic Chagas' Disease

Not all infected persons suffer such dramatic consequences of the acute phase. For most, the disease enters a chronic phase that can be asymptomatic for as long as twenty years. Approximately 50 percent of infected persons in serological surveys were asymptomatic in Brazilian research. The large percentage of asymptomatic carriers explains the very high transmission rate through transfusions. During the chronic phase, the probability of converting from asymptomatic to pathological is about 2 percent to 5 percent per year. Therefore, the likelihood of sudden death from cardiac arrest is not very high. Nevertheless, the leading cause of sudden death in Latin America (excluding accidents) is Chagas' cardiomyopathy. The public health problems of this stage include the spread of the disease by asymptomatic blood donors and the fact that some employers reject seropositive applicants who present no pathology, aggravating the economic conditions that contributed to the infection in the first place (Dias 1987, 74).

The remainder of chronic Chagas' carriers present symptoms of varying severity of cardiac, digestive, or combined chronic forms. Chagasic chronic cardiopathy has two forms, which affect between 15 and 30 percent of chagasic carriers: myocardial damage with progressive heart failure and complex arrhythmia syndromes (Dias 1987, 74). According to Dr. Castellucchio, about one-fourth of infected persons in Argentina develop cardiac symptoms, with a fatality rate of 70 percent (Goyoaga 1990, 10).

The digestive forms of chronic Chagas' disease, which can be present alone or in combination with cardiac forms, are present in another 10 percent of carriers. Swelling of the esophagus or colon, resulting in difficulty swallowing or blockages of the digestive tract, frequently require surgical correction and at times are fatal (Dias 1987, 76). Megacolon is the most common complication of intestinal Chagas' disease. Many times, surgery intended to correct blockages of the intestine is unsuccessful, and the condition persists unless corrected by additional, more elaborate surgery (Cutait and Cutait 1991, 188–197).

Human Ecology of the Endemic Areas

Macroenvironment of Ecological Disruption

The main vector for *T. cruzi* in Argentina is the *vinchuca*, which unfortunately is extremely well adapted to human dwellings and surrounding sheds, pens, and yards. The writings of missionaries in Argentina and Chile in the sixteenth century record the presence of the *vinchuca* in Indian dwellings, but the parasite apparently was moderately benign in that population, indicating a long period of coexistence of parasite and host (Dias 1985, 289). Evidence from Brazil suggests that the endemicity of Chagas' disease as a human affliction is a recent phenomenon there. The *vinchuca* existed in Brazil, but apparently it was not present in human dwellings since there is no indigenous word for the insect.

The insect and its parasite spread from the forest and brush in Argentina and Uruguay to human dwellings in Brazil, then back to Argentina. That spread resulted from the development of the coffee industry and the influx of laborers infected with the disease, as well as the ecological disruption caused by deforestation and cultivation. Although the parasite and its vector came originally from the wild, people created prime conditions for the vector by eliminating large mammal predators, which increased the number of vermin and small omnivores, such as rats, as cohosts of the parasite. Since agricultural development was accompanied by poor living conditions, especially poor housing for rural workers, the disease flourished over the past century (Dias 1987, 60, 64–65).

In the Argentine north, many areas have been damaged by irrational land management, heavy cattle burden, and the indiscriminate felling of trees, which have transformed the region into one of marginal goatherding (Ronderos and Schnack 1987, 91). The goatherding accentuates the exhaustion of plant life and of the soil (Dias 1985, 292).

The economy and the human ecology of northern Argentina is well suited to the Chagas' vector, which is able to colonize the wild, domestic, and peridomestic environments of rural areas and even penetrate urban ecosystems. The back-and-forth migration of people in the endemic areas maintains the parasite, even in urban settings. The combination of environmental devastation and bad housing apparently transformed an incidental parasite in the wild into one whose vector has as its primary focus human dwellings and peridomestic animal pens (Dias 1985, 291).

Microenvironment of the Poor Household

It is not simply living in the endemic zone but living in poor houses that exposes people to infection with Chagas' disease (Del Ray and Basombrío 1992, 4). The typical rural house and surrounding animal pens are an ideal niche for the *vinchuca*.

The *vinchuca*, like many bloodsucking creatures, is active at night. During the day, it hides in cracks and crevices, especially in the walls of precarious houses. It prefers the sleeping areas of houses, where it not only is less likely to be detected during the day but is best positioned for feeding at night, when it drops from its hiding place onto the face of the sleeping victim and bites. It lays its eggs in high-up cracks in the walls, where they are least likely to be detected.

Numerous studies have demonstrated the correlation not only of infestation of the dwelling with degree of infection but also the degree of infestation with the rate of infection in the human population (Piesman et al. 1985, 866–869). In

Mexico, it was found that the worst-constructed houses and those nearest forest and caves had the greatest degree of infestation (Rojas et al. 1989, 119).

In Bolivia, *T. infestans* and other triatomids (bedbug relatives) suspected of being vectors of Chagas' disease are found in poor housing, especially in valley areas, where nearly all the houses are heavily infested. The Sucre Health Project found that infestation was more widespread and complex than originally believed. All the communities studied were heavily infested. The bugs were an awful nuisance and kept people from sleeping. Some houses were so infested that the families had to sleep outside. The traditional construction in these areas allows little light or ventilation, and "even during the day *vinchucas* crawl across the walls" (Renshaw and Rivas 1991, 250). Of the insects studied in the Bolivian project, about 75 percent carried *T. cruzi* (Renshaw and Rivas 1991, 244–245).

According to a study of houses in the Chaco region of Argentina, "the roofs are a mixture of straw, branches, and mud, a complex interwoven structure. The walls are made of mud, being a discontinuous habitat, with holes and crevices distributed irregularly" (Ronderos and Schnack 1987, 86), providing the insects with an ideal environment. *Ranchos* are the most common form of housing, not only in the rural areas of the Chaco but throughout Cuyo and the Northwest as well. A large proportion of the houses in the towns and even the provincial capitals also are *ranchos* (visits 1987, 1989, 1991, 1992, 1993).

In a thorough study of the housing deficit in Argentina carried out for UNICEF, Susana Lumi found that about two million houses are precarious, are *ranchos*, or have other structural deficits. That constitutes almost 30 percent of the national housing stock. In the Northeast and the Northwest, 60 percent of houses fit one of those descriptions. In fact, about 95 percent of the houses that are precarious or *ranchos* are located in the areas of medium to high endemicity (Lumi 1990, 210). (See Chapter 3, "Housing and Health.")

The presence of domestic animals in the houses provides reservoirs for the parasite, and grain stored in or next to houses feeds populations of rodents that also serve as parasite reservoirs. The storage of firewood in or near the house adds to the favorable environment for the vector as well. The season with the highest incidence of acute cases of Chagas' disease is the harvest time because of a coincidence of host and parasite characteristics. The new generation of insects is most active; rodents and other hosts are displaced from the fields to the peridomestic setting; and domestic fowl are kept indoors to protect the harvest. The fact that rural houses are spread out in an area that is deforested and with low animal population encourages the blood-sucking vector to concentrate in houses. A family of six or eight persons can maintain a stable population of 2,000 to 4,000 *vinchucas* for many years (Dias 1985, 295).

The *vinchuca* also inhabits goatyards, where it generally lays its eggs lower down in the fences, where they are concealed in the mixture of sticks, feces, and goathairs. In the goatyard, the mud, sticks, and goat urine and feces create a warm, hospitable microclimate for the infected bugs, which feed at night on the goats nestled against the fences (Ronderos and Schnack 1987, 88, 93).

Chagas' disease, its insect vectors, and the parasites they carry also are prevalent in the precarious dwellings of every city and town in the endemic area. Dogs and cats in the cities, towns, and suburban areas throughout the entire region have been shown to be important reservoirs for the parasites. Those areas tend to be densely populated with dogs. Amamá in Santiago del Estero, for example, had an average of 2.6 dogs per house, with 95 percent of the households having dogs. Family size correlated with the number of dogs (with a range of from one to five dogs per house), and the human-dog ratio in the town was about two to one (Gürtler et al. 1990, 313, 315).

Another study of 28,000 urban and rural houses found 100 percent of rural houses in the La Rioja village of Villa Mazán *vinchuca* infested; of 8,000 houses in the provincial capital, 70 percent were infested. The insects were more numerous the more precarious the house (Ronderos and Schnack 1987, 90).

The higher the degree of infestation, that is, the more infective contacts per house, the greater the number of new cases of infection in the household (Rabinovich et al. 1990, 737–746). It also has been shown that houses with children under ten years old had higher degrees of infestation than houses without children (Giojalas et al. 1990, 439–442). Since the houses with children are more heavily infested, that means the outcome of infection is more likely to be acute Chagas' disease and death.

The *vinchuca* thrives best when the household temperature is stable, a condition that is more likely in larger households (Ronderos and Schnack 1987, 89). Since the number of household inhabitants tends to increase as family wealth decreases, the best environment for the vector tends to be the worst house with the largest number of inhabitants, in other words, the poor household.

Costs and Solutions

Accessible and appropriate medical attention to diagnose and treat Chagas' infection as early as possible would alleviate some of the consequences, but medical solutions to Chagas' disease are inadequate. Not only is medical intervention unable to prevent suffering and death, it also is economically unjustifiable compared to prevention. Dias reports on a number of cost-benefit studies that attempt to estimate the purely economic costs of ongoing Chagas' endemia. Pacemaker implantation is indicated in 0.5 percent of chagasics in Brazil, at a cost of $6,118 per unit. Each esophagus surgery costs about $3,500, and each megacolon surgery costs $4,412. Based on the prevalence in Brazil, an estimated $250 million would be required for those two treatments alone, funds that could build 200,000 new rural houses or spray 10 million houses. In addition, Dias estimates the loss of workdays to cost about $6 million and direct medical costs (hospital care plus drugs) to amount to an additional $250 million. Pensions for the permanently disabled run into the many millions of dollars (Dias 1987, 80).

Spraying

Although the disease and the parasite cannot be eliminated (there are at least 180 species of mammals that are also hosts for the parasite), it can be controlled and even eliminated from the human domestic environment. In the immediate short run, the only weapon against the *vinchuca* is chemical control or fumigation. Indoor spraying results in a rapid decrease in *T. cruzi* infection in dogs. Repeated spraying might be an effective strategy, since the average life of dogs in an endemic zone is 3.6 years. New populations of uninfected dogs would be achieved in relatively short time (Gürtler et al. 1990, 320).

The usefulness or immediate health impact of a specific spraying program can be shown in the rates of infection subsequent to eradication campaigns. A serological study conducted in seven Argentine provinces compared six towns that had been sprayed with seven towns that had not. The prevalence of Chagas' infection in various age groups in untreated areas was as follows: infants to four years of age, 17.5 percent; five- to nine-year-olds, over 22 percent; and ten- to fourteen-year-olds, 33.3 percent. Areas that had been treated saw the following prevalence of Chagas' infection: infants to four-year-olds, 2.6 percent; five- to nine-year-olds, 5.4 percent; and ten- to fourteen-year-olds, 6.2 percent (Chuit et al. 1989, 119–124). A study of infection rates in Venezuela before and after a Chagas'-control program showed a decrease in seropositivity from 47.8 percent to 17 percent, with the decrease most marked in children and teenagers, from 30 percent to 2 percent. The mean age of the seropositives increased from 35 years to 47 years. Both measures indicate that the transmission of the disease decreased after the national control program (Acquatella et al. 1987, 556–562).

In some countries, such as Venezuela and Brazil, continuous programs that focus specifically on Chagas' disease have been effective. In Argentina, more than thirty years of research, chemical control, and education have not resulted in an improvement in the endemic status. Administrative and financial impediments have prevented the continuity, intensity, and frequency necessary for effective vector control (Gualtieri et al. 1985, 320). Other shortcomings of the Argentine programs have been improvisation; lack of integration among technicians, administrators, and politicians; disincentive for innovation; and failure in the selection of personnel and in the definition of objectives (Dias 1985, 303). It would be helpful to involve residents of endemic areas in the campaigns, in particular by providing people with insecticides to spray their own houses. For that to be safe, however, the campaigns must make available insecticides that have low toxicity to humans and animals, have long residual action, are easy to apply, and whose cost is relatively low (Gualtieri et al. 1985, 320). A well-planned program of spraying could help eradicate other insect vectors as well.

Housing Improvement

Ronderos and Schnack maintain that insecticides are not an efficient and adequate way of controlling the *vinchuca*. Chemical control is expensive and requires an outlay of funds for fossil energy that poor people and poor governments do not have. Eliminating the pest and preventing its return to its ideal ecological niche in the precarious house and peridomestic environment would require continuous application, with probable toxic effects on humans. Much more cost effective, although initially requiring a longer startup time, would be to change the way rural houses and goatyards are constructed. New construction styles have been devised using the same locally acquired materials but arranged in such a way that they do not provide shelter for the massive populations of parasite-carrying *vinchucas* (Ronderos and Schnack 1987, 95). Eliminating the vector might require changes in house construction, in the layout and construction of sheds around the house, and in the types and locations of objects stored in the house. To eradicate some species of vectors, the key improvement in the house is replacing the palm frond roof. For other species, it is cementing the dirt floor or, especially for *T. infestans*, plastering the walls so the cracks do not harbor insects (WHO 1991*a*, 49).

In Venezuela and Brazil, the replacement of roofs was successful in reducing infestation. In some cases, however, it is not possible to replace a roof without rebuilding the whole house because the style of roof allows the release of smoke or the retention of heat. Rural families are conservative and often resist attempts to substitute traditional houses with entirely new ones. Architects often do not have experience with or do not understand rural needs, climate, family size, and lifestyle (Tonn 1985, 334).

The housing problem is aggravated by the extent of poverty in the national population. People are too poor for decent houses, and, because so many people are poor, there is a limited market for domestically produced construction supplies. Consequently, the price of materials is high, making it more difficult for the poor to reconstruct their homes (WHO 1991*a*, 50). A much simpler solution in infected houses would be bed nets. If the fabric is available, the nets can be made even without a sewing machine.

Spraying, combined with housing improvement (including depriving the insect of its hospitable niche in the dung and stick walls of the peridomestic environment) and removing domestic and farm animals to shelters apart from the house would have a more lasting effect on eliminating the vector than spraying alone. Experience has shown that giving people houses has very little effect on the Chagas' situation because doing so does not alter the way people live, particularly the lack of cleanliness in and around the home and the presence of animals in the home (Tonn 1985, 335). What is required is a successful educational program, one that alters the cultural perspective of the people through rural development. That, of course, would be desirable for many reasons related to the health and dignity of the people, including elimination of the plague of Chagas' disease, which drains the people of physical and emotional resources for a better life. Ultimately, improvement in housing and the socioeconomic level of the people is the only cure.

Health Education

One of the problems in eradicating the Chagas' vector is the invisibility of the health threat. People are well aware of the *vinchuca*; in some areas, as in the Bolivian villages, it is a serious nuisance. But given the many challenges people face every day for survival, the nuisance of the pest is a small concern. Because the health impact is not obvious, the *vinchuca* is not necessarily considered dangerous. In some areas, in fact, it is considered good luck.

Poverty creates other priorities that reduce people's receptivity to eradication campaigns (Tonn 1985, 337). It fosters a short-run view of life and its exigencies. Diarrhea, respiratory diseases, and malnutrition are much more immediate threats to survival. In the hierarchy of dangers that poor people face, Chagas' disease does not always seem important, despite its serious and incurable nature. Beyond that, in the face of crushing poverty, an endemic disease borne by so many of one's companions generates a certain amount of fatalism. It is hard to imagine being rid of the bugs that have always been there, or rid of the disease that has always been there, or being able to do anything with the meager resources available to combat something that seems inevitable.

Perhaps more than any other malady, Chagas' disease demonstrates that ill health for people in Third World countries is an economic rather than a medical problem. The only interventions that really are effective for Chagas' disease are the improvement of housing in rural areas and the modernization and sanitation of the human ecology of the rural house-corral unit. That has been known for decades. Carlos Chagas identified the ecologic niche of the vector early in the twentieth century. Hundreds of scientific studies since have verified the importance of the precarious house, the peridomestic environment, household pets, and domestic animals in maintaining the endemia. And the houses and the plague remain.

Five

Water, Waste, and Garbage

The water supply in the Juan Domingo Perón housing project in the Bosques section of Florencio Varela in Greater Buenos Aires produced a number of cases of poisoning in July 1990. Six children were hospitalized, 600 experienced gastric discomfort and 10,000 people were barred from drinking from the water supply. City Hall Civil Defense Chairman Roberto Dematei denied rumors that all kinds of garbage had been found inside the reservoir supplying the project, including bird feathers, dead mice and a human corpse. One hundred people witnessed the garbage being fished out of the water supply.

(Buenos Aires Herald, July 15, 1990, p. 4)

Every day, around the world, illnesses related to water supply, waste disposal, and garbage kill 30,000 people and constitute 75 percent of the illnesses that afflict humanity (Douglas 1990, 3). Contaminated water spreads many diseases, including typhoid fever, cholera, hepatitis A, trachoma, skin infections, and parasites. Even municipal water supplies are a hazard in many developing countries because of poor maintenance and rapid urban growth (WHO 1991*b*, 18).

Inadequate disposal of human waste also exposes people to numerous health problems, including infant diarrhea, gastrointestinal infections, cholera, and parasitic diseases. "Sewage and excreta seriously threaten public health because they have high levels of pathogenic organisms and organic and inorganic chemical substances, some of which may lead to toxic, mutagenic, carcinogenic, or teratogenic consequences. The pathogenic organisms in excreta, sewage, or improperly treated sludge, including bacteria, viruses, protozoans, and helminths, pose the greatest risks" (PAHO 1990*a*, 215).

Solid wastes, too, play a major role in the spread of gastrointestinal and parasitic diseases. People have direct contact with garbage in the streets and around their houses, as well as indirect contact with garbage through insect and rodent vectors, whose populations garbage supports. Garbage dumps also pose a threat of disease, injury, and poisoning for the people who live in and scavenge from the dumps and for nearby residents. Many kinds of domestic animals also scavenge on garbage in streets and in municipal dumps. Pets bring home disease, and food animals, especially pigs, feed off the dumps, thereby transmitting parasites to people.

The combination of contaminated water and contact with human and solid wastes produces a high incidence of morbidity and mortality from water- and vector-borne diseases, especially in a population whose health is already compromised by poor nutrition and by housing that is inadequate in so many other ways.

The Use of Water

The lack of water also fosters disease. Because water has to be carried long distances or purchased at high prices, people use too little to keep themselves and their homes clean. Sometimes it is not the objective difficulty of obtaining water that prevents good hygiene. Some people need health education to use water well and responsibly (PAHO 1990a, 215). Fecal-oral transmission, as in diarrheal diseases and infectious hepatitis, also occurs through food, hands, and eating utensils. A study in Greater Buenos Aires found that only 30 percent of the people wash their hands every day (*Buenos Aires Herald*, April 21, 1991, p. 6). Improvements in hygienic practices are important for the interruption of pathogenic transmission (Huttly 1990, 118). "It can take half a generation for people to acquire the habit of hygienically using water and for the rates of illness to begin to fall" (Douglas 1990, 7).

For some, the difficulties of life at the margin of society overwhelm what is a fairly universal tendency toward cleanliness among people in stable societies. Although the Buenos Aires housing project Ramón Carrillo has running water in every unit and sewer-connected waste disposal, doctors from Health Center Number 6 report that the children are filthy. The doctors go house to house teaching mothers how to bathe their children, but with little success. Skin infections, including scabies and mange, a serious problem for this population, are aggravated by inadequate hygiene (Dr. Norma Aprigliano, September 24, 1991).

Poor hygiene is not a condition of all of the poor. Going door to door (not always an accurate description when a house is made of blankets or plastic) in the Autopista section of Retiro *villa*, one can observe the dramatic differences between one family and the next. One mother emerges from a miserable shack, spotlessly clean, hair neatly combed, with her clean, healthy, inoculated baby. The mother next door, in similar circumstances, is dirty, unkempt, and with a dirty baby that reeks of urine, looks unhealthy, and has received no vaccinations.

With accessible water and hygiene training, people are better able to prevent ill-ness at the household level. Hygiene education also is important in protecting water sources from continuing contamination. Many waterborne diseases can be eliminated if the cycle of contamination of watercourses is broken.

Water Supply and Waste Management
Worldwide and in Latin America

In 1988, one-quarter of the urban population of the developing world did not have access to an adequate, safe supply of water, and one-half did not have an adequate excreta-disposal system. For the 75 percent with potable water, access is defined as having a tap within 100 meters of the house. In 1990 in Latin America and the Caribbean as a whole, 87 percent of urban dwellers had access to piped water; in rural areas, 50 percent of the population was served. Sanitary facilities served 81 percent of the urban population of the region and 22 percent of the rural dwellers (Douglas 1990, 5). Rapid urbanization coupled with lack of investment in the supply system has resulted in seriously inadequate coverage for the population in some countries. The daily drudgery of hauling water places an enormous burden on the poor, especially women, who are the chief water providers for the household, and takes time away from other work, child care, and food preparation (Brunstein 1986, 152).

Adequate treatment of human waste presents an even bleaker picture. "South America pollutes nearly eleven times more freshwater on a per capita basis than Europe" (PAHO 1990a, 221). In most countries, the sanitation systems them-selves are the worst offenders. They dump 90 percent of the region's sewage di-rectly into streams or rivers without treatment. The water supply systems are designed to work with intake water of much higher quality than the sewage-contaminated water they receive. The systems have not been adapted to remove the contaminants, so the quality of the water in municipal systems declines as the intake water becomes more sewage laden (PAHO 1990a, 218). The World Health Organization reports that "most urban centres in Africa and Asia have no sewage system at all, including many cities with more than one million [inhabitants]. Rivers, streams, canals, gullies and ditches are where most human excrement and household wastes end up, untreated" (WHO 1991e, 200).

Also, according to the World Health Organization, "garbage-collection ser-vices are inadequate or non-existent in most residential areas of Third World cities; an estimated 30 to 50 percent of the solid wastes generated within urban centres are left uncollected" (WHO 1991e, 199), and "in most cities, there is little or no separation of toxic wastes from those which can be safely disposed of in land-fill, and proper management of landfill sites is nonexistent" (WHO 1991e, 200).

Table 5.1 lists the percentages of rural and urban populations of selected countries with access to potable water, ranked by per capita GNP. Access to

_____ Table 5.1 _____

Access to Potable Water, 1985–1988, Selected Countries

Country	GNP per Capita 1989	Percentage of Population with Access		
		Total	*Urban*	*Rural*
Tanzania	$130	56	90	42
Somalia	170	34	58	22
Malawi	180	56	97	50
Nepal	180	29	70	25
Zaire	260	33	52	21
Rwanda	320	50	79	48
India	340	57	76	50
Haiti	360	38	59	30
Kenya	360	30	61	21
Pakistan	370	44	83	27
Sri Lanka	430	40	82	29
Angola	610	30	87	15
Bolivia	620	44	75	13
Honduras	900	50	56	45
Peru	1,010	55	73	17
Ecuador	1,020	58	81	31
El Salvador	1,070	52	68	40
Thailand	1,220	64	56	66
Chile	1,770	94	98	71
Costa Rica	1,780	91	100	83
Mexico	2,010	77	89	47
Argentina	**2,160**	**56**	**63**	**17**
Venezuela	2,450	90	93	65
Brazil	2,540	78	85	56

____

Sources: UNICEF 1991, 106–107; World Bank 1991, 204–205.

potable water is not a function, at least not solely, of per capita GNP. It is a result of policy decisions, as the data in the table show. For example, Kenya's per capita income is nearly three times that of Tanzania, but only 30 percent of Kenya's population has piped water, compared to Tanzania's 56 percent. Tanzania has per capita income one-sixteenth that of Argentina and has the same proportion of the total population with access to potable water and higher proportions for both urban and rural areas.

Seventeen percent of Argentina's rural population have access to potable water. That puts Argentina in the same range as Afghanistan, Angola, and Peru and significantly lower in rural access than Malawi, Burkina Faso, Niger, Somalia, Rwanda, Bangladesh, Tanzania, India, Haiti, Honduras, and El Salvador.

For the urban population, Argentina ranks with Somalia, Sudan, Haiti, Kenya, El Salvador and well below Mauritania, Rwanda, Angola, Pakistan, Egypt, Brazil, and scores of other countries (UNICEF 1991, 106–107). Only 40 percent of Argentina's urban population (the country is 86 percent urban) have sewer connection (PAHO 1990*a*, 216–217).

In Argentina

Census data for 1990 indicate the access to piped water supply by income class and the alternative sources people use. Table 5.2 gives the sources of water used by households in Greater Buenos Aires and Posadas, the capital of Misiones Province, for poor and nonpoor households.

In all of Greater Buenos Aires (the Federal Capital and the inner nineteen counties), the upper aquifer is contaminated and the groundwater is highly contaminated. Consequently, more than half the population take their water from unsanitary sources, including 75 percent of the structurally poor and 60 percent of the impoverished.

In Posadas, due to the almost impenetrable hardness of the basalt rock on which the city is situated, almost no one drills to the aquifer. Consequently, more than half the population take their household water from unsafe sources,

Table 5.2
Water Supply, by Poverty Level, 1990

Type of Water Supply	Percentage of Homes			
	Total	*Structurally Poor*	*Impoverished*	*Nonpoor*
Greater Buenos Aires				
• Piped water	47.8	25.8	40.2	54.7
• Aquifer	27.7	27.9	29.8	26.8
• Groundwater	20.1	28.3	26.3	16.2
• Public tap	2.5	7.7	2.0	1.7
• Truck, river, stream	1.9	10.1	1.7	0.5
Posadas				
• Piped water	45.2	16.6	37.5	67.6
• Aquifer	1.6	1.2	1.2	2.1
• Groundwater	27.7	35.4	31.9	20.0
• Public tap	16.7	39.4	16.6	3.5
• Truck, river, stream	8.9	7.3	12.9	6.8

Source: INDEC 1990, 347.

including 82 percent of the structurally poor and 61 percent of the impoverished. Those census figures may be a gross overestimate of piped-water access in Posadas, since another study found only 16 percent of the urban population of Misiones to have potable water in the house. In five cities in the province, there are even multistory apartment buildings without water. Posadas was found to have in-house access for only 12 percent of the population (Müller 1984, 46). In the five-city census study, Neuquén and Santiago del Estero had significantly better water systems than Buenos Aires.

Table 5.3 presents the waste-disposal methods for the five cities, giving the percentages of homes with a toilet, an outhouse, or no facility. In Greater Buenos Aires, over 2.5 million people have an outhouse or no toilet facilities at all. General Roca and Neuquén have higher proportions of households with flush toilets than Buenos Aires. Santiago del Estero has the highest percentage of people

_____ Table 5.3 _____

Excreta Disposal, by Poverty Level, 1990

	Percentage of Homes			
Type of Facility	Total	Structurally Poor	Impoverished	Nonpoor
Greater Buenos Aires				
• Toilet	76.9	31.2	68.4	88.5
• Outhouse	20.7	47.4	31.5	11.5
• No facility	2.5	21.4	0.0	0.0
General Roca				
• Toilet	84.6	49.1	83.0	95.5
• Outhouse	13.8	39.9	17.0	4.5
• No facility	1.6	11.0	0.0	0.0
Neuquén				
• Toilet	89.5	58.2	91.4	98.5
• Outhouse	5.9	12.1	8.5	1.5
• No facility	4.6	29.7	0.0	0.0
Posadas				
• Toilet	55.4	15.2	48.8	83.7
• Outhouse	39.0	62.4	51.2	16.3
• No facility	5.6	22.3	0.0	0.0
Santiago del Estero				
• Toilet	76.3	23.5	82.1	96.8
• Outhouse	8.9	7.6	17.9	3.2
• No facility	14.8	68.9	0.0	0.0

_____

Source: INDEC 1990, 348.

_____ *Table 5.4* _____

Homes without Any Bath or Shower, by Poverty Level, 1990

	Percentage of Homes			
Area	Total	Structurally Poor	Impoverished	Nonpoor
Greater Buenos Aires	21.2	69.1	28.7	9.5
General Roca	17.0	51.7	20.8	4.9
Neuquén	12.1	40.2	13.9	0.8
Posadas	41.8	84.0	50.3	10.9
Santiago del Estero	23.6	75.0	19.5	2.7

Source: INDEC 1990, 349.

with no facilities at all. Posadas presents the worst sanitary picture; only half the population and only 15 percent of the structurally poor have flush toilets. However, because Greater Buenos Aires is a much larger metropolitan area, it not only represents a larger number of people without access to decent sanitary facilities for an urban location but also a much more serious public health threat overall.

Table 5.4 examines the availability of bathing facilities. Often there may be a tap or well on the property but inadequate facilities inside the house. For each city, the table shows the percentage of homes without any bath or shower on the property. Over one-fifth of homes for all income groups in Greater Buenos Aires and Santiago del Estero and over two-fifths of homes in Posadas have no bathing facilities. In all the cities, between 40 and 85 percent of the structurally poor have no baths. The lack of bathing facilities in some nonpoor homes, particularly in Buenos Aires and Posadas, calls into question what the category "nonpoor" possibly could mean.

How people manage without baths can be seen in any *villa*. They stand outside their houses, in a place crowded with strangers, stripped as far as is decent, and wash from a shallow hand basin. (In Spanish America, unlike Europe, nudity is not practiced.) Taking a bath standing by a well pump is possible in a remote rural area, but carrying this practice to crowded slums means that personal hygiene suffers because of the bathers' modesty.

In Greater Buenos Aires

Although Greater Buenos Aires is wealthier than the rest of the country, the foregoing data show that the area has worse water and sanitation service than some of the outlying provinces. For that reason and because of its primacy

_____ Table 5.5 _____
Water and Sewers in Greater Buenos Aires, 1987

Jurisdiction	Urban Population (thousands)	Percentage Served by Water System	Percentage Served by Sewer System
Partido			
• Almirante Brown	399.4	12.3	8.3
• Avellaneda	329.0	86.5	33.7
• Esteban Echeverría	261.0	8.3	6.1
• Ezeiza	219.0	94.8	93.9
• General San Martín	403.5	48.2	35.6
• La Matanza	983.7	35.7	37.7
• Lanús	481.2	73.3	13.7
• Lomas de Zamora	590.0	51.4	27.2
• Morón	688.4	26.8	21.1
• San Fernando	138.3	49.4	23.2
• San Isidro	320.0	70.9	28.4
• Tigre	244.5	19.7	8.1
• Tres de Febrero	371.3	58.7	42.2
• Vicente López	296.0	95.2	92.8
Subtotal	5,725.3	48.7	31.9
Federal Capital	2,922.8	100.0	99.9
Greater Buenos Aires	8,648.1	66.0	54.9

_____

Source: Solo et al. 1990, 18, 27.

in the national population, its sanitary services deserve closer study. The ways people adapt to the lack of water and the diseases that result from inadequate waste disposal are detailed for Greater Buenos Aires, but they are representative of the rest of Argentina and developing countries in general.

Water and Sanitation. The sanitary infrastructure has not expanded as the population in the suburbs has grown (Solo et al. 1990, 9, 11). The largest increases in population have been recorded in the counties to the south and southwest of the city, where the sanitary deficiencies are greatest. In 1947, the water system served 94 percent of the population of the metropolitan area; by 1960, only 76 percent had piped water. In 1988, between 55 percent and 60 percent had potable running water, and between 30 and 35 percent had sewer connection (Brunstein et al. 1988, 13, 16).

Table 5.5 lists the proportions of the population served by water and sewer systems in the administrative subdivisions of Greater Buenos Aires (fourteen of the nineteen counties and the Federal Capital). The data overestimate coverage in several ways. First, only the urban population of each county is considered, so people living in suburbs and relying on wells and cesspools are not included. Second, the figures do not include the *villa* population, as is apparent from the figure of 100 percent for water and 99.96 percent for sewer connection for the Federal Capital. Only a small percentage of the *villa* population has water connection. Third, the five counties without any water and sewer service are not included in the data. Other large cities of Latin America have had higher rates of population growth and yet serve a greater proportion of the population with potable water from the system (Solo et al. 1990, 7).

Census data show another measure of sanitary risk in Greater Buenos Aires. The counties with more than 30 percent of homes at high risk (defined as those without flush toilets) are Moreno, outer La Matanza, Esteban Echeverría, San Fernando, Florencio Varela, General Sarmiento, and Merlo. The census defines homes at potential risk as those whose water supply is not from the water system and those without sewers. Counties with more than 75 percent of the homes at high or potential risk are General Sarmiento, outer La Matanza, Tigre, Esteban Echeverría, Almirante Brown, and Moreno (INDEC 1991*b*, 5, 11).

Sanitary experts find it remarkable that a densely populated metropolitan area with so many risk factors and without safe water or sewers has not yet had a sanitary catastrophe. One must assume that the population has taken on itself the cost of averting disaster by consuming bottled or boiled water (Brunstein et al. 1988, 33).

Alternatives to Piped Water. Nearly 100 percent of the legally constructed households in the Federal Capital and almost half of those in the surrounding fourteen counties of inner Greater Buenos Aires are connected to the water system. Even in the Federal Capital, however, large areas nominally served by the network get water only at night, and some, generally at the outer reaches of the system, do not get water all summer long. Some people have had to construct reservoirs in their basements, at their own expense, to compensate for the irregular service. There also are about 225,000 inhabitants clandestinely hooked up to the water system (Brunstein et al. 1988, 17, 22).

The approximately 50,000 people in *villas miseria* in the Federal Capital get their water in a variety of ways. A few houses in the oldest neighborhoods of Retiro have water from the municipality. Some have plastic-hose connections to the municipal water supply, while others carry water to their houses in buckets from public taps attached to the plastic-hose connections. In some *villas*, trucks bring water that is expensive and of dubious quality. Truck water costs the poor four times as much as a proportion of income as piped-water systems cost the rich (Wells and Klees 1980, 12). In Ciudad Oculta, hoses bring water to the neighborhood from the municipal system but do not connect to the houses (visit,

November 27, 1991). In Villa Fátima, in the block closest to the main avenue, hoses connect to the fire hydrant and are strung house to house (visit, September 24, 1991).

In Quilmes West, sixteen blocks are served by a clandestine grid connected to the city water supply. The entire grid and most of the taps are plastic. Defects in the joints and countless breaks in the hoses allow bacteria and parasites to enter and contaminate the water. The taps usually are not supported adequately and lie in puddles when not in use (Cuenya 1985, 108).

Although 61 percent of the people in Quilmes West have water from the plastic grid, only 6 percent have water connection inside their houses. Twenty percent have a tap on the lot, and the remaining 35 percent use a tap outside their lot (Cuenya 1985, 124). Every time the water is carried or transferred from container to container, there is additional risk of contamination.

Quality of the Municipal Water Supply. The city water supply is officially potable, but poor upkeep of the system makes that claim dubious. In response to the cholera and yellow fever epidemics of the nineteenth century, a system for water provision was instituted in Buenos Aires in 1868, expanded in 1895, and again in 1908. Obras Sanitarias de la Nación (OSN) was established in 1912, and in the 1920s the treatment plant in the Palermo neighborhood of the Federal Capital was expanded (Solo et al. 1990, 15).

In the early 1940s, the closest suburbs were included in the network. From 1943 to 1955, expansion of the distribution network lost out to decisions to keep down the price of water, subsidize plumbing installations in the houses of those already hooked up to the system, and increase salaries for OSN bureaucrats. The policy under Perón—to keep the price low and to maintain unlimited, unmetered use—led to an increasing deficit, decreased capacity to borrow, and an end to investment in expanded production and services (Brunstein 1986, 155–156).

Water quality continued to deteriorate from the 1950s to the 1980s (Solo et al. 1990, 16). The 1980s was called the Water Decade. As part of the World Health Organization's *Health for All by the Year 2000* program, governments pledged to extend water and sanitation service to their entire populations. Argentina was a signatory to the Water Decade convention, but investment in real terms in water and sanitation fell substantially between 1981 and 1985. Annual average investment (in 1960 pesos) was 41.4 million in 1966–1970, 55.6 million in 1971–1975, 54.2 million in 1976–1980, and 16.4 million in 1981–1985 (Loterszpil and Loterszpil 1988, 90–91). Investment in infrastructure for water and sewers fell from an average of 1.5 percent of gross domestic investment in 1966–1970 to 0.58 percent between 1981 and 1990, the Water Decade (Siglioccoli 1992, 9).

The lack of investment has led to a collapse of the system, with insufficient production, deterioration in quality, large losses in the network, and waste by the users (Cotic and Dascal 1988, 123). Average consumption per person is estimated to be 700 liters per day, compared to the international standard of 150 to 200 liters (Loterzspil and Loterzspil 1988, 91). Even compared to other large Third World cities, Buenos Aires uses twice as much water per person (Siglioccoli 1992, 9). That estimate is approximate because nobody knows either the actual production or the losses in the system because neither macro- nor micromeasurement exists.

The high usage results not only from consumption but also from breaks in the distribution network and in the water treatment plant. Eighty-three percent of the distribution network in the Federal Capital is more than forty years old, and 55 percent is more than sixty years old. There are about 100,000 reports per year of burst water pipes flooding surface areas. Losses "reach up to 40 percent of production, according to optimistic calculations" (Brunstein et al. 1988, 19, 22).

The Palermo water purifying plant, which in the 1950s was processing three million cubic meters a day, today can produce only 2.2 million cubic meters due to lack of maintenance and a failure to update the system (Solo et al. 1990, 19). "The state of abandonment of the plant is notorious: controls that do not work, deteriorated faucets and sluices, abandoned filtration basins where robust trees have grown" (Cotic and Dascal 1988, 123).

In the decrepit pump houses, maintenance is neglected on the turn-of-the-century pumps because workers consider it too dangerous to go into the basements, where the pumps are located. The bad state of faucets and sluices accounts for a loss of 5 percent of the treated water. The plant uses up to 10 percent of production to clean the system, which is far in excess of internationally accepted norms (Cotic and Dascal 1988, 123). A combined total of 55 percent or more of the treated water is lost in faucets, cleaning, and main breaks.

Since there is no macromeasurement of water intake, technicians have to guess the volume of water in the system and the amount of purifying coagulant to use. Experts figure there is a 5-percent error, which affects the quality of the water produced and raises costs (Cotic and Dascal 1988, 125).

A large part of the overall cost of the system is the coagulant, for which OSN contracted with San Juan province. The level of impurity of the San Juan supply is high and causes the filtration basins to fill up with manganese. The San Juan contract set very high prices, which determine the prices paid to other producers (Cotic and Dascal 1988, 124).

With losses of 55 percent or more of treated water, production is inadequate. Instead of blocking up the leaks, the waterworks pump underground water from wells in Greater Buenos Aires, adding approximately 370,000 cubic meters per day, or 19 percent of the total volume (Cotic and Dascal 1988, 127). The presumption is that the harmful effects of the contaminated well water from inner Greater Buenos Aires are lessened by dilution with the treated water.

Considering the dubious quality of the treated water, that seems a heroic assumption. The waterworks were privatized in 1992, but improvements, if they are
made, will take many years to complete.

Wells. The underground water resources of the Greater Buenos Aires
area consist of three levels: the groundwater; the epipuelche, which is the upper
level of the aquifer; and the hipopuelche, or lower level of the Puelche aquifer.
Almost all of Greater Buenos Aires sits above the Puelche aquifer. The groundwater in the entire metropolitan region is highly contaminated bacteriologically
and chemically from decades of industrial and domestic dumping into surface
water and cesspools.

According to the 1980 National Census of Population and Housing, there were
more than 700,000 wells in the Greater Buenos Aires region. The great majority
of the inhabitants of Greater Buenos Aires drink groundwater from wells about
sixteen to eighteen meters in depth that are highly contaminated. The poorest
people live in flood zones, so it is easier for them to reach the groundwater and
they can even use manual pumps (Brunstein et al. 1988, 16). Of course, in flood
zones the quality of the water is more vulnerable to contamination from nearby
and distant sources. Some people can afford to drill down to a depth of forty to
forty-five meters, to the upper aquifer, which is contaminated in all the inner nineteen counties. In some "countries" (as the residential country clubs are called),
the wells are drilled to the lower aquifer, at about seventy meters, at a cost of
$3,000 to $5,000 (Medina 1992*a*, 23).

When the poor do drill to the aquifer, they generally cannot afford to drill a
sheathed well *(encamisado)*. An unsheathed well not only produces contaminated water as it passes up through the subsoil and groundwater levels but
passes contamination downward to the aquifer by contact with the groundwater,
which has been permeated by the cesspools. A contaminated well and aquifer
cannot be disinfected; the damage is permanent.

People do not always know the water is contaminated. They judge by taste,
transparency, and smell, which are not accurate guides. Those most at health
risk, because of lack of good nutrition, poor housing structure, overcrowding,
and lack of access to health services, also are those most likely to be without
piped water or to have wells of inadequate depth and quality, thus exacerbating
the threats to their health.

The aquifer itself is threatened by the demands of heavy industrial use and
OSN pumping and by contamination. The aquifer has an average thickness of
twenty to thirty meters, but that is dropping by approximately one meter annually. Also, the aquifer is not recharging because of the presence of urban obstacles, such as pavement and buildings.

The dense concentration of cesspools infiltrates nitrates into the deeper subsoil and the aquifer. As well as generating higher extraction costs, the drop in the level of the aquifer creates cones of depression that are widening the saline front advancing from the south (Solo et al. 1990, 14). By the 1920s, salinization by suction had contaminated the aquifer in Avellaneda, Lanús, Lomas de Zamora, and Quilmes (Brunstein 1986, 159). Now the saline front is advancing 100 meters a year.

The cones of depression have the secondary effect of causing the disappearance of the groundwater and the suction of surface water, contaminated principally by untreated industrial effluents, through the groundwater level and into the aquifer (Brunstein et al. 1988, 23). All that remains to exploit is the lower aquifer, which is very expensive to do because of its depth.

Sanitation at the Microlevel: The Household

In the Federal Capital, virtually 100 percent of legally occupied dwellings are connected to the sewer system. For some, however, the sewers work in reverse. The system was supposed to work by gravity, but in some areas pumps have been added. When it is overloaded, the system pumps sewage into houses (Brunstein et al. 1988, 23).

In the *villas* of the Federal Capital, for example, Retiro, Ciudad Oculta, and Villa Fátima, houses are not connected to the sewer system. Outside the Federal Capital, 70 percent of households are not connected to the sewer system. They use cesspools or, in the case of squatters, shallow pits over which an outhouse is constructed. Those without latrines use that of a neighbor or nothing at all for excreta disposal.

In the *villas*, house water, such as from bathing, washing dishes or clothes, and night pails, is thrown into the dirt streets. Some houses have a drainpipe that runs an inch or two below the ground and carries the wastewater to the edge of the street, where the pipe opens out and the water creates a gully to the street. Housewater and rainwater collect in stagnant pools in the mud streets, mixed with garbage and human and animal waste. A few days of rain make the streets almost impassable, even on foot.

Many squatters are rural people, and they bring rural solutions to sanitation problems in the cities. Because of their lower population density, rural areas can accommodate a greater amount of filth than cities. (Solo et al. 1990, 5). The housing code requires a distance of eight meters between a well and a cesspool, but that is more than the size of the lot on which many people have built their shanties. Consequently, wastes directly contaminate many wells used for domestic consumption.

Table 5.6 shows the proportion of households in the five urban areas without access to a sewer network. As with other sanitary facilities, Greater Buenos Aires and Posadas are worst served.

_____ Table 5.6 _____
Urban Households without Sewer Connection, by Poverty Level, 1990

| | Percentage of Homes | | | |
Urban Area	Total	Structurally Poor	Impoverished	Nonpoor
Greater Buenos Aires	62.4	86.5	72.5	54.0
General Roca	41.5	69.8	51.9	26.8
Neuquén	49.1	80.7	54.5	33.6
Posadas	81.6	93.0	83.9	73.4
Santiago del Estero	49.6	88.6	59.4	24.8

Source: INDEC 1990, 328.

Sanitation at the Macrolevel

The Sewer System. Almost 40 percent of the households in Greater Buenos Aires (inner fourteen counties) are connected to the sewer system. Besides the inadequate coverage of the urban population, there are several problems with the sewer system: (a) the generalized deterioration of the system due to lack of investment in infrastructure; (b) saturation of the main sewer lines; (c) an inactive purification system; (d) the dumping of untreated wastes directly into the Río de la Plata or into its tributary, the Riachuelo, which passes through residential areas; and (e) location of the intake pipes for the water system near the outflow of the sewer system (Solo et al. 1990, 21–22).

The capacity of the trunk network has not been increased in more than forty years. The main sewers have reduced capacity for conduction because of blockages or breaks from corrosion and age. Principal and secondary pipes are blocked or banked by garbage (Cotic and Dascal 1988, 133). The pumps that are supposed to lift the raw sewage across the Matanza-Riachuelo River do not function properly, so the sewer contents are carried into the river system (Solo et al. 1990, 29). Overloading of the system and the lack of conduction cause pipes to overflow in parts of the city, especially after heavy rains (Cotic and Dascal 1988, 133).

Adding to the hazards of the system, in urban residential areas clandestine industrial operations dump toxic chemicals into the sewer system. Complaints are not investigated, although it is known that firms dispose of cyanide (used in chroming) and sulfuric acid (used by tanneries) in the metropolitan sewers (Pogoriles 1993, 49).

The decrepit condition of the sewer system adds to the hazards from illegal dumping, because many low-lying areas are flooded with every heavy rain. The lack of sewer covers has led not only to environmental damage but also to the disappearance of children in floods. In the past, floods meant rising water in streets and houses. Now, a sticky black liquid floods the streets and houses, staining the houses and leaving the streets and sidewalks slippery. A match thrown on the liquid ignites it immediately. The rising liquid also causes electrical outages and leaves streetlamps smoking (*Clarín*, October 24, 1993, pp. 48–49).

Waste Treatment. The southwest treatment plant in La Matanza was built in 1960 to carry out partial treatment of sewage. The liquid is spilled into the Matanza-Riachuelo River, while the remaining sludge is transported by impulsion pipes to the trunk sewer line. The trunk, however, is obstructed by debris. The treatment plant itself has numerous technical and structural problems that leave it paralyzed much of the time. Then the untreated sludge is pumped directly into the Matanza-Riachuelo River (Cotic and Dascal 1988, 135). Even when the plant is working, the system pumps forty-three cubic meters of untreated waste per second into the Río de la Plata (Siglioccoli 1992, 9).

The wastes are discharged into the river in the municipality of Berazategui, adjacent to La Plata, the capital of Buenos Aires province, which has a population of over half a million people. The intake for one of the water treatment plants for Buenos Aires is in the area of Bernal, upstream. A moderate southeasterly wind counteracts the current of the Río de la Plata and carries sewage wastes upstream, flooding all low-lying areas along the coast as far as the delta of the Paraná at Tigre, at the western edge of Greater Buenos Aires. The sewage discharge conduit was extended to 2.4 kilometers from the coast in an attempt to remove it from the influence of coastal currents, because the water intake was capturing sewage waste (Cotic and Dascal 1988, 135). The strength of a southeaster makes the success of that strategy questionable.

Outside the System. In addition to the five to six million people in Greater Buenos Aires who use pits or cesspools, contaminating the soil and their own water supply, a great many people have built clandestine sewer connections. One system of clandestine sewers was found in the fashionable neighborhood of San Isidro, in the suburbs of Buenos Aires. It connected to the storm drains and dumped raw sewage into the Río de la Plata (*Buenos Aires Herald*, February 12, 1992, p. 11). An elaborate system outside Greater Buenos Aires was linked up with the network of storm sewers that flow directly into the Río Guayleguaychú, a tributary of the Río de la Plata (*Entrerriano*, October 5, 1991, p. 20).

Another sanitary problem created by the existence of so many poorly constructed cesspools is that they have to be emptied frequently.[1] The extraction, transport, and dumping of wastes present environmental and sanitary hazards. Because of the lack of appropriate disposal sites and lack of government control, disposal companies often just dump the contents of their trucks into streambeds or semirural truck farms (Brunstein et al. 1988, 18).

The dumping of sewage wastes from the system or from trucks poses a serious health threat. In many Latin American and other Third World cities, primary effluent from sewer systems is used directly, without treatment, to irrigate lettuce, onions, tomatoes, artichokes, and other crops (PAHO 1990a, 215). Bacteria and parasites stay in the soil for months, contaminating food crops and causing disease outbreaks (typhoid, hepatitis, dysentery) (Douglas 1990, 5).

Industrial Dumping. An additional source of environmental contamination and a serious health hazard in Greater Buenos Aires and elsewhere in Third World cities is the dumping of industrial wastes in surface waters. The Pan American Health Organization special study of toxics in surface waters found that "[i]n Argentina, the Reconquista and Matanza-Riachuelo rivers, which flow through the Buenos Aires metropolitan area, receive huge amounts of heavy metals and organic compounds owing to the discharge of industrial wastes" (PAHO 1990a, 222).

In general, firms lack in-plant wastewater treatment and dump wastes directly into rivers and streams. Those that have purification systems are mostly for show. Consequently, all the rivers and streams in the Greater Buenos Aires area are dead (Medina 1992a, 23). In all, 7,300 factories toss 250,000 tons of toxic sludge and 500,000 tons of diluted solvents, as well as cadmium, mercury, and other toxic substances into the area's streams and rivers (Siglioccoli 1992, 9).

Scores of chemical industries, refineries, meat-packing plants, and tanneries dump untreated effluents into the Riachuelo. Sunken ships and other large obstacles in the river course block the river flow and the natural purification of the waters. Surface layers of oil and other contaminants block the sun's rays, which would increase oxygen levels (Pignotti 1993, 4). Correcting the situation is complicated by the fact that twenty-two public entities have jurisdiction over the Matanza-Riachuelo River (Medina 1992a, 23). Furthermore, penalties for dumping are so low that firms have no incentive to invest in environmental protection (Loterszpil and Loterszpil 1988, 89).

Garbage

Most people in marginal areas, certainly in *villas*, do not have garbage collection. Garbage sits in piles in the streets, a haven for disease vectors, flies, and rats. Cholera *vibrio*, for example, can stay alive on flies' feet for forty-eight hours. Dogs and cats scavenge on garbage and then bring diseases to their home. Edible animals pass tapeworm ova and other parasites to consumers.

Without garbage collection, people have to find solutions to solid-waste disposal. At the edge of Retiro *villa* which fronts city streets, people carry their trash to city dumpsters. The neighborhood, however, is large, and it is a long walk to the dumpsters, especially when mud tracks are difficult to pass after a rain. At the other side of the *villa*, I interviewed a young woman about her home and her family. She told me that she bagged her garbage and carried it to the dumpster, a distance of at least a half mile. Her house was neat and clean. But she gestured to her neighbor's enormous pile of organic and inorganic garbage, including soiled disposable diapers and food waste. Her neighbor, she noted, did not carry her trash. In Ciudad Oculta, there is no garbage collection. In Villa Fátima, the garbage is piled three meters high in one of the wider mud streets (visits, 1991, 1992).

Without collection service, people throw garbage into empty lots and abandoned houses, onto street corners, or anywhere a barricade has been thrown across a road. In empty lots, meter-high grass cannot conceal the piles of cans, plastic bottles, and bags of garbage (Gorban 1993, 8). Consequently, the city has been overrun with rats in spite of squads of ratkillers in Boca, Barracas, Constitución, San Telmo, and neighborhoods in the center and the periphery. Rats come out of the drains in bathrooms.[2] When the Riachuelo River rises in a storm, the rats come out of their underground city by the millions.

A 1990 study of the Buenos Aires rat population found one rat for every two square meters in the port, and 95 percent of them were parasite carriers. Rats transmit 243 different diseases, even when contact is not apparent, because scout rats mark paths from the dens to food with trails of urine. When evidence of rats is found, all food should be discarded, not just the part that has been gnawed. Not knowing how rats spread disease, poor people are reluctant to throw out all their food because of the expense of replacing it. Now that the city has let the rat situation get so bad, it will be very difficult to solve. A rat can have a litter of eight every twenty days. Even if the mother later dies of poison, the babies might be born with a resistance to the poison (Gorban 1993, 9).

Open-Air Garbage Pits

Disposal of collected garbage is another health problem. Open-air garbage dumps are used in 95 percent of the cities in Argentina, creating a permanent focus for infection. All kinds of animals, but especially pigs destined for human consumption, feed off the dumps and can bring serious health problems to the human population. Proper landfill management should include covering the garbage every day with impermeable soil so rain does not filter down and contaminate the upper levels of the water table, a practice not carried out in Argentine dumps (Gradizuela 1991, 21).

The mixing of various kinds of wastes in a single dump presents additional hazards. Domestic, industrial, chemical, and hospital wastes require different forms of disposal. Pathological wastes should be burned in special incinerators.

The La Tablada dump, which serves the Argentine city of Concepción del Uruguay in Entre Ríos, is typical. It receives every kind of waste since the city does not have ordinances for the special disposition of toxic industrial or hospital wastes, including pathological materials (Gradizuela 1991, 21).

Cirujeo

A special health hazard in all the open-air dumps is scavenging. Whole families make their living by practicing *cirujeo*, or "surgery," on the garbage. They pick over all the waste materials, looking for items that can be sold or eaten. At the La Tablada dump, twenty-five families reside around the dump and live off its contents (Gradizuela 1991, 21). In the Mendoza suburb of Godoy Cruz, a large proportion of the residents of the squatter neighborhood near the health center live off the garbage (visit to Health Center Number 149, Godoy Cruz, November 1, 1991). The dumps that stretch along the Camino del Buen Ayre (the ironically named Road of Good Air) in Greater Buenos Aires support a large number of families whose houses are perched right on top of the garbage. There is a continuous run of urban and suburban neighborhoods between Buenos Aires and La Plata. One of them, at the edge of La Plata, sits in a garbage dump. Two deep holes in the dump generally fill with water, making a lake of garbage. In the northern end of Greater Buenos Aires, the worst and most dangerous neighborhoods of San Fernando are situated on the dumps (visits 1991, 1992, 1993).

Living off dumps isolates those families in a particular and socially castigated lifestyle (Gradizuela 1991, 21; Dr. Roque Teixidor, November 1, 1991). In Mendoza, it was among the families living off the garbage dumps, surrounded by and isolated in filth, that the doctors and social workers reported an epidemic state of child sexual abuse within families. In other areas of Mendoza, according to doctors, child sexual abuse was rare. In the areas of the dumps, however, the incidence was so alarming that it was the first thing the doctors mentioned to me, without any prompting on my part (interviews, health centers in Godoy Cruz, Guaymallén, and Las Heras, November 1, 1991).

Living off garbage from the dumps is much more dangerous than picking garbage out of trash barrels in the city because of the variety of waste products combined at the dump. People find their food, as well as items to sell, in dumps that combine domestic, industrial, and hospital waste. In Buenos Aires, there is an ordinance that reserves all trash in barrels to the exclusive use of the municipal trash company. Consequently, people cannot legally scavenge where it is relatively safer and must do so in the dumps.

In 1993 a new law was introduced to address the garbage situation in the City of Buenos Aires (Municipalidad de la Ciudad de Buenos Aires, MCBA), but the order of magnitude assigned to various activities makes little sense. The fine for dumping sewage in city streets (as is done from trucks that empty cesspools) is

$100 or one day in jail. Parking vehicles so as to impede the cleaning of storm drains can result in a fine of $200. People who pick through city trash barrels can be fined $1,000 or punished with ten days in jail. Transporting hospital, toxic, or radioactive waste without authorization can lead to a $5,000 fine or fifty days in jail (Tucker 1993, 6).

Health Impact of the Unsanitary Environment

The consequence of the neglect of sanitary issues in Argentina is a rate of infectious and parasitic disease morbidity and mortality that places the country firmly in the ranks of the Third World. The numerous waterborne and garbage-spread diseases mean a heavy burden for the poor. Gastrointestinal diseases are the second leading cause of admissions to public hospitals in Argentina (Lumi 1990, 191). Intestinal infections have caused 80,000 deaths in Argentina in the past twenty-five years (*Clarín*, November 4, 1992, p. 20). (Chapter 11, "Stunted Development in Children and Adolescents," discusses the synergistic effect of intestinal diseases, parasites, and malnutrition on child growth and development.)

The difference in child mortality between houses with and those without sanitary facilities was recorded in the Inter-American Investigation of Mortality in Childhood. In Chaco, the death rate among children in houses with piped-in water was 9.1 per 1,000 compared to 21.0 per 1,000 for houses with water outside and 42.3 per 1,000 for those with no water on the property. Children who lived in houses with flush toilets had a mortality rate of 8.8 per 1,000, whereas those with outhouses had a death rate of 36.4 per 1,000, and those who lived in houses without any sanitary facilities had a mortality rate of 58.3 per 1,000 (Burke 1979, 31, 32).

Diarrhea in Children

In 1980, the number of diarrhea-associated deaths worldwide in children under five years of age was estimated at 4.6 million (13.6 per 1,000). In the period 1981–1986, diarrhea accounted for 38.5 percent of all deaths in children under five years. The average number of diarrhea episodes per child per year is highest in the Americas, at 4.6 per year, and in Africa, 4.4 per year. Diarrhea mortality as a percentage of child deaths, on the other hand, is slightly higher in Africa than in Latin America, reflecting the lower nutritional state and poorer access to curative facilities in Africa. Scores of studies from around the world have shown significant reductions in diarrheal morbidity and mortality rates among the under-fives resulting from improved water supplies and sanitary facilities (Huttly 1990, 120).

In studies of marginalized zones of Caracas, Venezuela, compared with other areas of the city, the rate of diarrheal pathology was much higher among children with poor sanitary facilities than among those with adequate water and sanitation (Castellanos 1984, 33). According to the Pan American Health Organization, the availability of water and basic sanitation services can decrease diarrhea morbidity by 35 percent (PAHO 1990a, 75).

A study of infant mortality rates in São Paulo State in Brazil demonstrated the importance of sanitation in improving health among the poor even in the face of falling incomes. In the years that were called the "Brazilian miracle" (1965 to 1973), GNP grew at a rate of about 10 percent per year but real wages fell. Public investment in sanitary infrastructure concentrated on central areas, and class differences in incomes and access to the sanitary infrastructure were accentuated. Infant mortality in São Paulo State increased from 70 per 1,000 in 1965 to 88 per 1,000 in 1973 (Oya-Sawyer et al. 1987, 90). Infectious and parasitic diseases as a cause of death increased from 22.5 percent of infant deaths in 1965 to 34 percent in 1973.

The Brazilian economy entered a recession in 1973, but at about the same time the government initiated a new sanitation plan, increasing access to running water in São Paulo from 71 percent of urban households in 1970 to 91 percent in 1980 and 98.6 percent in 1984. There was a dramatic decline in infant mortality during the recession years, from 88 per 1,000 in 1973 to 44.7 per 1,000 in 1983, with a specific reduction in deaths from causes avoidable by improved sanitation from 28 per 1,000 in 1975 to 6 per 1,000 in 1983 in the metropolitan area of São Paulo (Oya-Sawyer et al. 1987, 91).

Worldwide during the 1980s, there were significant reductions in infant and child mortality from diarrheal diseases, due in large part to the introduction of oral rehydration therapy. This specific and simple medical intervention has been extremely important in saving lives, but it is a remedy for the moment, not a long-term solution. Oral rehydration therapy reduces mortality but not morbidity. "The child that recovers finds himself immersed anew in the same not very sanitary conditions and succumbs to new episodes of diarrhea, a pattern which collectively weakens and atrophies the brain and body and quite frequently results in death" (Douglas 1990, 7).

Malnutrition exists in many countries that have adequate supplies of food, and the majority of malnourished children live in homes that have enough food. Diarrheal infections rob the child of the nourishment that is available and are possibly the principal cause of child malnutrition (UNICEF 1991, 10, 12). "The cure for malnutrition depends on water and hygiene more than on the supply of food" (Douglas 1990, 7). In sum, investment in safe water supplies and proper waste disposal, among possible health investments, has the greatest impact on the health of the population.

Helminths and Hydatids

Argentina has a high rate of infestation from various kinds of worms and parasites. The scandal is that such a plague is avoidable. The province of Mendoza does not have a helminth (worm) problem because of good enforcement of animal sanitary control legislation. However, its neighboring provinces, where the ecology is virtually identical, have such a high degree of infestation that a person can contract the worms merely by petting a dog (Dr. Roque Teixidor, November 1, 1991).

An additional hazard of improper waste management is the danger of hydatidosis. Inadequate sanitation around slaughterhouses and the feeding of sheep entrails to dogs result in the infection of humans by hydatids (cysts of tapeworms). The cysts can form throughout the human body but are most common in the liver and lungs and must be removed surgically. The Pan American Health Organization estimates that 1,500 cases are treated surgically each year in Argentina and Uruguay alone, two of the countries with the highest prevalence of hydatids in the Americas. Infection in dogs varies from 1 to 70 percent in studies in different areas of Argentina, and in sheep from 80 to 90 percent (PAHO 1990*a*, 182). This is not just a problem in the rural areas. In Greater Buenos Aires, Hospital Materno-infantil Gregorio LaFerrere children were treated for worm infestation.

Another serious problem is taeniasis in its various forms in the human host. Humans ingest the parasite in filth on food or in water or by eating pigs that have scavenged in dumps. The taenia is a liver tapeworm cyst; taeniasis is intestinal infestation with the adult tapeworm. Cysticercosis is tissue infestation with the larval stage of the worm. People can be affected either way. They ingest the eggs, which hatch in the small intestine. The larvae migrate to subcutaneous tissues (muscles, organs) and form cysts—in the eyes, the central nervous system, the heart, among other sites in the body. In the brain, the cysts can cause epileptiform seizures. The infestation causes serious disability and has a high case fatality rate. The cycle is continued when pigs range in areas contaminated with the excreta of infested persons, or when other food or water is contaminated with the eggs. The eggs remain viable in the environment for months (PAHO 1990*a*, 182).

Scores of waterborne illnesses cause serious disability and death in poor countries, including schistosomiasis (bilharzia), dysentery, and typhoid. The cycle of disease transmission can be interrupted by providing safe water supplies and by educating people not to contaminate watercourses. The transmission of river blindness is being stopped in Africa through education and the treatment of carriers.

Cholera

The failure of the Argentine government to respond to the challenge posed by the return of cholera to the Western Hemisphere is a study in miniature of many of the weaknesses of the social service net. The very establishment of the pandemic in Peru illustrates the important role that economics plays in health. Although no previous outbreak of the disease occurred in the Western Hemisphere in this century, the cholera *vibrio* did show up in various water systems and in surface water. In Argentina, it was found in samples of sewage discharged into the Río de la Plata in 1989 (Corrales et al. 1989, 71–77). The disease, however, did not establish itself until sanitary conditions had deteriorated substantially. Peru experienced a serious economic decline in the 1980s and did not invest in water and sanitation for the decade prior to the outbreak. At the same time, the population in Lima's shantytowns grew at a rapid rate.

Cholera is a high-ID pathogen, that is, it takes a large number of ingested organisms to constitute an infectious dose and cause diarrhea. Consequently, sanitary improvements are highly effective in eliminating or preventing cholera and other high-ID pathogens (Huttly 1990, 121). Conversely, a society can suffer quite a degeneration in its sanitary infrastructure before succumbing to such a disease. That was the roulette game that the Latin American countries played in the 1980s by allowing sanitary services to decline. In February 1991, the seventh pandemic of cholera, which had begun in Indonesia in 1961, broke out in Lima. At that point, doctors and other staff of the public hospitals in Argentina acted immediately to develop contingency plans to prevent the spread of the disease in Argentina. The government did nothing.

In May of 1991, the health minister of the province of Buenos Aires, Gines González García, said that 1,600 health centers were being built to combat cholera (*Buenos Aires Herald*, May 19, 1991, p. 13). In fact, none were built. In 1991, 1992, 1993, and beyond, La Matanza, a county of 1,200,000 people in the suburbs of the Federal Capital, remained without even one health center (numerous interviews and visits, 1991–1993). The only place to go was to the hospitals Gregorio LaFerrere, San Justo, and Diego Paroissien. (These hospitals are discussed in Chapters 8 and 9.)

Also in May of 1991, Mendoza Governor Bordón announced that between 200 and 400 hectares (up to 1,000 acres) of cropland in his province might be contaminated by cholera. Many crops already had been destroyed. The government promised compensation (*Buenos Aires Herald*, May 19, 1991, p. 13). When I asked doctors in public hospitals in Mendoza in November 1991 if sewage was used in the province to irrigate crops, some said they did not know that such a thing was done in Argentina, others said the practice had been stopped, and other doctors said that the practice continued (interviews at Hospital de Niños Emilio Civit, November 2, 1991).

In November 1991, it was suggested that something be done about the sewage treatment plant in the province of San Juan. In 1977, an earthquake had ruptured the plant and contaminated the groundwater in the province. With the cholera front advancing southward, repairs on the fourteen-year-old damage seemed timely (*Diario de Cuyo*, November 6, 1991, p. 6).

A full year passed between the outbreak of the cholera epidemic in Peru and the first case in Argentina. The advance of the disease north and south from Lima easily could have been predicted. The neglect of the sanitary infrastructure that had gone on for decades continued under the Menem government in spite of the encroaching threat (*Buenos Aires Herald*, February 18, 1992, p. 10).

In the early days of the epidemic, there was a 6 percent case fatality rate in Argentina, compared to 1 percent in Peru (*Buenos Aires Herald*, February 18, 1992, p. 10). The lack of primary health care was a major reason. Most doctors in Argentina are prepared only for secondary (hospital-based) health care and assumed they had to treat patients with intravenous therapy. Had they used one of the basic elements of primary health care, oral rehydration therapy, many more victims could have been saved by prompt action (Name withheld, November, 1993). The cholera appeared first among people living in remote rural areas. Cholera can kill within a few hours, so every minute counts in rehydrating patients.

After eleven people had died from cholera in Argentina, government officials made several statements. First, President Menem announced that cholera is not a disease of poverty. That did not influence the actual course of the disease, which has affected only the poor. Second, Menem announced that cholera would never reach Buenos Aires. It did. Third, the health minister announced that the government would send $4 million to dig wells and build water purification plants in towns in Salta. He said that in less than thirty days there would be running water in twenty-five Salta towns (*Buenos Aires Herald*, February 12, 1992, p. 11). The money never got there. As of the end of August 1992, nothing had been seen of a drinking water program in any of the towns most affected by the epidemic, the Wichi and Toba towns in the vicinity of Tartagal on the Bolivian border. The coordinator of the province's anticholera campaign said the Tartagal hospital had no money from the government to combat the disease. "The hospital is badly equipped, understaffed and in desperate need of repair. Paint is flaking off the walls and bloodstained sheets are left on beds" (Chandhary 1992, 4). Fourth, officials at the city waterworks in Buenos Aires assured the population that the city water was good, "unless the installations are substandard, allowing filtration from sewage, storm drains" (*Buenos Aires Herald*, February 10, 1992, p. 4). In a city with 100,000 water main breaks per year, that is not very reassuring.

It was also reported, and confirmed by the health minister, that wealthy landowners in Salta had pressured the government to downplay the epidemic lest their crops be embargoed in other countries, since "the victims were Indians" anyway (*Buenos Aires Herald*, February 10, 1992, p. 7). Another scandal that emerged was the sale of bogus bleach. The government staked its anticholera campaign on people adding bleach to their water supply. Several brands were found to be lacking the requisite strength, and a black market developed as people took advantage of the emergency to corner the bleach market (*Buenos Aires Herald*, February 11, 1992, p. 11).

Cholera first broke out in Argentina among the Indians who get their water and diet of raw fish from the Pilcomayo River that flows from Bolivia. Although cholera in Bolivia had been reported in the press and through PAHO bulletins to member nations, the Argentine government blamed Bolivia for the outbreak for not warning Argentina. When the groundwater and wells and fish in Salta were already infected, Argentina responded to the crisis by expelling 150 Bolivians and charging Bolivians $900 to enter Argentina (*Buenos Aires Herald*, February 21, 1992, p. 11). The situation in the north was made more difficult by heavy rains and flooding in December 1991 and January 1992, which left 10,000 homeless (*Buenos Aires Herald*, February 16, 1992, p. 1). The Formosa city of Clorinda remained under water for weeks. The only place for the population to live was on the shoulders of the raised roadway outside of town. Thousands made their homes on the narrow ribbons of land about ten feet wide between the pavement and the water below, and remained there for months (visit, September 1992).

Six percent of the schools in the province of Buenos Aires could not open after the summer recess due to unsanitary conditions (*Buenos Aires Herald*, February 12, 1992, p. 11). In the Federal Capital, concern began to mount over the high risk of infection when it was revealed that the main pipe of the city's water supply was choked with trash and infested with rats. The water main supplied residential neighborhoods in Palermo and the municipal Ricardo Gutiérrez Children's Hospital (*Buenos Aires Herald*, March 13, 1992, p. 11).

The cholera deaths in Argentina were preventable. The YPF state oil company compound is a mere seven kilometers from one of the epicenters of the outbreak in Tartagal. With careful attention to hygiene, the camp was able to prevent any cases of cholera (*Clarín*, March 19, 1992, p. 9). The same could have been done anywhere else in Argentina. Instead, the large farms in Salta made no modifications in the housing and sanitary facilities for migrant and permanent workers even after more than 1,300 cases of cholera and 24 deaths from the disease in that province. In August 1993, Salta health authorities announced that the farms still lacked "the minimum conditions of hygiene" in workers' housing, which had neither outhouses nor drinking water. The workers drank from the irrigation ditches. Fifty-seven of the sixty citrus farms inspected were found to be in violation of sanitary regulations. Only 65 percent of tobacco farms were found in compliance. There are an estimated 60,000 permanent rural workers in Salta, and the population swells at harvest time with migrants from other provinces and from Bolivia (*Clarín*, August 29, 1993, p. 46).

Government officials complain that the Indians are not adapting to the sanitary emergency. They still drink from puddles, they do not use the latrines that have been built since the crisis began, and they eat raw fish from the Pilcomayo (*Clarín*, September 20, 1992, p. 41). Although there are signs posted in Spanish about the dangers of drinking river water, the women still carry household water from the river (Fernández Guinti 1992, 40). The majority of the indigenous population, however, cannot even speak Spanish, let alone read it.

In May 1992, the U.S. Embassy became sufficiently concerned about the situation to ask twenty U.S. doctors to visit the cholera-affected region of Salta. The provincial and national health ministers were offended, insisting that there were enough doctors in the area to handle the emergency. The Salta-Chaco region has 3 doctors for 8,000 people spread throughout twenty settlements. "[E]ven if the area had more medical experts they would be hampered by the fact that the power generator at the Santa Victoria Hospital is broken and what little water is available there is contaminated" (*Buenos Aires Herald*, May 27, 1992, p. 11).

By 1996, cholera was well established in the northern provinces. Back-and-forth migration of northerners to pampean cities and towns ensures the spread of cholera to major population centers. Cases of cholera continue to appear in Buenos Aires (in Retiro *villa*, for example) and in suburban areas (*Buenos Aires Herald*, February 4, 1996, p. 4).

The cholera epidemic in Argentina exposes both the strengths and the weaknesses of the country. The foresight and heroic efforts of many of the country's public sector doctors and nurses, in the face of waves of illness pushed at them by an economic crisis and inadequate government support, reflect well on the intellectual preparation and the spirit of solidarity of a portion of the population. What they are up against is a national (and governmental) indifference to the conditions of the *negritos*, the Indians; decades of neglect of the infrastructure; an *ad hoc* rather than a planned approach to dealing with problems; denial of the nature of the problem (for example, Menem's insistence that cholera affects rich and poor alike, so that he need not admit that Argentina has more poor people than rich); the tendency to blame not only the poor (they should have read the signs) but also foreign people or entities (Bolivia should have warned Argentina about cholera); and the vicious opportunism that arises in every crisis (the adulteration and hoarding of bleach). There is a fatal synergy among poverty, a dysfunctional government, and a lack of concern for, even hatred of, the poor, which is the subject of the next chapter.

There is no refuge from filth for the poor. When plague broke out in Surat, India, in 1994, people searched for reasons. The editor of *India Today* wrote an editorial about the Indian situation, which could have been written about Argentina. The conditions of filth and official indifference are not unique to either country; they are a condition of the Third World and poor sectors of the First World.

A healthy rain in the nation's capital turns into a flood. Children are sucked mercilessly into the vortex of storm drains that have not been cleaned for the entire season, and adults sizzle to death in water electrified by exposed power lines. Cholera and hepatitis, meningitis and conjunctivitis, malaria and filaria. It's as if a medieval curse is upon us. But the hex is self-inflicted. Because we are the practitioners of filth. The emperors of garbage. . . . [The issue] is whether politicians and administrators care about how people live. . . . Delhi could well be Surat.   (Badhwar 1994, 23)

. . . or Caracas, or San Salvador, or Nairobi, or Buenos Aires.

Six

The Underdeveloped State

Underdevelopment is not just an economic condition. It can also describe the political or governmental apparatus. One of the political dimensions of Argentina's underdevelopment is the weak state. It might seem ironic to refer to a government that could cause tens of thousands of its citizens to disappear over a period of seven years (1976–1983) as a weak state. While the repressive state is strong in its extralegal capacity, it is weak in the conventional juridical and regulatory mechanisms that a moderate modern government carries out routinely.

In the industrialized countries, the safety of drugs and foodstuffs is closely monitored by the government. There is active debate in the scientific community about the safety of chemical additives and about the usefulness of certain pharmaceutical products, but the biological safety of foods generally is guaranteed. We assume that medicines administered in a hospital are real, subject to quality checks, and not just contaminated water. None of that can be taken for granted when the government has no mechanism of control over foods and pharmaceuticals nor over other commercial activities that affect public health and safety.

In very poor Third World countries, most of the food is unprocessed, and the main danger to health is mold. Argentina is more industrialized and has a large food-processing industry. Quality control is different for processed food because it can contain colorings, chemicals, and additives not readily seen. Similarly, in a very poor country, the poor either have no medicine or they use plants that they recognize from the forest. In a country that is half modernized, people take manufactured drugs that are generally available over the counter but that are not subject to quality control.

This chapter is about the weak regulatory apparatus of the underdeveloped state and the effect that has on public health through food and pharmaceuticals;

environmental, building, and zoning codes; traffic control; and protection of wards of the state.

The Need for Government Oversight

In neoclassical economic theory, in particular as enunciated by public-choice theorists of the 1980s, government regulations not only are an encumbrance on the efficient operation of markets, they also are unnecessary because people will not buy things that do not serve their interests, such as rotten food or fake medicines. That might be true in a market with perfect information. The market for food and pharmaceuticals in Argentina represents a case of market failure due to the large number of small firms selling nonhomogeneous products with little brand recognition.

According to the 1985 census, 51 percent of food-preparation establishments (2,839) in the Argentine formal sector had fewer than six workers and contributed 1 percent of the gross value of foodstuffs. In the manufacture of beverages, 53 percent of establishments (808) produced 3 percent of the value. In 1986, more than 112,000 businesses were engaged in the sale of food. Of those, 103,036 were small and sold 49 percent of the value (FIEL 1988, 107).

The presence of a large number of small firms works against self-regulation because suppliers "perceive a very low risk in the preparation and sale of foods dangerous to health. These suppliers are firms with very low investment of capital, without brandname investment, without a commercial reputation to protect and that can, consequently, leave and re-enter the market with low cost, generally under the shelter of informality" (FIEL 1988, 107). The costs of information to the consumer are prohibitively high; the only way to guarantee the safety of products is through regulation.

While regulation always raises the possibility of market distortion, the cost of regulation for a firm is not much more than what it would cost the firm to self-regulate by practicing proper hygiene (FIEL 1988, 111). The distortions to the market, therefore, are not great, and the benefits to society, while dispersed, are substantial.

Many other industries or services besides food and beverages require regulation because of the undeveloped state of the market, the weakness of consumer voice, the inclination toward rent seeking, the ineffective judiciary system in which aggrieved consumers cannot seek redress, and other reasons. The pharmaceutical industry has 351 registered manufacturers, of which about 50 are large firms (World Bank 1987a, 25). There are also many unlicensed firms. Even the drugs that are bought under brand names are not necessarily produced in factories. A woman I know works at home with her eight children, who range in age from fifteen to two, filling capsules with a diet drug for a pharmaceutical company. Their house has a dirt floor and the cesspool constantly overflows inside the house.

Food, Drugs, and Oversight in the Past

Argentina's pharmaceutical industry is the largest in Latin America. The industry is so powerful that it has been credited with the 1966 coup d'état that toppled the Radical government of Arturo Illia, who had proposed pharmaceutical regulation (*Buenos Aires Herald*, August 22, 1992, p. 11). Nevertheless, at that time, Argentina had a reputation among drug manufacturers of being a difficult country in which to get licensed. The multinational firm Pfizer, for example, ranked Argentina in the difficult category along with the United States (Arias 1992, 36). That was, no doubt, partly due to Argentina's high tariff and nontariff barriers to block imports of pharmaceuticals and protect its own industry. Argentina also liberally copies patented medicines from abroad and therefore would be less willing to license imported products. Still, in the 1960s, Argentines had the impression that their National Food and Drug Institute was protecting the population.

Over the years, that reputation has been tarnished by poor agency performance. Jobs in the Ministry of Health and Social Action, like those in other ministries, are filled on a patronage basis, top to bottom, without regard to professional qualification. There were five health ministers in the first three years of the Menem administration, none of whom had any background in the health field (*Buenos Aires Herald*, August 20, 1992, p. 10). In fact, it was not until the seventh minister, after five years of the administration, that someone with past experience in health was appointed.

The lack of professionalism on the part of appointees is facilitated by badly drafted pharmaceutical legislation. The lack of clarity of criteria and the variability of norms create a margin of discretion that encourages administrative corruption. Medicines have been authorized on the day of application "without any type of technical analysis. . . . There are virtually no controls over the production and marketing of medicines, owing to the lack of human and material resources in the agencies" (FIEL 1988, 119). In 1983, for example, 2,300 new pharmaceutical products were introduced into the Argentine market, while in the United States in that same year, only 14 new products were approved (United Nations 1984, 33).

Indications for medicines are overstated and adverse effects minimized. For example, in the United States, forty-two warnings are listed for Valium; in Argentina, there are five. Many products routinely prescribed in Argentina are proscribed or greatly restricted in other countries. Dipyrone is banned in the United States and Europe because it can lead to a fatal blood disorder, but it is one of the best-selling drugs in Argentina (United Nations 1984, 33) and is contained in sixty-seven products sold in Argentina (Battellino 1988, 474). Clofibrate is for sale in seventeen varieties, although its side effects are not mentioned in Argentina (United Nations 1984, 33).

The degradation of the regulatory mechanisms began in the 1970s because of the ideological opposition of the military *Proceso*. Much of the regulatory apparatus had served only to throw financial hurdles in the way of industry, providing opportunities for corrupt officials to collect bribes for their approvals. The military created the worst of both worlds. They annulled the protective aspects of the regulatory agencies but, because of their controlling, mercantilist mentality, left in place the licensing provisions that served only to feed corruption and encourage extralegal production in unsupervised labs.

The World Bank expressed its concern over the lack of oversight: "Since the late 1970s, the Government has relinquished its responsibility for the control of laboratory standards, pharmaceutical and food products, with costly results" (World Bank 1988, 21). The Pan American Health Organization also voiced its concern over the military government's default with respect to the control of the quality of the air, water, biological and pharmaceutical products, laboratory norms, and elimination of toxic wastes. Neither the provincial governments nor the private sector assumed those responsibilities. The 100 public research labs, 1,000 private labs in chemical, agroindustrial, and food preparation businesses, and the 10,000 labs in health centers, hospitals, clinics, and pharmacies are not coordinated or supervised, nor do they have any government lab to turn to for help (OPS 1989, 76).

De facto deregulation continued in the 1980s due simply to the lack of state funds in the economic crisis of the postmilitary years. The drug control agency has few personnel and lacks adequate equipment to carry out its responsibilities. By 1989 there were 13,400 registered medicines in Argentina, 1,500 of which we found in the market under 3,400 different names and with 7,000 different forms (OPS 1989, 77).

The government default of the 1970s and 1980s extended to food products as well. "The inappropriate use of preservatives, antibiotics and additives, and bacterial and chemical contamination, especially that produced by insecticides and herbicides, have occurred on production lines on a large scale. Unhealthy food products principally affect health in two ways. Each year there are several outbreaks of acute food poisonings . . . [and there are also] chronic intoxications, such as the accumulation of carcinogens and heavy metals in the organism, or the resistance to antibiotics," which are rarely investigated (OPS 1989, 78).

Although there were the remnants of federal and provincial agencies inspecting foods, drugs, food establishments, and the production of wine, the World Bank reported in 1987 that "[b]oth the Government and industry agree that quality controls should be reestablished to protect consumers and to help local manufacturers to obtain a satisfactory quality of products. . . . The absence of controls . . . also precludes any export [of pharmaceuticals]" (World Bank 1987*a*, 26).

The Dismantling of Oversight under Menem-Cavallo

In 1989, in the first change of government from one elected president to another since 1928, Carlos Saúl Menem took office. In 1991, Domingo Cavallo took over as his economy minister. Whatever intention the prior administration had to comply with the World Bank's suggestions were completely annulled under Cavallo. On September 2, 1991, by decree of Menem, Cavallo, and then–Minister of Health and Social Action, Avelino Porto, the agency responsible for the regulation of pharmaceuticals was reduced from a National Directorate to the obscure grade of department. Degrading an office lowers the grades and salaries of all employees. The department head faced a salary reduction from $31,000 to $13,650. The office also was assigned more tasks. By attrition, the agency was gutted. Requests to replace over 100 technical experts who had left during the Menem years were denied. The message to medicine controllers from Porto, Cavallo, and Menem was clear: in the unregulated market, they did not matter.

The dismantling of the state under the Menem-Cavallo administration has had a profound effect on public safety. Downsizing of government and deregulation was carried out to a degree that was irrational in a country that depends on exports of food, wine, and pharmaceuticals. National Medicine Institute head Alfredo Moro said that, due to the lack of investigators, the recurrent epidemics of poisoning in the 1990s were almost inevitable (*Buenos Aires Herald*, August 31, 1992, p. 7).

As funds were cut back and the number of health inspectors reduced over the years, the regulatory agencies stepped up controls on the easiest targets, the large firms, which already had the best quality control. They neglected the informal, local producers, "the segment of the market where the greatest health risk is found" (FIEL 1988, 111). The division that is supposed to inspect 150,000 food-service establishments in the Greater Buenos Aires area has twelve inspectors. Deregulation of other industries increases the need for oversight in foods, as is demonstrated in the almost daily newspaper reports of situations such as the storage of toxic waste imported from abroad in rotting containers alongside the central produce market of Buenos Aires (*Buenos Aires Herald*, November 20, 1993, p. 9).

The toll in morbidity and mortality has been growing since 1989. The quality of food has deteriorated generally in Argentina, but the greatest burden of death and disability has fallen on the poor, who buy non–brand-name products from bulk sellers and fly-by-night operators. Digestive problems account for 35 percent of patients in public hospitals, the majority of which result from the consumption of adulterated or spoiled foods (*Clarín*, December 22, 1991, p. 41).

The lack of oversight goes beyond food and drugs and extends into every aspect of consumer safety. No regulations cover elevator safety or require periodic inspections (*Clarín*, December 10, 1993, p. 18). The condition of sewers, storm drains, and gas mains, the dumping of toxic wastes, the application of pesticides, conduct on dangerous worksites, the facilities and procedures of hospitals, the installation of wiring, the construction of power lines, the maintenance of motor vehicles, including public carriers such as buses—all those things we might not even think of, year in and year out, either have no regulations or the regulations merely provide the opportunity for the collection of bribes on the part of officials.

Results of Dismantling the Regulatory Apparatus

The outcome of the intentional process of deregulation of every aspect of consumer protection might seem like something in a Monty Python script. The rosy picture of Argentina in the North American press in the 1990s is contradicted daily in a sick comedy of errors. Every few weeks, another scandal hits the newspapers, generally when numerous deaths have already occurred. The following is a sample of events that occurred during the first few years of the Cavallo-Menem regime.[1]

1991

April 11. Ten thousand bottles of fake mineral water were discovered; six bottlers operating thirty-two illegal factories were shut down.

April 20. Judge Llermanos closed two soda bottlers, one mineral water plant, and two juice warehouses for contaminated products (*Buenos Aires Herald*, April 21, 1991, p. 4).

August 2. A tomato cannery in the Greater Buenos Aires neighborhood of Lanús was closed when 1,700,000 cans were found to contain red paint used in construction.

August 29. Forty-five hundred kilograms of mozzarella cheese from seven clandestine factories were found to contain diesel fuel, fecal material, and a dead cat.

October 15. Authorities seized 62,500 kilograms of spoiled flour.

November 21. Forty-seven tons of spoiled powdered milk were seized.

December 10. Five hundred thousand kilograms of mozzarella were seized, containing fecal material, worms, mold, and bacteria (*Clarín*, December 22, 1991, pp. 40–41).

1992

August 4. Greenpeace added its voice to the protests of some Mendoza government officials that the National Atomic Energy Commission was endangering the population by leaving exposed nuclear waste from a plant that shut down in 1986. The waste covers eight hectares (twenty acres) seven meters deep and is open to the wind and rain. Cases of leukemia in children and cancer in adults are unusually prevalent in the area of the abandoned plant (*Buenos Aires Herald*, August 5, 1992, p. 11).

August 27. Judge Llermanos ordered a raid of the private Clínica D'Elia and impounded 600 disposable syringes that were suspected to have been reused numerous times and put back in wrappers. They had been used so many times that the brand names had worn off. The license of the lab doing the recycling had expired in 1988 (Míguez 1992, 32).

August. Twenty-three people died and another twenty fell seriously ill from the consumption of a contaminated batch of a tonic called *Propóleo* made from bee pollen. The tonic, generally consumed by poor people, was produced by Huilén Labs, which was not legally registered to sell health care products. The Minister of Health and Social Action, Julio Aráoz, announced that to correct thirty years without controls he would need $10 million to start up a National Administration of Drugs, Food, and Medical Technology. The minister said that 30 percent of medications sold in the country are phoney. He said that the death threats he received from the pharmaceutical companies to prevent the new legislation on quality control of food and drugs were from only *some* of the companies (*Buenos Aires Herald*, August 22, 1992, p. 11; August 26, 1992, p. 11; August 28, 1992, p. 11). The Health Ministry's Director of Regulation and Control, Angel Tulio, "admitted that 'we only have twelve full-time national inspectors in charge of controlling the almost 3,500 commercial brands sold as 9,000 different pharmaceutical products'" (*Buenos Aires Herald*, August 17, 1992, p. 7).

September 11. The Ministry of Health and Social Action banned the sale and use of a medication after the deaths of five newborns at a maternity hospital in Mar del Plata. Tests showed the product to be "unfit for use" (*Buenos Aires Herald*, September 12, 1992, p. 1).

September 30. Eleven children and one adult were seriously injured in a gas explosion in a school in Lomas de Zamora. A repairman had just fixed a gas leak, while the children remained in the room, and was reconnecting when the blast occurred from a buildup of gas between floors. Fire spread rapidly because the ceiling was made of styrofoam, which is highly explosive when heated (*Buenos Aires Herald*, October 1, 1992, p. 11).

October. A consumer protection group conducted a study of condoms available in the Federal Capital and found that 27 percent broke when tested to established limits and that 18 percent were punctured on purchase. Forty percent of the boxes contained condoms that broke when tested. Fewer than half the brands had instructions in Spanish (*Clarín*, October 25, 1992, p. 4).

October. Results of a study carried out in Buenos Aires showed that 76 percent of vehicles emitted exhaust that exceeded the legal limits for carbon monoxide (*Buenos Aires Herald*, October 6, 1992, p. 11).

1993

The year 1993 was one of repeated epidemics of poisoning from unregulated food and drink. Twenty-seven people died in February from methyl alcohol used to stretch wine from a San Juan winery. (They apparently meant to use ethyl alcohol.) The death toll was higher than expected because when the brand of the poison wine became known, wholesalers or distributors changed the labels (Soltys 1993*a*, 3).

The provincial court was "accused of siding with the vineyard owner" because it failed to seek the arrest of the prime suspect and wasted "valuable time during which the winery owner and his oenologist [technician] went into hiding and presumably were able to rid themselves of any incriminating evidence." The National Wine Board's inspector was the winery's technician (Tozer 1993*a*, 3).

August and September. Twenty-six people died from drinking jug wine that had been laced with methyl alcohol, apparently by distributors who had intended to stretch the wine with ethyl alcohol (*Buenos Aires Herald*, September 9, 1993, p. 11).

September 11. President Menem proposed a solution to the poisoning crisis, saying that those responsible for the tainting of the wine "should be put up against a wall and shot." House of Deputies member Héctor Polino said that the President was to blame for the poisonings, "since he has progressively dismantled the National Wine Institute" (*Buenos Aires Herald*, September 12, 1993, p. 4). (Cancel the firing squad.)

September 12. Investigations following the wine poisonings uncovered adulteration of vinegar, rice, juices, sugar, and pastas (*Clarín*, September 12, 1993, p. 20).

September. A formal complaint issued against the administrator of the National Health Administration (SENASA) said that there are 15,000 food products on the market that have no professional approval and for which "the minimum required health precautions have been ignored." The report said that 15 percent of all foods on the market are not "suitable for human consumption." Another 35 percent "do not contain what they are said to contain." The complaint listed 300 of the cases of food poisoning in 1992 and 1993 (*Buenos Aires Herald*, September 4, 1994, p. 4).

September 8. Four men died and a dozen were injured when a wall they were demolishing collapsed on them. The union said it had complained to the employers a month earlier about the possibility of the wall collapsing. Instead of securing the wall, the company offered the men bonus pay to work without protection. Given the lack of work elsewhere, the men accepted the $40-a-day rate (*Buenos Aires Herald*, September 9, 1993, p. 1, 11).

September 27. Seven people died from poison fumes leaking from a storm drain. Four died in their house, two medical personnel died from the fumes at the scene, and a third medic died after ten days in a coma. Neighbors said that two people had died from poison gases in the same area in October 1992, but their complaints to city authorities had not been followed up with investigations (*Buenos Aires Herald*, September 28, 1993, p. 1).

Although there was evidence that a warehouse owner had dumped cyanide into the city sewers from tanker trucks in his clandestine workshops, the judge dismissed the charges because the law limits responsibility if any other factor is involved, such as a fault in the sewer system or other chemicals with which the cyanide may have combined (Pogoriles 1993, 48).

November 7. Five people were treated for gas poisoning after breathing sulfuric acid fumes coming out of a sewer just four blocks from where the seven people had died in September. The privatized Aguas Argentinas water utility claimed it had "no responsibility" in the case (*Buenos Aires Herald*, November 8, 1993, p. 1).

November 19. An inspection of one of the newly privatized electricity companies found that Brazilian immigrants were working without work permits twelve hours a day, seven days a week, for $400 a month. The workers also were found to be welding and working with asbestos without masks. Their living quarters were unsanitary and dangerous due to faulty electrical installations (*Buenos Aires Herald*, November 20, 1993, p. 11).

November 20. Buenos Aires police discovered a gang that had been collecting spoiled meat out of dumpsters at meatpackers, rinsing it in bleach and selling it to grocery stores in poor areas. Investigators concluded that the practice had been going on for some time (*Clarín*, November 21, 1993, p. 18).

December 6. Fourteen tons of rotten cheese were found in a warehouse in San Justo (Greater Buenos Aires) after a warrant was issued by Judge Llermanos. Police also found a large quantity of spoiled canned goods and again found 6,500 kilos of the powdered milk from the mother-child food program that had been seized on previous occasions (*Buenos Aires Herald*, December 7, 1993, p. 11).

December 6. Five doctors in a hospital in Córdoba contracted hepatitis A from "lack of hygiene in the hospital's kitchens" (*Buenos Aires Herald*, December 7, 1993, p. 11).

December 7. Accumulation of toxic gases in the storm sewers of La Plata caused seven manhole covers to blow off when a child threw a firecracker down a storm drain. "Residents accused the municipal administration of failing to take action and even accepting bribes to cover up abnormalities committed by various manufacturers in the area. . . . [R]esidents charged that their complaints [had] gone unheeded for five years" (*Buenos Aires Herald*, December 9, 1993, p. 1).

December 8. Doctors at Garrahan Children's Hospital discovered that vials labeled as cancer medication actually contained only contaminated water (*Buenos Aires Herald*, December 9, 1993, p. 13).

December 8. Sixty residents of La Plata were sent to the hospital with symptoms of nausea, vomiting, and diarrhea from contaminated tap water. The water authority said the contamination could not have been in the system but rather occurred simultaneously in the individual domestic tanks of the neighborhood. Nevertheless, the authorities conducted tests and increased chlorination (*Buenos Aires Herald*, December 9, 1993, p. 1).

December 10. The near-year-end totals for deaths by elevator accident in the city of Buenos Aires were announced. One person every other day dies from elevator accidents, and hundreds more suffer mutilations of the hands and feet. According to figures provided by the fire department, 212 bodies were removed from elevators in 1992 and 181 in the first eleven months of 1993. "Lack of maintenance is the principal cause of these avoidable episodes, facilitated by the absence of any legislation that requires periodic inspection" (*Clarín*, December 10, 1993, p. 18).

December 20. At least seventeen teenagers were killed in a disco fire when 500 people tried to exit by the only door. Emergency exits were locked (*New York Times*, December 21, 1993, p. A3).

Feeble Response

In 1994, the government announced it would impose stricter controls on food, given the number of poisonings reported. The aim was to create a single inspectorate for standards, perhaps to reduce costs to the food industry because three different entities nominally checked food. Observers said the government's plans fail to ensure basic hygienic standards. Often, food is held so long for inspection that it is spoiled by the time it is released (*Buenos Aires Herald*, May 15, 1994, p. 4).

The problem of shoddy materials due to poverty and the shoddy oversight by the state extends to many services. A recurrent problem is the loss of power after every storm. *Buenos Aires Herald* reported a storm that hit the pampas on May 6, 1994. The nuclear reactor at Embalse went out of service the next day as a result of the storm; no explanation was offered. Main electricity carrier Transener said that nine towers carrying high-tension cables had been destroyed by the storm, which had winds of only sixty miles per hour (*Buenos Aires Herald*, May 8, 1994, p. 4).

A serious government takes oversight responsibilities seriously. Indiscipline in government ministries and corporate boardrooms puts into question the credibility not only of the government but also of the economy. Argentines are tired of living in a country where reading the paper is as good as watching a three-ring circus—people risk their lives making a living in one ring, while clowns and charlatans perform in the other two. The following sections highlight further the carnage that results when oversight is abandoned.

Treatment of State Mental Patients

Another area in which lack of government oversight has produced grisly results is in the care of those confined to state mental hospitals. The abuse ranges from neglect to the apparent murder of inmates to sell their organs for transplants. The latter charge has been made on numerous occasions in various parts of Argentina. The infamous Montes de Oca psychiatric asylum near

Buenos Aires repeatedly has been charged with organ removal, dating back to the days of the military regime, when political opponents were committed to the hospital.

Some experts argue that illegal trade in organs is impossible due to the demanding physiological requirements of transplant medicine. Incidents keep coming up, however, that lend weight to the accusations. The body of Marcelo Ortiz was found in a swamp on the grounds of the Montes de Oca Hospital with his corneas removed. The hospital authorities claimed that the patient had escaped. Ortiz was paraplegic (*Buenos Aires Herald*, March 11, 1992, p. 11). A BBC television documentary claimed in 1993 that Argentina was one of the main countries in the organ trade and the kidnapping of children for body parts. Official response was mixed, with some members of the government denying any Argentine connection. Others, including Argentine Ambassador to the United Kingdom, Mario Cámpora, acknowledged a certain amount of trafficking in body parts. The government confirmed that the traffic in organs and blood at Montes de Oca existed and that its director, Florencio Sánchez, had removed the eyes of dead patients (*Buenos Aires Herald*, March 7, 1992, p. 1). Sánchez, director of the asylum for seventeen years, was convicted for his role in the trade and died in prison in 1992. The government points to that conviction to say that the organ trade is under control (*Buenos Aires Herald*, November 23, 1993, p. 11).

When the government finally investigated after seventeen years of rumors and charges, the findings were sickening. From 1976 to 1991, 1,321 patients had died and 1,395 others had disappeared (Sánchez [no relation] 1992, 1; *Buenos Aires Herald*, March 15, 1992, p. 18). In 1990 alone, out of 1,000 patients, there were 110 disappearances and 87 deaths at Montes de Oca (*Buenos Aires Herald*, February 24, 1992, p. 7).

There had been investigations before. A doctor named Cecilia Giubileo went to work at Montes de Oca, reportedly to find two of her in-laws who had disappeared at the hands of the military. Numerous "disappeared persons" were confined at Montes de Oca, some healthy and some after irreversible brain damage due to blows to head. The day before she was to give evidence on the organ trade, Dr. Giubileo disappeared and has not been found. At one point, so many bodies were turning up on the grounds of Montes de Oca and another public asylum at Open Door that an administrative directive was sent out that at the end of each shift doctors should go out and round up missing patients or their bodies (Sánchez 1992, 4).

An investigative reporter named Enrique Sdrech noticed, as he was studying records of deaths in the asylum, that almost all the dead had Central European names. Why would all the patients with blue eyes die of cardiac arrest? Blue-eye corneas are better for transplant because they deteriorate less. Sdrech found that the asylum was a veritable chop shop for spare parts. The asylum also used the patients as a blood bank, sucking like a vampire more than the permitted amount of blood per month (Sánchez 1992, 4).

Dark-eyed patients tend to live longer, but their condition is abysmal. Only 20 percent of those at Montes de Oca get visits from relatives. The asylum has a budget of $25 million annually, $2,000 per patient, but the patients live in miserable conditions (Sánchez 1992, 2). There are forty doctors for the 1,000 patients. Investigators found $7 million worth of electronics (televisions, videocassette recorders) that had been purchased on the asylum's budget stashed in closets (*Buenos Aires Herald*, March 15, 1992, p. 18; Sánchez 1992, 2). Sdrech gained access to the asylum and found that many patients die of starvation; many are lacking clothes and are naked in all weather. There are sexual relations between guards and patients. Human excrement remains piled up in wards; a cheap stove burns grass for lack of wood. All that for $25 million. When patients die of starvation, the death certificate is altered to state the cause of death as cancer.

Another scandal broke in 1990 at the Braulio Moyano women's mental hospital. A report on the critical situation at the hospital was submitted to Minister of Health and Social Action Matilde Menéndez on January 18, 1990. Nothing was done about the starving of patients until the story reached the newspapers in July 1990 (*Buenos Aires Herald*, July 22, 1990, p. 18). It was found that 32 of the 1,650 patients (2 percent) had died of starvation in June. Menéndez said that was not true: there were only 28 deaths from starvation in June, about the same as in June of 1989. Investigators found that 30 percent of the inmates weighed between thirty and forty-five kilograms (sixty-six to ninety-nine pounds) (*Buenos Aires Herald*, July 1, 1990, p. 4). In mid-July, Minister Menéndez was fired over the Moyano deaths and because of the $40 million that disappeared during her stewardship. She was the seventh Health Minister in seven years (*Buenos Aires Herald*, July 15, 1990, p. 3). One week later, the new Health Minister, Eduardo Bauzá, swore in his team, but thirteen deaths were reported at Moyano mental hospital for the first three weeks of July (*Buenos Aires Herald*, July 22, 1990, p. 18). Menem then appointed Menéndez to head the enormous government pension and medical care fund for the retired, PAMI. She was compelled to resign from that post in 1994, after being implicated in a multimillion-dollar kickback scheme.

Traffic Accidents

Traffic accidents have become a leading cause of death and disability in developing countries, in spite of the fact that the number of cars per person and the number of miles driven per person are much lower than in industrialized countries. Because traffic accidents have their greatest impact on the young, each accidental death represents an average of thirty years of life lost, much greater than for most other leading causes of death. The recording of accidents often is inadequate, and traffic fatalities are underestimated since deaths that do not occur at the scene may not be included. The disability caused by traffic accidents overburdens the rehabilitation capacity of these countries and has important economic repercussions, not the least of which is the loss of productive labor (Bangdiwala and Anzola-Pérez 1987, 130, 132).

The reasons for the high rate of accidents are several and have much to do with the poverty of the people as well as the underdevelopment of the state. When a country is poor and the state regulatory apparatus is weak, the population as a whole assigns a lower priority to safety and prevention. Fatalism in the face of familiar hazards is part of the problem. Another aspect of the fatalism is the passivity of the population in not demanding better protection from the government. The mentality of accident prevention, just as any other kind of preventive health measure, is more common when the whole country is more affluent. To a large extent, this is a matter of education, not only through the schools but also through the mass media, as was done in the United States for seatbelt use.

The disregard for safety affects rich and poor alike. Even when people can afford seatbelts, they do not use them. They drive on superhighways with their children in the backs of pickup trucks. In Argentina, the press began to call attention to the carnage on the highways in the early 1990s, and seatbelt use became mandatory in 1992. A survey in 1993, fully a year after seatbelt use was mandated, found that fewer than 20 percent of drivers and even fewer passengers used them (Lamazares 1993a, 45). When traffic checks were instituted in beach resort areas in 1994, police found that nearly one-third of nighttime drivers were drunk (Soltys 1995, 3).

In most developing countries, the number of registered vehicles has increased greatly since the 1960s, as has the number of vehicles per inhabitant. At the same time, traffic legislation and education have not kept pace. Vehicle registration increased 135 percent in Argentina between 1969 and 1980 (Bangdiwala and Anzola-Pérez 1987, 131). "Part of the blame must be borne by the governments of the last half-century for an infrastructural neglect so total that even the legal speed limit of 110 kilometers per hour on intercity highways is positively dangerous" (Soltys 1995, 3). In addition to infrastructural neglect, enforcement of traffic laws is lacking as is responsible behavior.

Condition of Vehicles

Because of high tariff walls and decades of protection and subsidies, automobiles in Argentina are very expensive. Consequently, even used cars command five times the price they would in the United States, and there are no car cemeteries. Half the cars in the country—three million vehicles—are over fifteen years old. The average age of the approximately one million vehicles in the Federal Capital is seven years. In the interior, no one really knows how old the cars are. In the relatively prosperous province of Córdoba, the government does not even know how many cars there are, let alone the age of the vehicles. More than 25,000 drivers in the city of Córdoba have more than three tickets, but they cannot be located for collection. The beach resort city of Mar del Plata (Buenos Aires Province) has no data on the number of vehicles, but it is estimated that there are 180,000 vehicles, about one-third of them over twenty years old (Pogoriles 1992, 40). Only in 1991 did the city of Buenos Aires begin inspections of taxis and buses. Annual car inspections were initiated in 1992.[2]

Condition of Drivers

Some observers attribute the deteriorating state of traffic in Argentina to a breakdown in social conscience, a legacy of brutality from the Dirty War. The "almost savage individualism [of social life], applied to traffic, makes the common man think of the street as a no-man's-land, because of which each one does as he wishes: drive in reverse, double park, drive the wrong way on a one-way street, high speed, a bit of everything" (Lamazares 1993a, 44). The problem, however, is more fundamental: there never has been a concept of shared citizenship in Argentina to support a level of civility on the street.

The other key element in the pandemonium on Argentina's highways (and this could be said of many other Third World countries) is the disregard of laws—life is lived always on the brink of chaos. There is no accepted notion of right-of-way. At every intersection, right-of-way has to claimed by toughing it out, with or without eye contact. Drivers on side streets fly through intersections with main streets, maybe blasting their horns as they approach the intersection, unless the main avenue drivers display more macho. (Use of the term *macho* does not imply that women cannot play the game. Indeed, with a little practice, and an inuring, every-day exposure to death, anyone can.)

The outcome of all this is that Buenos Aires now ranks as the city with the most traffic deaths in the world, five to six times the number in Rome, Paris, or Madrid. Nationally in 1990, there were 1,200 fatalities per million vehicles; in Italy, there were 241; in the United States, 229; and in Sweden, 192 per million vehicles (Lamazares 1993b, 44). The newspapers were reporting public concern over traffic fatalities in 1991, when 1,358 deaths per million motor vehicles were counted, compared to 278 per million vehicles in the United States (*Buenos Aires Herald*, September 12, 1991, p. 11).

In 1992, alarm over traffic fatalities over the three-day Easter holiday weekend surfaced once again, when accidents claimed forty-three lives. In fact, the Easter weekend toll was below the 1992 average of twenty deaths per day. In the first quarter of 1992, there were 100,000 accidents, with 1,800 deaths and 120,000 injuries (*Buenos Aires Herald*, April 21, 1992, p. 10). Public outrage was raised by a particularly grisly bus accident in which the driver was going between 120 and 130 kilometers per hour (75–80 miles per hour) in spite of dense fog (*Buenos Aires Herald*, April 19, 1992, p. 4).

In 1994, there were over 9,000 traffic deaths in Argentina, ranking it among the five worst countries in the world. Traffic deaths in 1994 exceeded the official count of those killed during the military regime's Dirty War. The main cause of death for Argentines between the ages of five and thirty-five is traffic accidents. There is one death for every 350 cars in Argentina, compared to one death for every 7,000 cars in Sweden (*Buenos Aires Herald*, April 30, 1995, p. 4).

The most notorious issue in 1994 was bus accidents. As things stand, "[B]us transport is simply not a public service. The bus companies blatantly place speed and profit ahead of safety with the complicity of the authorities" (Soltys 1995, 3). The government's response was more show than substance: 10,000 policemen were assigned to ticketing parking violators and impounding the motorcycles of riders without helmets. The deaths continued unabated.

In spite of much publicity about the government safety campaign in 1994, the situation worsened. In the first quarter of 1995, there were 2,883 traffic deaths, an increase over 1994 and 1993 (*Buenos Aires Herald*, April 2, 1995, p. 4). In the city of Buenos Aires, there was a substantial surge in traffic accidents in January 1995. In the first twenty-five days, there were 745 accidents, with at least twenty-five deaths, compared to 265 accidents in all of January 1994. The city announced that all buses would be equipped with automatic door locks to keep drivers from driving with their doors open (Sims 1995*a*, A11). Considering that every bus at rush hour speeds along with four people hanging out who would not fit if the doors were closed, that could save lives, but the devices probably would be disabled.

The death toll is multiplying. Early 1996 returns showed a 40 percent increase over 1995. In January 1996 alone, there were 1,200 deaths on highways and city streets, 38 per day, almost twice the daily rate for 1992 (*Buenos Aires Herald*, February 4, 1996, p. 4).

AIDS

The same factors that make Argentine highways, hospitals, and asylums unsafe threaten to precipitate an epidemic of AIDS of frightening proportions: a lack of government oversight, disregard for rules and standards of practice, lack of concern for prevention, indifference towards others, rent seeking, and corruption. All those factors have played their part in the spreading AIDS crisis in Argentina. Cultural factors also foster the disease, including the still common practice of fathers bringing their sons to prostitutes for initiation (Pignotti 1992*b*, 9). The unequal status of husbands and wives and the keeping of mistresses also contribute to higher risks of spreading infection.

When I interviewed doctors in Mendoza in November 1991, I asked each one what protection they had against AIDS. They all assured me that AIDS was a big-city problem, maybe in Buenos Aires, but not in Mendoza. In a public clinic there, doctors performed internal gynecological exams without having sterilizing equipment for instruments. The latest official estimates are that 1 out of every 400 people in Mendoza is infected with AIDS. The disease has gotten a foothold in all the towns throughout the province (*Buenos Aires Herald*, May 15, 1994, p. 4).

As early as 1990, the *Buenos Aires Herald* warned of the threat of AIDS in Argentina, but its message went unheeded. Although the number of AIDS cases at that time was thought to be few, poor hygiene in hospitals and the overall crisis in public health constituted a dangerous breeding ground for the spread of the disease. Dr. Pedro Cahn, chief of infection control at Fernández Hospital said that part of the problem of AIDS in Argentina was that many people denied the country's drug problem (Ulanovsky Sack 1993, 20).

The prevalence of AIDS in the Federal Capital is 2 per 1,000, but the composition is changing. In 1985, when Fernández Hospital opened its outpatient clinic for AIDS, two-thirds of patients were homosexuals and 20 to 25 percent were drug addicts. In 1992, heterosexuals were 47 percent of the patient population, 30 percent drug addicts, and the rest homosexual men (Ulanovsky Sack 1993, 20). As is common in less developed countries, sexually transmitted diseases are an important cofactor of heterosexual, urban spread of AIDS. The number of women in developing countries with AIDS tends to be about equal to that of men. No woman was diagnosed in Buenos Aires until 1987. By 1993, 207 female cases were reported. In 1988, there were more than 12 men for every woman with AIDS, but by 1993, the ratio had dropped to 4 to 1 (Quistgard 1994, 4). The data on child AIDS mortality is difficult to collect because a child dying of AIDS looks much like a child dying of diarrhea, malnutrition, and respiratory disease. A child who is immunocompromised is very likely to die of measles, and the underlying AIDS might go unnoticed (*Buenos Aires Herald*, May 27, 1990, p. 17).

Buenos Aires, but not the rest of the country, began to wake up to AIDS in the early 1990s with, as often happens in Argentina, a scandal. A judge asked Interpol to capture the president and the auditor of a reputable private hospital for reusing disposable needles (*Buenos Aires Herald*, April 29, 1990, p. 13). Concern also spread because thirty patients in a renal dialysis unit contracted AIDS in 1990.

Then, in 1991, the extent of the AIDS epidemic in the prison population began to surface. Figures released by court sources indicated that 40 percent of the Olmos prison population (3,050 persons) carried the AIDS virus (*El Día* [La Plata] also reported that many inmates have mange, hepatitis, and measles.) The Buenos Aires Penitentiary Service denied that number and said it had detected only eighty AIDS-infected prisoners, not more than 15 percent of the total. The Service also admitted, however, that there was no systematic disease control plan in effect. Penal judge Hector Decastelli visited the prison and found that its hospital ward lacked disposable materials, medicines, and sheets. The bathrooms were abysmal, and the building was falling apart (*Buenos Aires Herald*, October 17, 1991, p. 11).

Sources at the Penitentiary Service admitted that 30 of the 150 minors held in Unit 16 of Caseros prison in 1991 were sick with AIDS, but they did not know how many healthy carriers there were because they lacked the funds to test them (*Clarín*, January 5, 1992, p. 37). Seventy percent of drug addicts are estimated to be HIV positive, and the average age of nondeclared carriers is thought to be fifteen (*Diario de Cuyo*, November 5, 1991, p. 3).

The initial response of the government to AIDS was a disaster. "A glaring example of massive testing turned havoc were the checks on conscripts in Buenos Aires provincial Army barracks . . . most of the youths who tested positive and underwent severe psychological shock were later found out not to have AIDS" (Pignotti 1992*a*, 17).

The government does almost no public education about AIDS (or any other public health issue) on the television station it owns, unlike other Latin American countries. When the public station aired a program about AIDS, it was a twenty-five-hour marathon rather than ongoing reporting and education. The government announced a huge campaign, made sweeping, unsupported statements, spent $10 million in the first six months, and came under heavy criticism for apparently not consulting any recognized experts (van der Horst 1992*b*, 40).

Government officials are not well informed about AIDS. In October 1992, when concern was rising about the quality of blood products, Alfredo Miroli, director of the National Program for the Fight against Human Retroviruses—AIDS, claimed that testing covered 100 percent of blood donors (van der Horst 1992*a*, 40). Health Minister of the Month Conrado Storani claimed, "Blood-testing regulations went into effect in Argentina in 1986. Under the guidelines all hospitals and clinics were required to test all blood and blood-derived products such as Factor VIII plasma for the presence of HIV antibodies" (*Buenos Aires Herald*, November 2, 1992, p. 11). In fact, until 1988 it was not obligatory to test blood or blood products for HIV in municipal hospitals of Buenos Aires. In the provinces, testing was not required until 1991.

The procedures for blood testing increase the dangers. In the Federal Capital, there is a two-month wait for free HIV testing at Muñiz Hospital (Quistgard 1994, 4). Because tests at blood banks were free and fast, homosexuals and drug addicts in great numbers went to give blood. Blood banks gave the potential donor a confidential questionnaire about sex and drug habits. The validity of the questionnaire depended on candid answers, but the high-risk donors had gone to the blood bank specifically to learn their current HIV status. The screening method greatly increased the risk for blood recipients because the proportion of donors who were high risk was great and because of the "window," the time before the virus produces antibodies that show up in blood tests (Clivaggio 1993a, 42).

Even after the 1991 legislation that requires testing, 50 percent of Argentine hospitals were not equipped to detect AIDS-contaminated blood donations, according to Israel Stolovtizki, President of the Multidisciplinary Association against AIDS. He said that the government does not have the political will to launch a coherent anti-AIDS campaign (*Buenos Aires Herald*, May 19, 1991, p. 13).

After the August 1992 raid of another private hospital that netted 600 shop-worn needles, the implications of some of the statistics of health care dawned on investigators. The world average for the number of needles and syringes used annually is 10 to 15 per person. In Argentina, it is 3 syringes and 1.5 needles per person. The factory-new ones are supposed to be sterilized at National Atomic Energy Center in Ezeiza, but there has been an alarming drop in shipments to Ezeiza (Míguez 1992, 33). The government figured out, somewhat belatedly, that the shortfall of about 300 million syringes meant not that the country was getting healthier but that syringes and needles were being reused. In fact, according to the data, most were being reused.

In spite of the government's reassurances in 1991 that all blood supplies were "100 percent" safe, people were still becoming infected in 1993 and 1994 due to sloppy work that was covered up. In investigating the source of infection of an eighteen-year-old patient who had died of AIDS, a doctor found that the blood bank supplying the patient had not tested the blood of approximately eighty donors and then had destroyed the records of those donors (*Clarín*, September 19, 1993, p. 38). Even after that scandal, new infections from transfusions continued in 1994. Two babies died and two were sick as a result of receiving contaminated blood in the Córdoba Children's Hospital (*Buenos Aires Herald*, May 8, 1994, p. 4).

Faced with a potentially huge number of carriers in Argentina (estimated as high as one-half million, or 1.5 percent of the population), the response of the health care system seems chaotic at best. Doctors at Felipe Heras Hospital in Concordia, Entre Ríos, filed a labor complaint that they had gone fourteen days without the necessary reagents to perform AIDS tests for blood transfusions. Subsequent investigation uncovered the AIDS-testing equipment in a bathroom, along with three vials of plasma infected with AIDS and some cleaning and maintenance equipment (*Entrerriano*, October 5, 1991, p. 5). (You just have to know where to look.)

The hospital responded to the union action by removing the complainant as head of the intensive care unit. The person named in his place was out on maternity leave, so that left intensive care without a director. When the hospital director was asked about the AIDS-testing equipment being kept in the bathroom, he replied that it was a "vocational" problem—if a medical worker is afraid of catching any disease, that person should stay home. Two workers at the hospital were identified as HIV carriers, a nurse and a cleaning person (*Entrerriano*, October 5, 1991, pp. 6–7).

By 1992, some doctors specializing in infectious diseases were becoming alarmed. Fernández Hospital was receiving between fifteen and twenty-five new cases of AIDS a week, and doctors there were calculating the multiple risk factors the country faces. "'Argentina is a country with a high risk rate for the spread of AIDS because drugs circulate, sexuality is expressed in a plural way and in the last ten years nothing had been done to prevent the epidemic from expanding,' said Dr. Cahn" (*Buenos Aires Herald*, May 5, 1992, p. 11).

Many doctors were slow to respond to the public health threat. "'Many physicians are unwilling to relearn what they already do with ease,' says Leonor Nuñez," AIDS specialist and psychologist. "Thus dentists may refuse to use rubber gloves because they find them uncomfortable, to name one of many such examples. Proper sterilization also is essential but not always available and blood transfusions are still a source of risk" (Pignotti 1992a, 17).

A positive outcome of the crisis is that doctors are giving more thought to the desirability of transfusions and are using them only when absolutely necessary. Between 1988 and 1993, the number of transfusions was cut in half (Clivaggio 1993a, 42). Nevertheless, the health biweekly *Consultor de Salud* estimated that by the year 2003 40,000 people will have died from AIDS in Argentina. Forty percent of new victims are under the age of thirty (*Buenos Aires Herald*, June 6, 1993, p. 4).

Due to the attention given AIDS by the press, the public is understandably concerned. Blood banks in Argentina are down to 40 percent of their usual supplies, because people are afraid of getting AIDS as donors. Specialists say the fear is unjustified because blood bags and the needles that are incorporated in them can be used only once, but people know that in Argentina disposable syringes are reused (*Clarín*, April 26, 1992, p. 40).

In an attempt to reassure the public, Dr. Laura Astarloa, director of the National Plan for the Fight against AIDS, pointed out that tests now available can be conducted for only $1.50. In remote areas without specialized equipment, the testing would cost only $2.00. She added, reassuringly: "In sum: if someone has an accident in a less populated area, and is taken to a particular station to receive medical help and receives blood contaminated with HIV, that is only possible because someone wanted to save two dollars *and violated the National Blood Law, which requires testing for Chagas' disease, brucellosis, syphilis, hepatitis and—finally—AIDS* in the blood that is used for transfusions" (*Clarín*, April 26, 1992, p. 41, emphasis in original).

Well, how reassuring is that? People poison their fellow citizens with methyl alcohol for less than two dollars and then change the labels so sales do not fall off. There are countless other examples: selling meat out of dumpsters, providing spoiled milk for the child nutrition program, putting red paint in tomato paste, even kidnapping children for organ transplants. Will the National Blood Law stop them if it is not enforced? Lack of oversight, in fact, the abandonment of the regulatory obligation of the state, has greatly expanded the opportunities for adulteration and careless production. In a society in which the concept of neighbor is eclipsed by hatred of the "other," where the anonymous consumer is equivalent to an enemy because he or she is unknown, moral restraint is weak.

Even more widespread than the consciously criminal activity of those who sell adulterated products is the generalized lack of seriousness and even lack of awareness on the part of health practitioners and the public. Six months after the article about the National Blood Law quoted above was published, I brought a student to a private clinic for stitches. I had to insist that new needles be gotten from the pharmacy instead of recycled ones for his suturing.

Part III

The Medical Response

Seven

Divided Economy,
Divided Medicine

Part II examined how the physical and civic environments of the poor produce so much suffering and premature death. Poverty is the cause of most of the diarrhea, acute respiratory infections, Chagas' disease, worms, malaria, severed limbs, burns, leprosy, tuberculosis, meningitis, and exposure to toxic substances. That tidal wave of illness and injury is independent of the medical system. The solutions are cleaner water and food, better housing, and safer transportation. Nevertheless, medicine is not irrelevant. An effective medical system, with both preventive and curative capacity, could do much to alleviate the health problems of the poor. That is especially so in a country such as Argentina, which has relatively high GDP per capita and a substantial medical infrastructure.

What facilities exist to address the health of the poor are the subject of Part III. Chapter 7 examines the organization of the medical industry in Argentina and the interactions among its three components: private medicine, social security, and public medicine. Chapters 8 and 9 offer a detailed look at the public sector. Chapter 8 examines primary health care. Chapter 9 is about secondary care in public hospitals.

Argentina spends 9 percent of GDP on medicines and medical care, has more CAT scanners per person than the United States, and more doctors per dollar of GDP than any other country. Argentine performance is mediocre in infant survival and maternal survival, and the population is burdened with many debilitating diseases. Why does a country with so many resources produce such dismal results? The organization of the medical market and the collapse of the public system provide part of the explanation. Preventive primary health care is almost completely lacking, and curative facilities increasingly are concentrated in a private sector that fewer and fewer citizens can afford. There is excess supply in urban areas and unmet demand in suburban and rural areas, duplication of highly technical services in the private sector, and absence of basic equipment, supplies, and personnel in the public sector (Arce 1988, 102).

Medical services are provided in three different systems in Argentina. The private sector includes numerous private hospitals, health plans, practitioners, and clinics, including fraternal, for-profit, and religious organizations. The social-security sector consists of more than 350 union and trade association health plans, called *obras sociales*, which are funded by a payroll tax but which have autonomous spending power. The public sector consists of a national Ministry of Health and Social Action, twenty-four provincial health authorities, and municipal authorities that have some autonomy from provincial and national governments. Decision making is dispersed, and there is no mechanism for coordinating policies. Even within the public sector, decisions are made in the context of successive governmental policies that often are contradictory (OPS 1989, 61).

In recent decades, the medical industry in Argentina has developed almost exclusively in response to market forces. In any economy, supplier-induced demand impedes the operation of a medical market because the supplier (doctor) decides what services are needed. Consumer decision making is inhibited by lack of information about the merits of treatment, resulting in market failure. In the Argentine economy, encumbered by oligopoly, rent seeking, special interests, and corruption, the market failure is exacerbated.

Even aside from that weakness, the private sector cannot be expected to provide the health care needed in a developing country. The services needed by the poorer half of the population are not profitable. Limited spending power keeps the poor from influencing the market for health services. Public health care, primary and secondary, is a necessary investment because the market does not protect the health of the work force.

Because medicine is increasingly market driven and the once prestigious public sector is in disarray, the system produces results that are anomalous and that impede national development. By 1992, there had been an estimated 80,000 silicon implants performed in Argentina, 4,000 in 1991 alone (*Clarín*, February 16, 1992, pp. 32–33). Argentina is said to be the best in the world in liposuction (Wright 1995, 5). Yet in 1991, I was told that there were only two public hospitals in Buenos Aires performing cardiac surgery, one of which (Gutiérrez) had a three-year wait for nonemergency surgery due to the lack of funds for disposable materials (Name withheld, 1991). There are, however, fashionable sports medicine clinics, with glossy brochures, not only for elite and professional sports figures but also for recreational athletes. Meanwhile, a judge forced the closure of the maternity hospital of San Francisco Solano because neglect of the cesspool repeatedly caused "water and waste to flow out of the drainage grates in the floors of the consultation rooms, wards and delivery rooms" (Kreplak 1991, 32).

Argentina has the resources to provide both sports medicine and safe delivery rooms, but the 9 percent of GDP that goes to medical care is badly spent and the Argentine population badly served. UNICEF calculates that a basic package of preventive health care, including vaccination, oral rehydration therapy, women's education, monitoring of child development, family spacing, and food supplements would cost no more than $20 per person annually (Bustelo 1989, 62). Even if the costs were substantially higher, it would be far less than Argentina's per capita annual spending of about $180 (Arce 1988, 102). Sri Lanka, Costa Rica, and Chile spend about $45 per person annually and have lower infant mortality rates than Argentina (Bustelo 1989, 63). And the situation for Argentines is worsening. Argentina is one of very few countries in which the steady downward trend in infant mortality of the past three decades has been reversed (Abalo 1989, 68).

One of the reasons the health budget is spent so badly is that there is no system of evaluating—or even recording—huge categories of budgeted funds. Payments of as much as $250 million can be made without any indication of payee or purpose (Bustelo 1989, 66).

Another reason for the disappointing results is the gigantism that afflicts both the private and the public sectors. The focus is on the big solution, which overemphasizes curative hospital care and neglects primary care. Doctors bemoan the lack of a vaccine for AIDS, but inexpensive, even commonplace preventives such as childhood vaccinations are neglected. The medical profession focuses on the past. Honoring the memory of Argentina's Nobel prize winners has been an obstacle to developing a health system that fits the epidemiological profile of this Third World country. From a cost-benefit perspective, indirect methods to better health, such as nutrition and urban sanitation, improve efficiency and lower costs considerably. Cost-effective innovations, such as ambulatory surgery and endoscopy, and preventive measures are neglected, leading to higher costs in all three sectors (Pampliega 1991).

Gigantism and fame seeking also afflict the public hospitals, which are now even less able to provide highly technical services. The teaching hospital of the University of Buenos Aires, Hospital de Clínicas General San Martín, offers free *in vitro* fertilization (*Buenos Aires Herald*, November 15, 1992, p. 13). But by 1993, the neonatology ward at Clínicas, because of lack of funds, was turning away 71 percent of the critically ill infants referred to it (Dr. Isabel Kurlat, August 26, 1993).

The governor of Buenos Aires announced that the province would provide transplants for all residents. Even when he later reassured citizens that he meant only for those who needed transplants, his goal of 700 transplants a year and a special transplant hospital seemed unrealistic (Veltri 1992, 32). It is disingenuous of the government to cut health budgets and promise greatly expanded and expensive medical procedures. To promise transplants when so many die of simple causes like vaginal infections and diarrhea reflects the obsession with appearing First World. The transplants that are now carried out are not successful. Multiple-organ transplants grab the headlines. The organs are removed in the public hospitals and transplanted in the private facility, with plenty of publicity. The death of a patient a few days later does not make news (Werthein 1991, 28–29).

Grand designs but frustration with detail lead to the abandonment of a workable infrastructure. Instead of repairing an old structure, a new hospital is built, at the greatest cost possible (Arce and Roncoroni 1987, 33). Such was the case of Garrahan Children's Hospital, proclaimed to be the best equipped in the world, while the formerly prestigious Ricardo Gutiérrez Children's Hospital languishes thirty blocks away, with a thousand doctors, no medicines, and few supplies.

Market Structure in Argentine Medicine
The Private Sector

Ten percent of the Argentine population depends on private out-of-pocket payments or private insurance plans for medical care (World Bank 1988, 15). The private hospitals expanded greatly in the 1970s and 1980s, in spite of the small number of private patients, because the largest financer of medical care, the social security system *(obras sociales)*, relied increasingly on the private sector to provide services. The *obras sociales* turned to the private sector because of the new technology it was acquiring. The contracts with the *obras sociales* in fact provided the financing for the technological enhancement of the private sector.

The economic policies of the *Proceso* favored the expansion of private sector technology with tariff concessions and the price code, the *Nomenclador Nacional*, which assigned higher prices to the use of technology than to doctors' services. When the overvalued peso made imports cheap, Argentina bought thirty CAT scanners, twenty-eight of them for private hospitals (De Genaro 1989, 242–243). Of approximately 150 sonogram machines, 90 percent are in the private sector (Dr. Pablo Muntaabski, June 26, 1992), as well as 55 to 95 percent of medical technology in other categories. About three-fourths of heavy technology is concentrated in the Buenos Aires metropolitan area, which has about 35 percent of the national population (Arce 1988, 103).

There is an excess of advanced equipment in the private sector in Argentina. In developed countries, there is one CAT scanner for every 1.5 million inhabitants. In Argentina, there is one for every 400,000 (De Genaro 1989, 242–243). Combined with the oversupply of doctors, the excess of private-sector equipment accentuates the supplier-induced demand for both expensive advanced medical care and sophisticated technology (World Bank 1987a, v). To cope with the excess supply, doctors resort to overbilling, charging the *obras sociales* for services not actually rendered (Tafani 1989, 10). They also overuse diagnostic tests, which not only raise costs but also can have serious iatrogenic effects (Alonso 1990, 566).

Another response to excess supply is specialization. The generalist "offers an undifferentiated product and behaves as a 'price taker' . . . [whereas the specialist is] a 'price setter' and impedes the natural tendency of prices to fall in the face of the growth in the supply of professionals" (Katz and Muñoz 1988, 86). A further step in the process is the development of the microspecialty; for example, a doctor works in pediatric endocrinology, without ever having had a residency in either pediatrics or endocrinology. One of the results of self-defined specialization is the enormous increase in medical malpractice suits because the doctors are not adequately prepared for the specialty they choose. At present, about one out of every twenty doctors is facing a lawsuit in Argentina. Surgery generates 80 percent of the suits (*Clarín*, December 29, 1991, p. 42).

Supplier-induced demand in the private sector has attracted some attention but little action. "To raise their incomes, professionals encourage patients' visits and use expensive X-rays or laboratory tests and high-tech procedures in dubious cases. In the absence of suitable standards and monitoring, abuses have reached large proportions, raising repeated medical association concerns" (World Bank 1988, 18). There are duplication and overlap in more profitable areas (X-ray, lab testing, renal dialysis, CAT, echography, etc.) and severe gaps in less profitable areas (World Bank 1988, 19).

"Quality of care, in the private sector, varies widely. Many of the private-non-profit hospitals are considered as models of care. Private-for-profit hospitals generally offer the best amenities, but profit considerations often interfere with the quality of care" (World Bank 1987a, 32). There are as many cardiac bypasses in relation to the population in Argentina as in United States. This issue is not one of epidemiology, it is the choice of the physicians. Almost all the excess surgery is performed in private hospitals (Dr. Eduardo Mele, August 26, 1991). (Dr. Mele is head of the cardiac intensive care unit at a major private hospital in Buenos Aires.)

The competency of hospital staff varies in the private sector. Some private hospitals have a quality advantage because they can recruit qualified personnel from the public sector. In public hospitals, auxiliary nurses who have completed primary school plus nine to twelve months in a hospital course administer medicine. In Sanatorio Anchorena, a private hospital, only university-trained nurses perform that task (Dr. Eduardo Mele, August 26, 1991). Other private hospitals use personnel who would not be considered qualified in most public sector hospitals. They hire residents with a minimum of specialized experience from the public hospitals to staff their intensive-care wards nights and on weekends (Dr. Alberto Schwarcz, August 21, 1992). At one private hospital, a pediatric resident reported that she was paid $250 per shift and an additional $30 for every patient admitted. Of the thirty patients admitted on her shift by other residents, only four needed to be admitted. The resident also reported that the doctors charged for numerous medications that were not given (Name withheld, 1992).

The Argentine private sector has one of the highest rates of Caesarean-section deliveries in the world. A 1985 audit found that 35 percent of deliveries in private hospitals paid for by social security were by Caesarean section (World Bank 1987*a*, 32). A later investigation reported by then-Health Minister Eduardo Bauzá found that private clinics serving the *obras sociales* have a 46 percent rate of Caesarean sections. In Japan and Holland, 7 percent of births are by Caesarean section. Fifty percent of Argentine mothers have had a C-section. Under the old price system, the main incentive for doctors was saving time: C-section takes only forty-five minutes. Now that the private clinics can charge 65 percent more for C-sections, there are both price and time incentives. The disadvantages of unnecessary surgery are serious. Caesarean sections in Argentina are an important cause of maternal mortality. One-third of women have postoperative infection, and the babies are born depressed from drugs. Norberto Larroca, president of an association of private clinics and hospitals, admitted the higher costs of Caesarean sections but said that doctors do not want to give up a whole Saturday waiting for a birth (Canepa 1991, 18).

Drug Dependence. Another segment of the private health sector is the pharmaceutical industry. An oversupply of pharmaceutical products and "a prescriptive attitude on the part of professionals" has led to overmedication and suppression of symptoms rather than treatment of underlying causes (Arce 1988, 105). Thirty percent of total spending on health and 57 percent of direct household spending on health goes to medicines (González García et al. 1987, 81). Argentines spend $1.5 billion a year on medications, $50 or more per person per year. That is more than three times what Brazilians spend and more than four times what Mexicans spend (Zicolillo 1992, 8). Argentines spend more than four times as much per capita as Chileans and in the hemisphere are surpassed by only the United States, Canada, and Puerto Rico in per capita spending on pharmaceuticals (OPS 1988, 190).

The reasons for the high rate of spending include the custom of writing prescriptions *de favor* (on request), the availability of almost all drugs without prescription, the presence in the market of many badly trained doctors who prescribe too much, extensive advertising by pharmaceutical companies to the medical profession and to the general public, and abusive self-medication with tranquilizers, analgesics, laxatives, and diet pills (Zicolillo 1992, 8).

Argentina has the highest number of psychiatrists in relation to population of any country in the world, and the population is heavily sedated (although you wouldn't guess it in traffic). In the month of October 1991 alone, Argentines spent $28 million on tranquilizers, of which half was spent on one drug, Lexotanil. It is the third biggest selling drug in the country and doubled its sales from 1989 to 1991 (Aulicino 1992, 4), the years of the hyperinflation.

In spite of the $1.5 billion spent on medicines in Argentina yearly, the only drug for the treatment of Chagas' disease has been withdrawn from the market because those who need it cannot afford it. There is a lack of effective demand in a population of which perhaps as many as 13 percent nationally are infected with that degenerative and fatal disease (Aulicino 1992, 1).

Actually, spending on medications exceeds the estimate of $1.5 billion and is closer to $3 billion because of the many tonics and unlicensed medications taken, particularly by poorer people, such as *Propóleo*. According to the World Health Organization, developing countries consume $34 billion worth of drugs annually. If that figure is accurate, then Argentina (which has less than 1 percent of Third World population) consumes almost 10 percent of all the drugs in the Third World, or 5 percent of the value of licensed pharmaceutical sales (Aulicino 1992, 2). For 1985, total spending on drugs amounted to 2.4 percent of GDP.

The role played by the pharmaceutical companies in the Argentine medical industry affects health at all levels. Medical research deals only with the uses of new drugs because all the funds come from pharmaceutical companies (Agrest 1990, 560). Promotional expenditures amount to 25 percent of total sales value, unduly influencing choice of therapy. Firms distort the regulatory process by submitting labels and booklets that are not the ones actually used when the product is marketed (United Nations 1984, 85).

The pharmaceutical industry also distorts the political realm. The industry is said to have been behind the 1966 coup that overthrew Radical president Illia and the death threats to Health Minister Aráoz in 1992, both times because of proposed changes in pharmaceutical regulation. (See Chapter 6.) In 1995, the continuing dispute between the United States and Argentina over intellectual property rights was commandeered by the pharmaceutical industry. The dispute could cost Argentina dearly in trade sanctions, entry into the North American Free Trade Agreement (NAFTA), and investment, but the Argentine drug copiers defeated Menem's attempts to accommodate U.S. patent holders. Charges of enormous bribes and, of course, death threats again accompanied the Congressional override of Menem's veto of an inadequate patents bill (Murdock 1995, A15).

The Social Security System (Obras Sociales)

The principal financer of health care in Argentina is the social security system, which accounts for 39.2 percent of total spending on health. The private sector is the principal provider of medical attention to affiliates of the *obras sociales* (Arce 1988, 103). Workers contribute 4 percent (including retirement health contribution) and employers contribute 4.5 percent of the wage to the union or trade association health and pension plan. Most unions do not have their own medical facilities but subcontract to private insurance companies and keep 50 percent of the tax revenue. Other unions contract directly with private health care providers. The unions collect billions of dollars a year from the payroll tax. The Alfonsín government attempted to launch a national health system, like Canada's, but the unions defeated it.

The social security system is an organizational form that Latin America borrowed from Europe. It was designed for a European population, which is mainly urban and employed in industry, civil service or, at least, stable employment (Ugalde 1985, 115). In Argentina, however, especially in the interior, a large segment of the work force is not covered because they are not wage or salary workers. Only 19 percent of the population of Formosa, for example, has health care coverage (González García et al. 1987, 51).

By 1993, it was estimated that half the population were outside the *obras* and the private programs and had the public system as their only recourse. The proportion of health care spending does not reflect the distribution of the population that uses each sector. Of the 9 percent of GDP going to medical care, 2 percent goes to the public sector and 7 percent goes to the private sector and *obras sociales* (Soltys 1993*b*, 3, 17).

The economic crisis and endemic corruption led to the bankruptcy of the *obras sociales* in the 1990s. The decrease in the real wage, the contraction of salaried employment and consequent increase in self-employment, the impunity of firms in nonpayment of their contributions, and the increasing practice of paying workers under the table to avoid contributions were among the causes (Belmartino 1991, 30). The Labor Ministry estimated in 1991 that one-fourth of the national work force, three million workers, may be employed in illegal conditions and paid undercover by employers who evade contributions to social security and pensions (*Buenos Aires Herald*, November 21, 1991, p. 11).

There is great disparity among the obras. The twelve largest *obras sociales* account for more than half the covered population, and the fifty largest account for 93 percent. The remaining 7 percent of the covered population are divided among the 254 smaller plans. PAMI, the health plan for the retired, has over three million beneficiaries and accounts for 30 percent of total revenues of the more than 300 *obras* (World Bank 1988, 29, 30).

Of 353 union health care plans, 203 had revenues of less than $50,000 a month, and 57 had monthly revenues of less than $1,000 in 1993. The top ten health plans receive about half of all wage contributions, which amounts to between $2.5 billion and $2.7 billion a year (*Buenos Aires Herald*, November 2, 1993, p. 5). Each of the *obras* has its own rules about what is covered, and each has its own paperwork. Hospital billing departments have a nightmare job following the different rules of the 353 different plans (Dr. Eduardo Mele, August 26, 1991).

"Unlike most other [countries'] social insurance systems, the OS [*obras sociales*] system does not merge the funds it collects so there is a wide gap between the benefits from OSs serving low-wage industries and those serving such groups as business executives. The inequity of the system is exemplified by per capita health expenditures which are nine times higher in the most affluent OSs than in the poorest ones" (World Bank 1988, 19). A Redistribution Fund was created to assist the poorer *obras*, but it works in reverse. The poorer funds do not offer many services, do not pay for disposable surgical items or intensive care, and limit extent of coverage and length of stay. The larger, richer funds cover everything for their members but spend without regard to income. At the end of the year, the fund balances end-of-year deficits, and the poor subsidize the rich (World Bank 1988, 19).

For most *obras*, bad management, a bad choice of the health package to offer, little control of quality of care, and the absence of any choice of provider for the captive customers has meant seriously deficient care. "Over the last 20 years, the quality of health care has declined markedly. Since 1970, when membership in social insurance funds (OS) became compulsory, consumers have been unable to choose their insurer and are limited in their selection of a provider. The necessity to go through uncoordinated and time-consuming procedures has led to inefficiencies, lower quality service and serious delays" (World Bank 1988, 15).

The Menem-Cavallo administration announced that workers would be able to choose their health coverage freely but backed down on that promise in exchange for union support for an amendment to the constitution that would allow Menem to be re-elected. "Responsible employers simply write off this 9 percent as a tithe to labor [unions] and take out private insurance for their staff, effectively doubling the cost of health care in Argentina" (Goñi 1992*b*, 2).

The Public Sector

The public sector is administered by many different entities, including the national government, the provinces, and the municipalities. At all levels of government and all levels of care—primary, secondary, and tertiary—the public sector has lost its key role in its triple job of treatment, teaching, and research. The public sector has deteriorated because of limits on operational hours, unsatisfactory quality in the delivery of services, lack of medicines and materials, lack of trained personnel in the provincial hospitals, bad maintenance and obsolete and deteriorated physical plant and equipment, care based on hospitalization, failure to innovate, and the failure of *obras sociales* to pay public hospitals for services (OPS 1989, 62).

"The fragmented organization of the sector and its weak coordination and supervision create severe problems of quality and efficiency. The services available to the population not covered by insurance are seriously deficient and rapidly deteriorating ... [with] striking inequalities between the services enjoyed by the rich and the poor" (World Bank 1988, 15). "The service provided by this huge number of physicians, many working extra hours, is notoriously low in public institutions. Low efficiency is attributed to piecemeal duties, part-time jobs, long commuting times, insufficient staff, outdated equipment, in addition to low salaries and morale. Public sector physicians earn much less than their counterparts in the OS system and private sector and perform many nurses' functions" (World Bank 1988, 17).

Leadership in public health is undermined by frequent turnover in the Ministry of Health and Social Action (MSAS) in key positions, leading to inconsistent policies and uninformed officials. Overstaffing, promotion by seniority, not performance, and lack of management training also waste public sector funds (World Bank 1988, 20). In dollars, the budget of MSAS, which is two-thirds of federal government spending for health fell 41 percent between 1986 and 1988 (OPS 1987, 109). Generally, of funds budgeted, only 30 to 50 percent is actually spent. "Over the last two decades, the Federal Government has transferred some 200 hospitals to the provinces and today it retains only long-term hospitals serving the entire country in such special fields as psychiatry, burns, ophthalmology, dentistry, leprosy and the care of the mute and deaf, the blind and the severely handicapped, that no other provider would accept because of the heavy burden of long-term care" (World Bank 1987a, 29).

Within the provinces, health administration is varied. In some, such as Mendoza, all hospitals are provincial, whether in the city or in the rural areas. In other provinces, including Buenos Aires, there are also municipal hospitals. Different counties in the same province spend different amounts on health care. San Isidro, in the suburbs of Buenos Aires, has half the population of Morón and Quilmes combined but spends as much as the other two on health care (González García et al. 1987, 44).

Clientele of the Public Sector. In the past, the public sector was used by people of all income groups, especially for secondary care. In the interior, public hospitals still serve all classes because of the lack of private sector hospitals. With the expansion of the *obras sociales* in the 1960s to 1980s and the private sector in the 1970s to 1990s, public hospitals now serve a narrower, but still substantial, range of patients. The following are among those served:

- the 50 percent of the population not served by *obras sociales* or the private sector
- people who do not want to pay the copayment charged by their *obra social*

- emergency cases
- people with chronic or expensive conditions, which the private hospitals and the *obras sociales* refuse to treat because of low profit margin, such as AIDS, cancer, high-risk births, severe burns, and intensive care
- people who need the specialized, high-level care that is available only in the public sector, including the special hospital for burns and Ricardo Gutiérrez Children's Hospital's respiratory ward for cystic fibrosis

The specialty hospitals treat nonpaying patients regardless of origin. Burn patients come from all over southern South America, although the entire budget comes from the Municipality of the City of Buenos Aires (MCBA). Because of the severe shortage of hospitals in the province of Buenos Aires, the city hospitals also take those patients who cannot be treated in the province. Provincial hospitals also lack the expertise that city hospitals have and therefore send referrals of special cases to the capital, as do hospitals from around the country and neighboring countries. Gutiérrez Children's Hospital receives 70 percent of its patients from outside the capital.

In the Hospital de Quemados (burns), almost none of the pediatric cases are covered by *obras sociales* or private insurance. Almost all of those cases are from very poor families, from *villas*. Adult injuries tend to be spread across classes, resulting from car accidents, attempted suicides, and homemade suntan potions, so Quemados has a more varied social spectrum than most public hospitals. About 50 percent of adult patients there have *obra* coverage. The hospital also provides nonburn plastic surgery for major reconstructions. The high-profit, high-turnover cosmetic surgery work is done in private clinics. The reconstructive work done at Quemados rarely is paid for by a health plan.

Public Subsidies to the Private and Social Security Sectors

The interrelationships among the three sectors are complicated, but all lead to the same thing: deterioration of the public sector. The technological advantage of the private hospitals, the declining infrastructure of the public facilities, plus sizable kickbacks to the union administrators of *obras sociales* have caused the *obras* to contract with the private hospitals for their services. So the private hospitals' investment in equipment is paid for with lucrative contracts from the *obras*. The *obras* send to the private hospitals all the high-turnover, high-profit cases, such as normal deliveries. To the public hospitals the *obras* send zero-profit cases, including the chronically or mentally ill and AIDS patients (interviews at Fernández Hospital, September 9, 1992). "[T]he free use of public hospitals by *obras* deprives the hospitals of a substantial part of their income, leading to further deterioration of publicly provided health care services" (World Bank 1988, 29).

The overvalued currency, which helped the private sector buy equipment, also contributed to the ruin of the economy, which sent many more patients to the public hospitals. The shrinking base in the formal sector led the *obras sociales* to cut benefits and institute copayments for the remaining members, further burdening public hospitals.

Forty percent of patients in public hospitals have *obras sociales* coverage but do not report it and are treated free. The *obras* collect the tax, pay it to the private system, but the private hospital does not treat the patients. The public system bears the cost of treating them. It is equivalent to a subsidy from the public sector to the private sector (World Bank 1988, 18). The proportion of patients who have coverage varies among the hospitals, depending on the type and the location of the facility. At Gutiérrez Children's Hospital (MCBA), 60 percent have no coverage or say they do not. At Diego Paroissien Hospital (La Matanza), only about 5 percent have their stay paid by an *obra social*. The other 95 percent have no coverage or say they do not, because they mistakenly fear they will have to lay out the money and wait to be paid back, which is no small matter in an inflation-prone country. They may know their coverage does not include the treatment they need (Dr. Alberto Schwarcz, August 21, 1992). Finally, there are the *obras* that collect money from their members but pay the public hospitals late (this was especially true during the hyperinflation and generalized high inflation of the 1980s). The 100 australes billed in August 1987 and worth $100 were worth only $1 when paid in December 1987. (The austral replaced the peso between 1985 and 1992.) In the country with the longest sustained high inflation in the world, paying late is an art form.

Another cost to the public sector is the training of medical students, residents, and nurses at public expense who leave immediately for the private sector or, better yet, for the United States. And who can blame them? Doctors cannot support themselves, let alone their families, on the $600 to $700 a month they receive for full-time work at the public hospital. Nurses train in the public hospitals, but leave for the private hospitals, where they earn twice as much, $400 instead of $200 a month.

The public hospitals also support the reputations and public relations of the private hospitals, as well as the fees charged to the *obras*, by providing the organs for the attention-getting transplant operations performed in the private sector.

Problems Facing the Public Sector

Finance. The problem facing the public sector that has been the subject of the most discussion is that of finance. Doctors and administrators face waves of new patients—those without coverage, those with too little coverage, accident victims, AIDS patients, lepers, mental patients—with ever shrinking budgets. In Argentina in 1978, 2.24 percent of the federal budget went to health; in 1984, only

1.09 percent of spending was on health. Chile spent 6.8 percent of its 1982 budget on health even under the military *junta* of Augusto Pinochet. Another country with a federal system, Brazil, spent 7.82 percent of the federal budget on health during the crisis years of the early 1980s (OPS 1988, 9, 10). Including provincial and municipal spending, the health sector's share of public spending in Argentina fell from 5.5 percent in 1978 to 1.8 percent in 1984. In real terms, federal health expenditures in 1984 were only one-fourth that of 1978 (World Bank 1987*a*, *iii*).

About 10 percent of public hospital costs are recovered from third-party payers. Hospitals have little incentive to identify *obra social* patients and recover payments; the costs of recovery fall on the hospital staff, but the funds go to the treasury. The plans for decentralization should help some hospitals because they will have the incentive to collect from those patients who have social insurance or private plans (World Bank 1988, 17). Decentralization also will be desirable in large provinces, which need to develop their health programs locally because the local community knows its own health problems (Romero 1987, 225). In the past, hospitals had little control over their expenditures: salaries, supplies, food, drugs, service procurement, and maintenance—all were decided centrally (World Bank 1988, 16).

Decentralization of the public system should improve efficiency because it lessens the opportunity for waste and corruption. Much of what Argentina spends on health is wasted in top-heavy administration. La Plata, for example, has a ministry of health thirty times the size of that of Madison, Wisconsin, although the population of La Plata is only three times that of Madison. The public sector also spends much more on medicines and supplies than needed (Dr. Raúl Mercer, August 31, 1993). (There is a similar problem in education, where 40 percent of the budget is spent on administration, not on teachers, schools, and supplies.)

The disadvantage of decentralization and the charging of fees is that some hospitals serve populations that have no coverage and cannot pay. Different public hospitals offer different levels of service and quality within the public system. In La Plata, there are two public hospitals, a few blocks apart. One (Rossi) accepts only patients with *obra* coverage. The profits made from those third-party paying patients are split among the doctors in the form of higher salaries. Any public patients who show up are sent to the other public hospital (Gutiérrez), five blocks away. That hospital is in terrible shape because it cannot charge its patients. It has no medicine, no equipment, and hardly any staff. Each hospital is meant to pay its own way, but those that receive no paying patients obviously cannot provide adequate care (Name withheld, 1993).

The public hospitals have managed to survive somewhat by private foundation funds and *cooperadores*. The latter arrangement allows corporations to contribute money to hospitals in lieu of paying taxes. Fernández Hospital, for example, receives many corporate contributions because it is located in affluent Barrio Norte.

Some doctors in the public sector believe that the intention of the inadequate funding and low pay is to close the public hospitals. They believe that keeping nurses' salaries so low is part of the plan to force them out of the public sector. But the plan for converting health care into a private enterprise does not address the 50 percent of the population that cannot afford private care. The public hospitals already cannot absorb all the demand. Cutbacks in public spending only aggravate the composition of the labor force, which has 20 percent unemployed, 11 percent underemployed (and probably in the informal sector), and another 20 percent in employment without health coverage.

Corruption. Of the pitiful amount of money budgeted to health, a significant proportion, perhaps most, never does any good for public health because it is stolen along the way. The stories of corruption in Argentina would fill a library. Following are a few cases that show how corruption interferes with health care delivery.

When Matilde Menéndez had to resign as Minister of Health and Social Action because it was learned that she did nothing about the starvation deaths of state mental patients that had been reported to her, $40 million was found missing from her budget. (See also Chapter 6. Menéndez also resigned in disgrace as director of PAMI, the national *obra social* for pensioners, because of a kickback scandal in which she was implicated.)

At every level, from national to municipal, funds disappear. The $50 million that the city of Buenos Aires owed the trash collection firm MANLIBA disappeared, so the firm stopped collecting trash and cut back its janitorial services at Muñiz Hospital for Infectious Diseases (the AIDS hospital), and at two other hospitals it used skeleton crews (*Buenos Aires Herald*, October 18, 1992, p. 4). The city claimed that normal cleaning services and staffing were in place, but admitted that trash was piling up in the patios of the city hospitals (*Buenos Aires Herald*, October 20, 1992, p. 11).

Diego Paroissien Hospital in La Matanza was built in 1984 and had always been run by a board of directors elected by the staff. In March of 1992, the province (Buenos Aires), leaving no stone unturned, imposed a new board, all friends of the provincial government. Immediately, systems of procuring materials that had worked for eight years were undermined by the new board. The board asked for kickbacks of 30 percent on infant respirators. Funds for running the hospital seemed to vanish. For two months, March and April, it was difficult for the staff to get any of the supplies they needed. Only after the staff sued the board in court did the funds start to flow (interview, name withheld, September 1992). The new directors are still unable to oversee a large hospital because they have no experience in health. They are just cronies of someone in the provincial government.

Lack of Norms and the Cult of Personality. The quality of care available in the medical sector, both public and private, is uneven, in the same jurisdiction and even more so between jurisdictions. Factors affecting the quality of care include the infrastructure, the level of funding, and personalism. There is no uniform code for equipping, funding, or managing the various entities within a jurisdiction. Consequently, the outcome in a given hospital depends very much on the status of a particular branch of medicine in the profession, on the political importance of an area, and, finally, on the individual personality of the person in charge.

Perhaps the most important factor in determining the quality of care in a public health facility is the personality of the unit chief, whether it be the ward in a large hospital, a health center in a *villa*, or the whole facility if it is a small hospital. In a society without a strong sense of the importance of rules, in a system without standards of care, in a system where corruption is rampant, personalism plays an important role. In fact, everyone expects that a strong person is needed for anything to be accomplished. The journal of epidemiology of the Ministry of Health has a photo of Ramón Carrillo on the front page of the few issues it has published. Doctors who were not even alive when Carrillo was Minister of Health still talk about his days with an "if only" intonation.

The role of the leader is crucial in a system in which morale is low, and it adversely affects the treatment of public patients. It is due in part to the racism that exists in Argentine society against those who are called *negros* or Indians. It is also a class bias, since the doctors of the urban middle class find little in common with their poor patients from the countryside. But even leaving aside the bias, doctors are paid so little for their work in the public health sector, $600 to $700 a month for full-time work, their first priority is feeding their own families. Unless they have an unusually well-developed sense of social responsibility for religious, political, or other reasons—and many of them do—they cannot be concerned about the people they treat. The difficulties of operating in ramshackle health centers or emergency rooms without funds, time, personnel, supplies, or medicine make the whole operation so unpleasant day after day that it is hard for the staff to be anything but ugly with the patients. It is here that the leadership of the department head and the spirit of the team make all the difference.

The unstructured nature of the system, especially in conditions as difficult as those that the doctors face in the public health centers and public hospitals, means that the provision of quality care depends on the person in charge of each unit. What is required is a person of extraordinary commitment and extraordinary capacity for both management and compassion, and that is the biggest failure of the public health care system. It should be structured in such a way that the services to be offered, the quality of care, the materials to be used, and the manner of acquiring them are so clear that people of ordinary talent and ordinary commitment are able to provide excellent care to the people who come to them for help.

Medical Education

The turmoil of the *Proceso*, the restoration of democracy, and twenty years of budget cutbacks have taken their toll on medical education and, consequently, on medical care in all sectors—private, social security, and public. The repression of intellectual life during the *Proceso* led to stagnation in many fields, including medical education. Since the 1970s, Argentine medicine has been less open to influence from abroad. Training in epidemiology and statistics is completely lacking. Teaching and research are narrowly specialized. The pedagogy, like that in all fields and levels of Argentine education, emphasizes passive learning and memorization and lacks opportunities for practice and research. The training discourages the development of an aptitude for scientific thinking, leading to methodological weakness, naive ideas, acritical impressions, "proof" by analogy in clinical as well as in "scientific" work (Neri 1982, 171–173). The *Proceso* also abandoned the fields of epidemiology and public health. Through the price system and the tariff structure, they promoted a highly technological emphasis in medicine, which led doctors to ignore the prehospital phases of disease. Residencies reinforced that bias (Mera 1988, 37).

The emphasis on memorization, the narrow specialization, the absence of epidemiological focus, and the lack of research survived the military regime. Into the scholarly void, an aggravating factor was introduced. The new civilian government reinstated open admissions at the universities, including the medical schools. (Medicine is an undergraduate course in Argentina.) Vast numbers of students chose to go into medicine because it seemed to offer a secure career in a very uncertain time (Dr. Eduardo Mele, August 26, 1991). Consequently, by the 1990s, the medical school of the University of Buenos Aires alone was accepting 8,000 students a year, and other schools around the country had similarly burgeoning enrollments. The Faculty of Medicine of the National University of La Plata is one of nine medical schools in Argentina. In 1988, seventeen percent of all students at La Plata studied medicine. Medicine was the largest of any academic unit, with more than 12,500 students (Pérez Arias and Feller 1990, 23).

The open admissions policy does not change the class composition of the student body. It does not mean that poor students can become doctors—the poor drop out in primary school or high school. The open-admissions policy enables less capable middle- and upper-class students to be admitted (Mera 1988, 36). The doctors who are being certified today are badly trained and cannot solve problems. The city of Buenos Aires in 1987 decided to carry out a study of graduates taking the residency exams, since there was no other method of quality control. Of the medical school graduates of the University of Buenos Aires in 1986, half took the residency exam. Of that half, 30 percent got more than 60 percent correct. So only 15 percent of medical school graduates demonstrated even a 60 percent competency (Etcheverry 1987, 184–187).

Basic science, clinical disciplines, laboratory practice, and public health training have all deteriorated (World Bank 1988, 18; interviews with numerous doctors in public and private institutions). "Doctors graduating from medical school are technically unprepared to serve in the present health care delivery system" (World Bank 1987*a*, 39). Classes increased tenfold with no more teachers or funds. By 1987, there were only 7 teachers for every 1,000 medical students (Etcheverry 1987, 190).[1] There are so many students that they do not see patients, they see pictures of patients. The students no longer go on rounds, and they read notes, not books (Dr. Lucía Saracco, August 21, 1992). Clinical supervisors in many hospitals complain that students read abstracts and summaries. They come out of school unable to read a scholarly article or judge its validity (Dr. Isabel Kurlat, August 26, 1993).

The dean of the medical school at the University of Buenos Aires says the whole education system suffers from "flight forward." For medical students, it is hoped that whatever is not taught in university will be covered in residency, but only 10 percent of graduates do residencies (Etcheverry 1987, 189). The other 90 percent graduate from medical school with a five-week practice, in obstetrics for example, and at graduation are licensed even to perform surgery (Canepa 1991, 18). With decentralization, the training of doctors will suffer because only Córdoba and Corrientes have residency programs (Mera 1990, 42).

When it seemed that medical education already was as bad as it could get, cutbacks in the University of Buenos Aires undermined the residencies in the medical school's teaching hospital (Clínicas). In 1993, the university, in an attempt to limit the expenses incurred from the hospital, decreed that the hospital could admit only one public patient for every paying patient. Since the patients in pediatrics had been almost all nonpaying, the new rule effectively emptied the ward, vitiating its teaching capability. Since fixed costs predominate, particularly in a teaching ward, and variable costs are minimal, the order made no economic sense.

Before the decree, the pediatric ward was bustling with activity.[2] Residents gained experience in a great variety of cases, including meningitis, pneumonia, leishmaniasis, eye trauma, serious fractures, ruptured appendicitis, and rare genetic disorders. They also learned a tremendous amount about the people served by the public sector, since whole families took advantage of a child's hospitalization to move in off the street or out of their hovels to the warmth and comfort of the ward. When the residents got lice from the babies they handled, they learned the importance of hygiene in and out of the hospital. By August 1993, however, doctors and residents far outnumbered the four child and adolescent patients, all of whom were in the terminal days of cancer. The variety and complexity of a fully functioning ward have been replaced by a hospice. The best graduates of the medical school are going through the motions of a residency that is empty of meaning. For the children out in Morón or La Matanza with meningitis or pneumonia, who now will not be admitted to Clínicas, the decree is a death sentence.

Continuing Lack of Education

The poor training in medical schools and the failure to inculcate a respect for knowledge leads to diagnostic errors, even among doctors who have acquired a certain amount of experience (Werthein 1991, 28). There is a dearth of reference libraries for doctors. Even where they do exist, few doctors look for information on unfamiliar conditions.[3] They let what they believe pass for what they know. Study is considered unproductive idleness and is not compensated (Agrest 1988, 100). The paucity of research means a generalized lack of data. Clinicians as well as health administrators have no information to inform their diagnoses and decisions. There are some specific studies, for example, of anemia in Buenos Aires or of measles in Misiones, but no one is conducting studies over time or of overall health.

Decline of Vital Statistics and Stagnation of Public Administration

The neglect of epidemiology, research, and medical surveillance and the cuts in budgets have had a serious impact on the compilation of vital statistics. Argentina had a reputation, at least in Latin America, for the quality of its birth and death records. On the presumption that the data continue to be good, it appears that the health situation in Argentina is reasonably successful. In fact, Argentina's vital statistics are in disarray, with both birth and death figures incomplete. In 1989, in one outbreak in Greater Buenos Aires, thirteen children died of whooping cough. Due to the attention given to the outbreak in the press, it was discovered that in the official records only one child was recorded as having died, because the other twelve had not been entered in the birth statistics. The children most likely to die are the poor, whose births are least likely to be recorded, so the gap in mortality data could be quite significant. In a recount in the Federal Capital, investigators found more than 100 cases of congenital syphilis that were not recorded. Data on maternal mortality and problems of pregnancy and the postpartum period consist of anecdotes and a few studies done in individual hospitals. Therefore, neither doctors nor administrators have any idea of the magnitude of problems (Werthein 1991, 28, 29). The degeneration of vital statistics not only masks the increase in the infant mortality rate that has occurred since the 1980s but also the estimated 30,000 deaths or more (of persons fifteen to thirty-five years old, for the most part) during the Dirty War of the 1970s and 1980s.

Public administration in health is backward, discredited, and bureaucratically routinized. Information is gotten from newspapers and political channels rather than from direct observation by people working in the field (OPS 1989, 101). In-adequate information is an obstacle to basic primary health care. The doctors do not even know how many lepers there are in the backyards of health centers. No agency oversees the quality of secondary facilities. If health units were inspected in Argentina, 60 to 70 percent of them, both public and private, would be closed for lack of equipment (Moreno 1992, 39).

Responses to health problems are rigid and stereotyped. In the absence of in-formation, from operational and epidemiological research, the health systems seem to bet that the health problems of the people will remain constant and can be dealt with by repetition of the same programs indefinitely (OPS 1989, 101). In many areas, the lack of information undermines curative care as well. The progress of transplant surgery is impeded by the lack of a computerized archive of donors, rapid communication such as fax or computer, transport, a network to unify provincial centers, and trained personnel (Pazos 1992, 41).

Neglect of ongoing study and lack of information on particular patients are the sources of much of the medical malpractice in Argentina. Out-of-date doctors are often the ones who fail. The corporatization of medicine in *obras* has weak-ened the doctor-patient relation, which can lead to mistakes. Because of inatten-tion to data and inadequate clinical histories doctors in large systems are treating patients without adequate information on their conditions (Spinelli 1992, 4). That is true for the country as a whole. Decisions about the future of medical care are made without adequate information on the health conditions in the country.

Medicine in Argentina in the 1990s is in disarray. The private sector has most of the facilities and receives most of the funds, but the quality of service is uneven. Profit drives decisions over choice of treatment, leading to avoidable iatrogenic injury. Most of the *obras sociales* are collapsing because of shrinking employment in the formal sector and corruption in the funds. The public sector faces increasing demands from a growing population of poor who lack health coverage. Since the *Proceso*, the public health sector has received a smaller and smaller share of the federal budget. Structural adjustment in the Menem admin-istration consists of slashing health and education spending while other areas continue to soak up government funds. Government cutbacks affect the poor most, but they also endanger the health of all Argentines. Medical education and epidemiology have deteriorated drastically over the past thirty years to the detri-ment of all health care.

Eight

Primary Health Care

The starting point for a health care delivery system is in primary health care. It is at the primary level that preventive care and education for healthy living can be carried out. It is also the entry point to the health care system, in which 90 percent or more of diseases or disorders can be resolved (Bergel 1989, 18). Finally, it serves as a referral station for those who need more complicated medical intervention, which is available in secondary care facilities (hospitals with in-patient care).

Health for All

The idea of a system of primary health care, with referral to secondary care, as a national program for developing countries became the banner of the World Health Organization conference in Alma-Ata (Kazakhstan) in 1978. In its simplest form, the program of *Health for All by the Year 2000* has been reduced to (1) breastfeeding; (2) oral rehydration therapy for diarrheal diseases; (3) prenatal checkups; and (4) vaccinations. The goals of Alma-Ata, in fact, require much more comprehensive national programs, including the extension of water and sewer systems to the whole population. The Water Decade of the 1980s was to have accomplished that goal, but many countries, including Argentina, have fallen short of complete coverage. (See Chapter 5.)

Health for All by the Year 2000 is a schematic way of describing medical coverage, health education, and, hopefully, changes in the environment that creates disease. Coverage means reaching all the needy population, not only for the spontaneous demand that arises from earaches and diarrhea but also the preventive elements of primary care. Among the services a primary health center should offer, if the *Health for All* program is to be effective, are prenatal checkups and referral for risk factors; vaccinations for all children and expectant mothers; Pap smears; breast cancer screening; TB tests, treatment, and follow-up; dental care; and well-baby care, which includes growth and development monitoring. The education component at the local level includes advice and help with breast-feeding for employed and at-home mothers; family planning classes; instruction in oral rehydration therapy; information about the dangers of smoking and alcohol and drug abuse; and community education about AIDS and seasonal health threats, such as meningitis. At the national and provincial levels too, there needs to be a program of public education on tobacco, alcohol, drugs, AIDS, cholera, Chagas' disease and other endemic and epidemic problems.

The proclamation of the goal of primary health care for all raised a storm of controversy among public health specialists around the world. Some of the issues were practical; others were political. The World Health Organization intended to replace verticalist programs in public health with primary health care. Verticalist programs focus on a particular health problem, such as malaria or Chagas' disease. They generally are organized nationally and tend to be executed in a top-down approach. The *Health for All* agenda criticized verticalist programs for not addressing broader health problems of the population. Public health workers, however, soon realized that abandoning verticalist programs exposed the population anew to endemic diseases. Many public health experts now support a compromise program that combines primary health care with focused verticalist programs to maintain protection from endemic problems.

The second controversy was more intractable because of the ideological issues it raised. The argument made against primary health care was that it is "primitive" health care, that the poor are offered only minimal care while the rich have access to all of modern medicine. Part of the problem here is one of path dependence. Critics of "primitive health care" generally agree that what they call the hegemonic model of big medicine is irrational. Modern medicine generally is curative, hospital based, and invasive. Even the rich have less than optimal preventive care. But because the affluent already have big medicine, the critics of primary health care seem to be arguing for the same irrational solution for the poor. The best program for all would stress prevention, with referral to secondary care as needed. On the other hand, critics probably are correct in their suspicions that some countries will not, in fact, offer an adequate range of educational, nutritional, and preventive medicine programs and access to high-quality secondary care to the poor.

The third controversy addresses the issue of whether medical personnel can have any meaningful, beneficial role when the fundamental threat to health is not microbes but poverty. It certainly is true, as this book attempts to demonstrate, that poverty and national indifference are the greater menace. Nevertheless, the argument that medical personnel can do nothing to help or, in fact, that by virtue of their profession they are part of the problem is defeatist. The public health field in Argentina has many ideologues who take that essentially fatalistic tack. It is ironic that those who think they are criticizing Argentina's systemic flaws reflect them so well. Those public health philosophers argue that until the revolution nothing can be done. Fate has determined that. Only the "big solution" offers any hope. Argentina lacks a history of reform or cooperative movements.[1] Consequently, the mentality of the *tirabombas* (bomb throwers) dominates social and political criticism. Reliance on the *caudillo* and the cult of the personality dominates their thinking. The era of Ramón Carrillo is remembered as the last days of promise for health care for the masses.

The argument, ultimately, is opportunist because it allows those doctors, educated at national expense, to sit around smoking, drinking coffee, and talking about the futility of primary health care. Meanwhile, in other health centers, less ideologically "enlightened" doctors and nurses work like ants in an ant hill providing primary health care, educating, vaccinating, preventing disease, and giving loving attention to the poor who come to them burdened with physical and emotional injuries. If that care is clumsy and paternalistic, as judged by the critics, the patients do not mind, because their children will live to see another birthday.

Even so, there is some truth to the "ultra-left" argument. Doctors are not farmers or sanitation engineers. Their job is to repair the damage done by the economic system. They are trying to face a tidal wave of health problems with inadequate personnel, supplies, and equipment. They can only meet the spontaneous demand. Their ability to actually prevent disease is hampered by inadequate health facilities and even more by the living conditions that foster disease. The answer for people trained in the curative arts, however, cannot be to refuse to serve in the hopes of heightening the contradictions. In fact, curing people and helping them stay healthy are in themselves potent political acts because healthy people are less fatalistic and more able to shape their own lives.

Primary Health Care in Argentina

Argentina does not have a system of primary health care. There are *some* public clinics in *some* neighborhoods providing primary health care against great odds and thanks only to the ingenuity and determination of their staffs. There is no national system; only the province of Neuquén has made a concerted effort over twenty-five years to provide primary care under public (provincial) auspices. This chapter evaluates the availability and the quality of primary health care in the public system, to the extent that it exists.

The focus of public health expansion in the Perón era (1945–1955) was on physical infrastructure, especially hospitals. Ramón Carrillo's aims for integrated health centers throughout the country were halted by the coup of 1955. In the

1960s, the quality of medical education and research was emphasized. The coup of 1976 nullified the emerging interest in epidemiology and public health and reinforced the already prevalent bias in favor of curative, hospital-based medicine (Dr. Pablo Muntaabski, June 26, 1992). (The efforts of the military *Proceso* to eliminate the public health sector were outlined in Chapter 7.) As several World Bank studies of the health sector in Argentina have pointed out, perhaps belatedly, "Heavy reliance on curative medicine and little concern for preventive care raise costs unnecessarily" (World Bank 1988, 15). The emphasis of the military years was on private health care and within that on highly technical fields. During the *Proceso*, a number of public health centers were built in Buenos Aires but were never staffed. Many clinics built by community groups were harassed by the military. Public health and community workers, including doctors, nurses, nuns, and priests, disappeared as the military attempted to stamp out all grassroots organizing.

The revival of the public health sector (if, indeed, there was any governmental will to revive it) was inhibited by the economic crisis of the 1980s. In the face of government neglect and paralysis, community organizations all over Argentina established *salitas* (little wards) to offer primary care.[2] Later, some of those *salitas* were incorporated into county systems. For example, the center in San Francisco began in a two-room house and is now part of the county system of Florencio Varela in Greater Buenos Aires. Others, such as those in La Matanza, after initially positive results in prenatal and well-baby care, closed for "political" reasons. Unproductive ideological battles within the health centers left the community without primary care.

The *salitas* that remain have the support of various government entities, municipal, county, or provincial. In the outlying areas, there are not enough doctors, in spite of the doctor "surplus" in the country. There is also a shortage of supplies, although there is no apparent shortage of administrative personnel. The satellite health center at Huaco (Mendoza) has thirteen administrators but only one doctor and no medicines or supplies (*Diario de Cuyo*, November 6, 1991, p. 6).

Primary health care encompasses a wide range of services. The problem for those who run local health centers is that there are no guidelines as to how to run a center, what services to offer, or how to make contact with the community. The extent and the quality of care depend entirely on the personality of the center director. As will be seen in the descriptions of some centers, that means very different care from center to center.

It is in primary health care that the lack of norms and oversight and the paramount importance of personalism take their greatest toll. Hospitals are more visible and involve large sums of money. They are part of power chains and career ladders, part of university structures, and are interconnected through referrals and the interchange of staff and residents. They vie for status within the municipality and nationally. Argentine hospitals once enjoyed international recognition, at least in Latin America. It is in the hospital that the tradition of medicine in the footsteps of the Nobelists resided. So, in spite of the lack of oversight, the lack of norms, and the current lack of funds, a certain homogeneity of practice might be expected in the hospitals.

The peripheral health centers, on the other hand, are isolated, without facilities, and without prestige. Extraordinary care can be delivered in a health post, but it goes unnoticed. In another, because the head is a visible political figure, the care is applauded, although it is of indifferent quality.

With the worsening crisis and the provincialization of hospitals, the differences among satellite centers have grown. In Formosa, due to the lack of fuel, doctors' rounds have been eliminated for many villages. In many provinces, there are no pens, paper, or forms for registering health statistics. Vaccination programs are irregular, due to the scarcity of vaccines and syringes. Salaries go unpaid (Fontán 1991, 34).

The infrastructure of the health centers also is uneven. Some large centers have many specialized rooms, even furnishings for dental care, X-rays, and labs. Others, such as the health center in the *villa* of Retiro, are small and without equipment. The centers are on their own in securing the necessary equipment. In one health center in Mendoza, the director proudly told me that they were already conducting fifteen pelvic exams a day in the gynecology room and that very soon they were going to buy an autoclave to sterilize the equipment.

Even under such difficult conditions, it would be a mistake to think that people are not helped by the attention offered in most centers. Peripheral health centers are like leper colonies. Doctors work there either out of great dedication or because they have no alternative. Motivation makes all the difference in the quality of care, since there is neither uniform equipment nor uniform practice.

Primary health care in Argentina has not been the subject of systematic inquiry. The only comparative discussions of the problems of primary care around the country are contained in the transcripts of an annual conference of public health workers that has been held in Buenos Aires since 1987 *(Jornadas de Atención Primaria de la Salud)*. To convey how the centers operate, what primary health care is available, and how it is offered, I describe several centers that I studied in depth.

Outpatient Clinic, Hospital Materno-infantil Gregorio La Ferrere

Gregorio La Ferrere is a neighborhood at the far edge of the Greater Buenos Aires *partido* of La Matanza. It is a very poor area in which the great majority of the population live in precarious housing and have unstable work, no medical coverage, and little education. The people are migrants from the provinces or from Bolivia and Paraguay.

The hospital at Gregorio La Ferrere offers maternity services and emergency care. It is supported by the Buenos Aires Province and receives medical residents from the pediatrics residency of the University of Buenos Aires (Hospital de Clínicas General San Martín), who spend a month seeing children in the outpatient clinic that operates five mornings a week.

The hospital wraps around a walled, unpaved parking area, with the emergency room on one side, the outpatient area on the other, and the maternity area behind the emergency room. There is also a little bungalow outside the hospital in which vaccinations are given two mornings a week. The mud from the parking lot gets tracked into both the outpatient area and the emergency waiting area. The smell from the hospital cesspool, which overflows frequently, dominates both areas. The waiting room in the outpatient area is not heated and is very cold in the winter. There is no bathroom for outpatients in obstetrics or pediatrics (there was one, but the toilet bowl was broken off at floor level some time ago). The doctors have a bathroom, which is kept locked.

The emergency room is open twenty-four hours a day. Patients who turn up at the emergency room for nonurgent care are not directed to the clinic (for example, for a health certificate for school). Patients who still are unattended after a long wait in the emergency room are not sent to the clinic, even if doctors are available there. One morning, a small child had been vomiting in the emergency room for three hours. By 10 A.M., nothing had been done, and she was having trouble breathing. At the time, there were doctors in the outpatient clinic who were not occupied (November 3, 1992).

There are three examining rooms in pediatrics, but only one is ever used. There are two examining tables, two chairs (for the doctors), a desk, a heater at each doctor's feet, and a radio that plays all the time. With two doctors, a helper, sometimes the residents' supervisor, two patients, and two parents, the room can be quite crowded. Patients are taken in order of arrival, regardless of age, gender, or condition. Consequently, a twelve-year-old boy and an eleven-year-old girl are questioned, undressed, and examined at the same time, with the father of the boy and the mother of the girl also there and the young people looking quite uncomfortable. All the while, two examining rooms sit empty (November 3, 1992). Another group of patients taken together were a girl of eleven years with scarlatina, a baby with sores and inflammation of the face, and an infant for a well-baby check (November 4, 1992). There was no need to expose a well infant to scarlatina or a skin infection.

The medical residents get a wealth of experience working at the clinic because of the variety of diseases and injuries. A typical patient roll included numerous cases of mumps (many with complications), parasites and helminths, a new case of Chagas' infection, meningitis, pneumonia, diarrhea, skin diseases, and a twelve-year-old whose sister brought her because she thought the younger girl was pregnant. At the clinic, the residents have some exposure to the most marginalized of the poor. The children are dirty, their clothes are dirty, they smell dirty, and very few seem robust or well cared for.

The clinic is staffed by a director, a staff doctor, and three residents on month-long rotation. The director, Dr. Nilda Chávez, helped the residents when they encountered unfamiliar conditions. The individual doctors at La Ferrere had very different responses to patients. The director was competent and compassionate. Some doctors, however, gave indifferent care to their patients. One doctor was quite sullen with the patients. He did not look at them, nor did he converse with them. Even when patients were lined up outside, sometimes he just sat idle. When he permitted them to enter, he was rude. The mothers tried to be considerate to waiting patients by hurrying out, taking their babies into the freezing waiting room undressed. The doctor would just sit there anyway and not call the next patient.

The medical residents tried to talk with the mothers and practice some health education, but they were not prepared to do so, nor was the situation conducive. There were no chairs in the room for the mothers. One resident asked the mother of a six-month-old with diarrhea why she had given up breastfeeding. She said she had no milk. He had neither the education in breastfeeding nor the will in the face of the alienating, impersonal situation to pursue the matter beyond chiding her.

Although the residents were supposed to work every morning, they would show up only three, sometimes four, days in a week. When the residents were there, the director did not attend to the patients, but she helped. When the residents did not show up, she saw the patients. If she could have counted on the residents to show up, her time could have been spent on health education, or she could have attended to the patients and sent the residents into the community.

Health Center Number 21, Villa de Retiro

The squatter community of Retiro had 8,000 residents in 1992, mostly in precarious housing without water or sanitary facilities. (Some of the area has since been bulldozed for a highway.) From the *villa*, affluent downtown Buenos Aires can be seen and heard, although the reverse is not the case. The health center in Retiro is a satellite of Fernández Hospital. Although Fernández is a public hospital, it is quite good, because it is situated in the fashionable neighborhood of Barrio Norte, which supports the hospital through *cooperadores*, or voluntary contributions. Because the Retiro clinic depends on Fernández, it can get hand-me-down furnishings and medicine, although it gets much of what it does not need and often not what it does need.

The center was rebuilt in 1990 from the remains of the one destroyed by the military. When Dr. Pablo Muntaabski took over as director in 1992, he conducted a survey of the health needs of the community and then proceeded to make up a plan for the center to meet those needs. When he presented the plan to his superior, he was told that no director of a *salita* had ever submitted such a plan.

Assessing the health needs of the community was made difficult by the chaotic state of data storage at the hospital. Fernández keeps three different clinical history files. A patient could be put into three different books on three different visits. A story I was told may be apocryphal: a woman who had twins brought one baby in for a checkup. Where was the other? With three clinical history files, the doctor did not even know that the child was a twin.

The center at Retiro is small and rickety. It is packed with supplies and jammed with people. Sometimes so many mothers and children are in the waiting room that it is impossible to squeeze by. Everyone is good natured in the crush. The cleaning women work all morning, but the mud keeps getting tracked in from the neighborhood. The toilet does not work and floods the bathroom and the lab, and the mess is tracked into the examination rooms.

There are rooms for reception, general medicine, pediatrics, and gynecology, a lab-kitchen-office, and a bathroom. The pediatrics room has two cots, for examining two patients at a time. The rooms are very plain, not attractive, but as clean as possible, and stacked high with supplies. Next door is a soup kitchen for children of the *villa*. In addition to the director, there are three pediatricians, two psychologists, two child development specialists, and two social workers. The clinic is open all day but has different hours for different specialties.

The winter of 1992 was a good time to visit the Retiro health center. I had already visited a center that was very well organized (Number 6, in Villa Soldati) and one that kept no records on the patients. From June to September 1992, Dr. Muntaabski was carrying out the plan he had devised for the *villa* by organizing a data system for all the patients. He wanted to have a file on each patient that included not only individual history but also family risk factors, such as the type of house and the condition and whereabouts of parents and siblings. A three-month-old baby had just died in the Autopista neighborhood of an upper respiratory infection. The baby was of good birth weight and her individual clinical history indicated no particular risk factors. If the survey had been completed, however, her history would have included the wretched condition of her house (one small room, with plastic sheets for the roof) and the fact that she was the fifth child of a twenty-six-year-old alcoholic mother who worked nights.

To complete the surveys, the clinic staff enlisted the aid of teams of nursing students from a private hospital. One week in July and another week in September, the teams came and canvassed the neighborhoods, conducting a census and vaccinating any children who were not up to date on their shots. In the four older, more settled neighborhoods, a vaccination center was set up at a central location. In Autopista, however, the teams went house to house. Different populations require different approaches.

Even though the health center in Barrio Güemes is less than half a mile away, some women in Autopista did not know it was there, had had no prenatal checks, and did not know they should. There were mothers with no vaccination cards for their children, although the cards are required by law. Our teams were well received, no one refused our interviews, and everyone was cordial. Some of the mothers clearly were dysfunctional. One eighteen-year-old mother of three had a year-old boy with an inch-wide dirty gash all the way down his shin. She could not keep straight the names of her two girls, complicating the question of what vaccinations each might require. It was also a challenge for the team to have a vaccination campaign when there was no water in the whole neighborhood. On the second day, the nurses came equipped with alcohol for hand washing.

The nursing students had worked for years with only on-the-job training and were now completing three years of coursework to become professional nurses. Part of the training was to go into the neighborhoods and see cases they would not encounter at a private hospital. The nursing students did not want to be there: they walked very slowly to their starting points, did what they could to avoid approaching the doors or the people, and did not split up to cover more territory or more people. Their reluctance to embrace the *villa* is understandable. Some of the plots reek of human feces in the yards, some of the people smell, some of the children are filthy and badly cared for. For the students, this life is strange but not distant enough. Because they are empirically trained nurses, that means they come from families not very much wealthier than these *villeros*. The specter of slipping to this way of life haunts the working class.

The team came with one box of vaccine. They vaccinated one pregnant woman and her child for tetanus, and then they were out of vaccine and went back to the center. Not exactly a campaign.

The second day, when we had gone to a few houses, we came upon a child who needed a measles shot. The nurses said they did not have any measles vaccine and would come back after the weekend. (In the middle of a measles epidemic—95,000 cases—and health-care workers went out on a vaccination campaign without measles vaccine.) Then we spent a great deal of time returning vaccination cards that had been taken the day before to be stamped at the center. So a group of twenty or so nurses and instructors wandered around doing a job one person could have done. The others could have set up a hygiene post, with information about breastfeeding, AIDS, and diabetes.

We met one very messy, very young woman who had a three-year-old and a twenty-month-old and who was nine months pregnant. She had had no prenatal care; she had gone to the center for a checkup, but it was the wrong day for obstetrics. The health center was a very good one that with more staff could have had obstetrical care every day, increasing the chances that the poor could enter the system. When the population is as marginalized as this, it takes a very energetic program to get them started doing something successfully in their lives. A system that responds only to spontaneous demand is not sufficient to care for dysfunctional, pregnant fifteen-year-olds.

A Health Center in Greater Buenos Aires

The neighborhood of this health center in Greater Buenos Aires includes a *villa brava* that has a young population of about 8,000 with a relatively higher proportion of drug addicts and delinquents than other *villas*. Doctors there estimate the infant mortality rate to be 108 per 1,000. The health center serving the *villa* and surrounding neighborhoods is located in an abandoned building. Windows are missing in most of the first floor and all of the upper floors, and the clinic often has no water. This center is open from 8 A.M. to 4 P.M., Monday to Friday. There are three doctors on the staff.

The health center gets some of the medicines it needs from the city, but not the equipment. There is no x-ray machine. Dentistry is offered for adults but not for children, which means only extractions are performed. AIDS is epidemic in this neighborhood, but the doctors have no protection, not even water. They do have sterilizing equipment for gynecological instruments.

The doctors in the center say it is not possible to do preventive care in this environment. They cannot prevent infection from developing in dirty houses or tuberculosis from spreading in houses that consist of one room for eight people. Doctors cannot do preventive care when the hallway is full of sick children. These doctors say that the World Health Organization guidelines for primary health care are appropriate only for populations with reasonable living conditions. They also say they cannot go into the community because they would be in danger.

Observers sympathetic with the center say the doctors there are depressed. "The center is in crisis. Its hospital does not support it. They are overwhelmed with spontaneous demand. They do not have time to go into the community." On the other hand, the head of the center says that to go out into the community is "*asistencialismo*," or social work. *Asistencialismo* is a key word for critics of primary health care, who say it is social work to go out and look for patients. The center's doctors risk their lives every day working in a building that does not even have water in a neighborhood where AIDS is epidemic but seem too demoralized or too ideological to make more of the opportunity.

When I asked an official of an international organization if he thought primary health care was impossible under such conditions, he replied that if doctors can practice primary health care in Africa, they can certainly do it in Buenos Aires. He said that the doctors at the center just do not bother to go out and look for patients. They also keep no files on patients. They write a new record every time a patient comes in. He also said that it is not the case that the doctors would be in danger if they went into the community, even though it is a *villa brava*—the gangs would punish anyone who hurt a doctor. (It should be noted that these criticisms were made from a comfortable office downtown.)

It is not clear if the doctors at this center have the resources they need to practice primary health care under such difficult conditions. It is clear, however, that the doctors are ideologically opposed to aggressive primary health care and lack the organizational motivation to produce a plan for the neighborhood and collect and store the data for a primary care approach. Center Number 6 provides a stark contrast.

Health Center Number 6, Villa Soldati and Villa Fátima

Health Center Number 6, directed by Dr. Norma Aprigliano de Schnitler, serves three quite different neighborhoods: a high-rise zone of apartments, a new public-housing project with many severely marginalized people, and a *villa* of hardworking Paraguayans and Bolivians. In the two and a half years the center had been open as of September 1991, they had attended to almost 19,000 people. The center never charges a fee, Dr. Aprigliano explains, because she cannot spare staff to do accounting.

Patients get a number as they enter, and no one is turned away. This method greatly reduces the inconvenience and tension for patients. In many other centers, patients must keep their place in line beginning at four in the morning. They may wait all morning and still not be seen by a doctor.

Dr. Aprigliano has arranged that every baby born in the area hospital (Piñero) is reported to the center, so the staff can make follow-up visits to the home and ensure that the child's vaccination schedule is carried out. Every person in the community has a file with all pertinent data on family health, special risk factors, and vaccination record. Because every household has a file, Dr. Aprigliano can use teams of medical students and medical residents effectively in house-to-house follow-up. The center printed flyers to tell the neighborhood what services are available and clearly indicate the hours for each specialty. Neighborhood women with little education have been trained to be public health educators to their neighbors. When Dr. Aprigliano and I met the women on their rounds, their broad smiles revealed not only the absence of almost all their teeth but also their enormous pride in the work they were doing.

Dr. Aprigliano's base hospital sends her everything she needs. She has medicine from the hospital and from samples that she hoards. At the center, they administer the more common antibiotics and anti-inflammatories that generally are available. All the medicines dispensed at this center are free. The center has stark, bare walls but is clean. There is no dust or dirt. There are sheets (albeit dirty ones) on every bed. Chairs and a very plain table are in every room, to facilitate doctor-patient discussion. For example, when I visited, a gynecologist was sitting with a patient explaining postpartum contraception.

As we went on the rounds of the center and the neighborhoods, Dr. Aprigliano kissed and hugged the patients and community workers. She does not distinguish between social work and clinical work. After the lootings (during the hyperinflation) in 1989, she went into the neighborhoods and asked people why they were looting. They said they were hungry, so she encouraged them to build a soup kitchen. It started under a tree with food begged from the local stores. Now the kitchen also houses a day care center and rooms for adult education. When I visited, the room was being used for a class on responsible fertility. The gynecologist comes to the people because the center is a long distance away.

County of Florencio Varela, Greater Buenos Aires

Florencio Varela is the poorest county in the Greater Buenos Aires region. It stretches from an urban zone to a rural area where the poor live by sharecropping. Florencio Varela has made public health a priority and has thirty local health centers, which are open mornings and afternoons. There is also a new hospital, which was completed in 1993.

The health centers and the hospital deal with a wide array of medical problems: violence, bus accidents, tuberculosis, acute respiratory infections, diarrhea. Because there is a network of primary care, with referral to the hospital, the doctors find that adult patients arrive at the hospital not already in the terminal stages of disease (Dr. Raúl Mercer, August 31, 1993), as they do at Diego Paroissien Hospital in La Matanza (Dr. Lucía Saracco, August 21, 1992), where there are no *salitas*. Diarrhea is a serious problem year-round in Florencio Varela; all the groundwater is contaminated, and only 30,000 of the 250,000 residents have piped water. Parasites are also a common problem. In winter, respiratory infections are the most common threat. Among adults, hypertension, alcoholism, and abortions are serious health problems. In Villa Mónica, the center started an HIV self-help group, and in the first two months, the group had fifty members.

The county is divided into four health regions, each with a main health center. The goal is to have a twenty-four-hour emergency room at all four regional centers. The first all-night emergency room was set up at the health center at Barrio Pepsi (near the Pepsi plant) because it is a *barrio bravo*, with many drug addicts and social problems.

The regional health center at Villa Mónica attends to 18,000 people in its vicinity and supervises nine satellite centers. The day I was there, there were almost no medical staff because it was payday. To get paid, each person on the staff has to travel to Quilmes, which takes all morning, so on payday, there is no medical attention. The satellite centers are small. The center in San Francisco, which consists of two small rooms, attends to a community of 10,000 people. It is flooded with patients because of high unemployment.

Large centers and small have no disposable supplies. Gloves are washed in bleach and hung to dry and reuse. They do have sterilizing equipment. In the winter of 1993, center directors reported that they were not receiving the medicine they needed nor the equipment. The municipality of Florencio Varela was still paying its share to the centers, but the province of Buenos Aires was not. The new hospital is draining funds, it appears, from the centers, because it was a huge expense and is expensive to run. The old hospital was run down, and the new one obviously was needed, but it is diverting funds from primary to secondary care.

The hospital and the centers are limited in how much of the community they can canvass, even in their immediate vicinity. Adolescent girls still arrive to give birth totally unprepared, without having had any prenatal checks. When I visited Florencia Varela Hospital, the neonatal ward was caring for a baby whose twenty-year-old mother had died. The woman was attended in the birth by her mother, who considered herself a midwife. She did not realize that her daughter was carrying an undelivered twin. Two hours after the birth of the first child, the young woman died of hemmorhage and the second baby died with her. They lived two blocks from the hospital (*Mi Pueblo* Hospital, neonatal intensive care unit, August 31, 1993).

The Basic Elements of Primary Care

Many problems remain. Among the services that should be available in a primary health care program are prenatal checkups, well-baby visits, vaccinations, oral-health care, surveillance and treatment of infectious diseases, education, and data collection for epidemiological studies.

Prenatal Care

One of the most cost-effective programs the public sector could offer is adequate prenatal care. When Diego Paroissien Hospital in La Matanza opened in 1984, Dr. Alberto Schwarcz conducted a study of neonatal mortality in the area. That in itself was unusual. Up to that time, only the Sardá Maternity Hospital had maintained records of neonatal mortality. For the area of La Matanza served by Paroissien, the neonatal mortality rate was 24 per 1,000 live births. The doctors found no correlation with the mothers' education, parity (number of pregnancies), age, or type of delivery. What they did find was that mothers who delivered with no prenatal care at all had a neonatal mortality rate of 60 per 1,000 (Schwarcz 1987, 545).

At Paroissien, Schwarcz and his colleagues conducted some of the only studies in Argentina of the causes of neonatal death. They found that most were the result of prematurity due to infection. Mothers get an ordinary vaginal infection, but because they do not go for prenatal care, it remains untreated. The infection spreads to the uterus, causing premature birth by rupture or sepsis (Dr. Pedro de Sarasqueta, September 25, 1991).

Because the cause of death so often is in the untreated pathology of the mother, the staff at Paroissien has been unable to bring down the rate of perinatal deaths. Initiation of a neonatal intensive care unit at the hospital has reduced neonatal deaths there to about 15 per 1,000. Stillbirths, however, continued unabated and outnumber neonatal deaths because the doctors cannot intervene to influence the conditions that cause them (de Sarasqueta 1988, 52). Among women with no prenatal care at Paroissien, the neonatal death rate is still 40 per 1,000.

Drs. Schwarcz and de Sarasqueta also investigated why mothers do not go for prenatal care. They expected to find that the women did not know that they should go. On the contrary, they found that women knew that prenatal care was important but that their experiences in the medical system were so negative— counterproductive, in fact—that they did not go for prenatal visits in subsequent pregnancies (Schwarcz 1988, 500). Women had to line up at four in the morning to be seen by an obstetrician and then had to come back another day for a sonogram and yet another day for lab work (Schwarcz 1989, 34). Other studies confirmed those findings. For example, the wait for attention in the outpatient clinic at Ramos Mejía Hospital in Buenos Aires generally is two hours. To see the gynecologist, however, a woman must take a number to receive a date for an appointment thirty to forty-five days hence (Viladrich 1990, 25).

The doctors have found that when adequate prenatal care is accessible, the women not only take advantage of it they bring in every mother in the neighborhood (Schwarcz 1987, 554). It might be argued that the perfect mother would come back for prenatal care regardless of the inconvenience and insulting treatment by medical staff. However, no country can afford to provide care only for "perfect" people. The next generation of workers is being born under conditions that impair their performance for their whole lives.

Another irrationality of the lack of prenatal care that causes enormous expense and has tragic outcome is the failure of the system to screen for Rh incompatabilty. This factor can be dealt with successfully by immunizing a mother after either an abortion or the birth of an Rh positive baby. Because Rh incompatibility is not adequately prevented in Argentina, the mother has to be rushed off to Fernández Hospital for a risky (and expensive) high-tech birth (Dr. Isabel Kurlat, August 26, 1993). Other causes of infant mortality are discussed in Chapter 10.

Well-Baby Care and Vaccinations

Regular monitoring of infant and child health and development can avoid costly and tragic results. (Chapter 11 considers this topic in detail.) What also is important in the well-baby visits is the opportunity for educating and supporting mothers for healthier children.

_____ Table 8.1 _____

Immunization Coverage in Argentina

Vaccine	Percentage of Infant Population Covered
Poliomyelitis	91.0
Diphtheria/pertussis/tetanus	62.0
Tuberculosis	61.0
Measles	60.0

Source: World Bank 1987*a*, 10.

Vaccination coverage is an important element of primary health care. Healthy, well-nourished children are likely to weather childhood diseases without dangerous complications, while malnourished children are at much greater risk. High levels of vaccination coverage reduce the rate of transmission and lengthen the cycle of epidemic recurrence, thereby protecting even the unvaccinated in a vulnerable population.

Although it would cost only four million dollars to vaccinate all Argentine children for seven immunopreventable diseases (polio, diphtheria, pertussis, tetanus, measles, rubella, and tuberculosis), the level of vaccination coverage in Argentina is poor (Marcelino Fontán, December 10, 1991). Reports published by the Pan American Health Organization reproduce the Argentine government's rosy but inaccurate picture of vaccination coverage (PAHO 1990*a*, 81). A confidential World Bank country study, however, indicates serious deficiencies. The percentage of infants fully immunized before one year of age is given in Table 8.1.

The percentages listed in Table 8.1 are based on the number of doses of vaccine. "Taking into account losses and deterioration of vaccines, real immunization rates, as shown by field surveys, are sometimes unacceptably low (a 40 percent coverage for measles in one province) or not completed until the child's second or third year, as evidenced by the 1984 epidemic of measles" (World Bank 1987*a*, 10).[3]

The neglect of vaccination for measles is just one scandal in Argentine public health. Measles was uncontrolled in Argentina, with epidemic peaks every two years, until 1971, when regular vaccination began. For four years, incidence was low, but in 1976 and 1977 it increased again, since there had been no mass vaccination in 1975. From 1978 to 1983, incidence again decreased. A serious outbreak in 1984, with a rate of 112 per 100,000, coincided with low vaccination coverage, the average for the country being 75.4 percent (Manterola et al. 1987, 45).

Epidemiological studies amply showed the relation between failure to immunize and outbreaks, as well as the high mortality rate for the malnourished.

Measles could be eradicated, just as smallpox has been. Its epidemiological characteristics are similar: it is easily recognizable clinically; it has no carriers besides humans; the vaccine is effective in only ten days; and the period of incubation and transmission is compatible with the timing of the vaccine. Since only the poor die of measles, the political will to eradicate it has failed to materialize. In 1990, Argentina was the only country in the world not to buy vaccines, according to a UNICEF official. The government applied the emergency law banning government purchases to vaccines. UNICEF intervened with President Menem and finally he relented, but it was too late. The cycle of measles outbreaks depends on vaccination coverage. With 80-percent coverage, an outbreak comes around every five years or so. After the serious epidemic in 1984, an outbreak was expected in 1990. When it did not materialize, Argentina played roulette with measles and did not buy any vaccines. In 1991, there were 95,000 measles cases, avoidable with an expenditure equal to about 0.002 percent of GDP that year.

Another shameful story is that of neonatal tetanus. The neonatal tetanus vaccine is 99.9 to 100 percent effective, but in Argentina it is not universally used. In fact, Argentina is the only country in southern South America that does not have complete vaccination for neonatal tetanus (Werthein 1991, 28). This is not a country with a high percentage of home births, nor do they put cow dung on the umbilical. Nevertheless, infants still are being lost to tetanus. Tetanus is also a problem for adults. In 1996, there was a rash of tetanus deaths at a Buenos Aires cosmetic surgery clinic. (*Buenos Aires Herald*, June 9, 1996, p. 4).

There are ways of achieving satisfactory levels of vaccination coverage, when a means is sought. The maternity hospital at Del Viso, Greater Buenos Aires, has managed to achieve a high rate of vaccination by working through the schools. The hospital educates the teachers, and the teachers educate the children and send notes home in the copybooks, and the kids get the parents out for the campaigns. A notice from the clinic to the parents, on the other hand, has little effect (Jorge Sparvoli, September 3, 1992).

Oral Health

Oral health in much, but not all, of the Third World is abysmal. In most of the health centers I visited, if there was dental attention at all, it was for what was called "adult dentistry." That meant no prophylaxis, only extractions. One exception was the outpatient clinic at Gregorio La Ferrere Hospital, where the dentist proudly noted that they performed preventive as well as extractive dentistry. She explained, however, that the Argentines in the neighborhood came in only for extractions. They do not want to be bothered with dental care. The Bolivians from the same *villas* did come for preventive care. She attributed it to different upbringings (Hospital Gregorio La Ferrere, November 3, 1992). A very low percentage of the population, especially the poor, have been to the dentist. Whereas from 69 percent (Neuquén) to 89 percent (Santiago del Estero) had, at some point, been to a doctor, only 0.5 percent (Santiago) to 8.4 percent (Neuquén) had been to a dentist. In Greater Buenos Aires, 2.7 percent of poor people reported having been to a dentist. Perhaps more astounding is the range among nonpoor in the five cities surveyed. Four percent of the nonpoor in Santiago del Estero reported having been to a dentist, 5.4 percent of the nonpoor in Greater Buenos Aires, and, at the high end of the range, 12.8 percent in Posadas (INDEC 1990, 200). Only 35 percent of all eighteen-year-olds in Argentina have all their teeth. By age fifty, one-fifth of the population lose *all* their upper teeth (PAHO 1990*b*, 16).

Surveillance and Treatment

Argentina has serious problems with diseases that could be eradicated or reduced to very low levels. An effective primary care system would maintain surveillance of these infectious diseases, treating those infected and exposed and consequently eliminating the source of spread. Argentina's performance in leprosy control is particularly derelict, all the more because it is not a highly contagious disease and effective treatment exists. Humans are the only carriers of leprosy, and, with effective therapy, control of the disease is possible (*BEN* 1990*a*, 60–64). Reported coverage with multidrug treatment for leprosy in countries of the Americas illustrates the low priority given to this disease of poverty in certain countries: the Dominican Republic reportedly treats 100 percent of lepers; Ecuador, 90 percent; English-speaking Caribbean countries, 80 percent; Paraguay, 46 percent; Argentina and Venezuela, 30 percent; and Brazil, 4 percent (*Boletín de la Oficina Sanitaria Panamericana* 110(2) 1991, p. 166). Treatment of lepers in the early phases of disease not only would be humane, it also would save the $13 million Argentina spends annually for the Sommer Hospital for lepers (Lauro 1992, 24).[4]

Tuberculosis is another disease for which surveillance and a dedication to treatment is particularly important. Since 1986, with the neglect of case searching and the deterioration of notification procedures, there has been an increase in infant tubercular meningitis. Argentina has higher rates of tubercular meningitis than Cuba, Uruguay, and Venezuela, among others, because of underreporting of adult TB and late application of BCG vaccine to infants. Tubercular meningitis is fatal without treatment, and the survival rate with late diagnosis or treatment is only about one out of three. More than half of survivors have serious neurological consequences. Vaccinating an infant for TB costs 68 cents. Treatment for an adult with TB costs $157. Treatment for an infant who is infected, which in about three-fourths of cases is by a family member, is $1,900 (Miceli 1990, 31–33).

Another health problem that requires surveillance of the population is women's health. The correlation of cervical cancer rates with income, housing, education level, and job status is well established (Poletto and Morini 1990, 201–205). Gynecological exams and Pap smears are a cost-effective way of avoiding enormous expense and suffering and are procedures that can be done even by briefly trained community workers. When this was practiced in La Matanza, provincial health authorities protested that doctors could do the test better. The response from the community was *era eso o nada*, it was that or nothing, since doctors were not available (Schwarcz 1989, 33).

Education: A Two-Way Street

The primary health care system should provide health education. That means medical personnel teaching the people, but it also means the medical community learning from the health profiles seen in the health centers. The centers, through their surveillance and regular record keeping, should be providing epidemiological data to central offices. The response of the medical community has been severely hampered by the lack of data. In 1992, doctors in Mendoza's best hospitals were unaware that AIDS had already made grave inroads in the local population. (See Chapter 6.)

Reporting on infectious diseases is essential. Meningitis outbreaks, for example, are an annual occurance in Argentina. Unfortunately, if the government is indifferent to the health threat, reporting is futile. In the 1993 outbreak, amid 2,000 cases and 170 deaths, the federal government still dismissed a request by a senator for information on the disease, responding that "the meningitis outbreak was not important and measures to provide information would be taken if it spread" (*Buenos Aires Herald*, September 27, 1993, p. 7).

The other side of the education trade is in bringing useful information to the people. Women, particularly those who work outside the home, need information on how to maintain successful breastfeeding. That means the doctors need to be educated and need to encourage women who have had happy experiences with breastfeeding to participate in classes for new mothers.

The two-way exchange of information also needs to be carried out in the case of parasitic diseases. The neglect of public health has allowed the threat of yellow fever and malaria to return to Argentina's northern provinces. The health centers should be monitoring the vectors' progress and also advising people on how to avoid infection, that is, the clothes to wear and the times of day to be careful. Because yellow fever and dengue had been eliminated in Argentina, very few people have antibodies to these diseases, which are now returning (Alonso et al. 1987, 551).

Nutrition information also is needed. When there were health centers in La Matanza, diet classes were available for diabetics. Now they are offered only at the Diego Paroissien Hospital. The nutrition staff of the hospital is completely inadequate for taking the classes out to the people in their neighborhoods (Laura López, August 21, 1992).

Crisis, Adjustment, and Primary Care

The collapse of the Argentine economy that began in the 1970s and the austerity measures of the Menem government have had a dramatic effect on health in Argentina. Doctors report that patients come to the hospitals in much worse shape than before. Once, doctors only read about kwashiorkor, now they are seeing it. Doctors used to say that cavitary tuberculosis did not exist in children, but now they see it. People cannot get to the hospital because they do not have the bus fare, nor can they do what the doctor prescribes because they cannot afford the treatment. Middle-class patients can no longer go to private doctors and are moving into the public sector. That is creating a bottleneck, and the charging of fees is expeling the very poor from the system altogether (Spinelli 1991, 30).

The commitment to primary care, in this situation of extreme need, is lacking in the Ministry of Health. According to key informants, the situation worries the international organizations of technical cooperation, such as the Pan American Health Organization and the World Health Organization. In spite of international agreements, to which Argentina is a party, for the strengthening of primary care and local health systems as strategies to improve coverage and equity in health care, the political orientation of the government since the early 1990s is toward reform of the health sector, by which it means the consolidation of the market in health care. In this effort, the government neither needs nor solicits international cooperation for the development of primary care. The government states that Argentina is an economically developed country and does not have problems of health care coverage, nor does it need international help. A key concern of the international organizations is that in Argentina very few doctors work as generalists in primary health care. The emphasis on specialization, which is promoted in medical school, does not lend itself to satisfying the health needs of the population (interviews, names withheld, 1993).

Because of the lack of primary care in Argentina, if you ask people what they want in their neighborhoods, they say they want a twenty-four-hour emergency room. They do not want primary health care or health promotion. "They want a 24 hour emergency room because the people feel unattended, unprotected and because they don't have anywhere to go because coherent, round-the-clock care does not exist" (Schwarcz 1988, 501–502).

This chapter has described some of the few centers available for primary health care for the poor. La Matanza, in the suburbs of Buenos Aires, is fairly typical. It has 1.2 million people. Not all of them are poor, but most of them are. There are no *salitas* there. Mothers and children can go to the hospital at Gregorio La Ferrere, if they do not mind the cold and the smell. Mothers and children can also go to the hospital at San Justo and line up for hours from the early morning trying to keep their place, menaced by barking stray dogs in the hallways of the hospital. At neither place can they use a bathroom. Adults can go to the Diego Paroissien Hospital, if they are already in the terminal phase of a disease and do not mind if their house is stolen while they are gone.

This system throws at the public hospitals premature and low-birth-weight infants from mothers who have had no contact with the system before the birth. They come already in transition, already with fetal distress, with ruptured membranes or undiagnosed *placenta previa*, septic, or in the expulsive phase. The babies are born oxygen deprived and brain damaged and fight for life in neonatal intensive care units, if they get there. The children who survive the lack of prenatal attention and inadequate birth environment are not inoculated and return to the hospitals suffering from the combined effects of malnutrition and immunopreventable diseases or from diseases of bad water and bad food.

The system also delivers adults in terminal stages of tuberculosis, cancer, emphysema, and diabetes. The victims of bus accidents, work accidents, and occupational exposure to toxins; infants with acute respiratory infections from living in plastic-bag shacks; cardiac patients with Chagas' disease; lepers; AIDS patients; burn victims; and the mentally ill—they all end up in the public hospitals, to which we turn our attention in the next chapter.

Nine

Public Hospitals

Argentina's medical system depends, for the most part, on curative, hospital-based care. In the 1950s and 1960s, the public sector provided that care reasonably well. The agenda of successive governments, from the Liberating Revolution of 1955 to the *Proceso* of 1976 to 1983, was to dismantle public medical care, distribute facilities to the provinces, and foster private medical care as a part of the wage package in the *obras sociales*. In the 1970s by design and in the 1980s by design and default, the public hospital was progressively weakened as a provider of medical care. The weaknesses of the public hospitals stem from budget insufficiency but also from the failure to institute norms of procedure that would safeguard medical practice even in times of crisis.[1]

Staffing

In spite of the large number of doctors in Argentina, one of the main problems in the public hospitals is a lack of trained personnel, arising from both demand and supply factors. Higher salaries in the private sector have caused doctors, nurses, and support staff to leave the public hospitals. Most of those who stay do not supply the hours for which they have contracted.

On the demand side, in spite of critical shortages of personnel, hospitals are not hiring. Since 1989, shrinking budgets and self-financing have led hospitals to ban new hiring, even for replacements (Dr. Alberto Schwarcz, August 21, 1992). Dilapidated physical plant, inadequate equipment, lack of norms and oversight, and low morale reduce productivity and exacerbate the staffing shortage.

Doctors and Residents

Until the 1970s, doctors accepted the low salaries because of the prestige attached to medical research and teaching in the public sector. They could work mornings in the hospital and have a more lucrative second job in the afternoon. A number of factors have combined to diminish the appeal of the public hospital, including inflation, which widened the salary gap with the private sector, and the technological backwardness and changing clientele of the public sector. As the middle and upper classes moved to the private sector, the public hospital became the caretaker for the poor only, lessening its prestige.

The monthly salary for fully trained physicians (postresidency) in the public hospitals is $600 to $700, but the cost of living in Argentina is now more than in the United States. Most doctors who have full-time positions in the hospital, in fact, work two or three jobs. They put in only four hours at the hospital, and work afternoons and evenings in the private sector or for an *obra social*. They also work twenty-four-hour shifts in the emergency rooms or intensive-care wards of private hospitals as often as once a week.

The economic crisis of the 1980s and 1990s virtually emptied hospitals of doctors. The low salaries spawned a tolerance for absenteeism and idleness (Kreplak 1991, 32). The principle has become that little is paid and little is expected (Dr. Pedro de Sarasqueta, September 25, 1991). Given the low morale and waning credibility of the public hospitals, the new Garrahan National Children's Hospital attempted to recruit staff with exclusive dedication to the hospital. Even at $2,000 a month, the salaries are inadequate and doctors have to work another job.

Consequently, the hospitals are left without trained personnel for much of the day, all night, and the weekend. When I visited Mendoza's Lagomaggiore General Hospital, we found, much to the chagrin of my host, that all the doctors had left the neonatology ward, although it was not yet noon (October 31, 1991). Until the next day, the nurses, who had no formal training, would be in charge.

In Hospital de Clínicas General San Martín (University of Buenos Aires), the job of the professors is to make the morning rounds, checking on each patient and consulting with medical residents. The attention they give is excellent, but at 11:00 or 11:30, their job is done. Only residents and nurses are left to attend to patients for the next twenty-one hours.

After four in the afternoon, the two pediatric wings, accomodating forty children, are staffed by one third-year resident, two first- or second-year residents, and sometimes nurses. The residents in Clínicas and the other public hospitals are the best in their class. But they come through a medical school with open admissions, large classes, virtually no clinical training, and even inadequate basic science. The first-year residents are particularly ill prepared to attend to patients on their own. An infant death in neonatology at Clínicas during the time I was there would not have occurred had a trained person been available. During the entire weekend when the infant died, like all other weekends, only residents were on duty (Dr. Isabel Kurlat, August 26, 1993).

The crisis of trained personnel is not confined to the public hospitals. The higher death rate at night and on weekends is, if anything, worse in the private hospitals, where less qualified residents work. Higher mortality also follows the change of tour for residents, because the new class coming in really has no preparation (Katz and Maceira 1990, 186).

The shortage of doctors in the public hospitals has other repercussions on the quality and even availability of medical care. There is a significantly higher prevalence of intrahospital infection in the pediatric wards of public hospitals in Buenos Aires that have a high patient-doctor ratio (Manterola et al. 1989, 22). In provinces with more severe doctor shortages, there is no one to replace a doctor who calls in sick. In the hospital in Sáenz Peña, in Chaco Province, an entire outpatient specialty has to be shut down if the doctor in charge does not report (*Norte*, April 15, 1992, p. 14).

Nurses

"Nursing is the most critical area in health manpower in Argentina, not only because of the shortage, but also because the growth of this professional category appears to have stagnated" (PAHO 1990*b*, 22–23). There were fewer nurses in 1988 than there were in 1979.

There are about 65,000 nurses (of all classes) in Argentina, or about one nurse for every doctor. In developed countries, the ratio is three or four nurses for each doctor. Clearly, medicine is practiced very differently in Argentina than in the United States and other industrialized countries (Katz and Muñoz 1988, 110).

Distribution of Nurses by Training. There are four categories of nurses in Argentina: university trained, professional, auxiliary, and *empírico*. University-trained nurses, comparable to registered nurses, number fewer than 400 in the entire country (PAHO 1990*b*, 23). They generally do not work directly with patients but are directors of nursing at the private hospitals.

Professional nurses are similar to licensed practical nurses, having completed secondary school and a course of study of one or two years. There are about 16,000 professional nurses in Argentina, about one-fourth of the total, and 300 graduates a year (PAHO 1990*b*, 23). In 1984, there were 4.7 nurses (with post–secondary school training) per 10,000 population, the lowest ratio in twenty-five years. In the United States in the same year, there were 83 registered nurses and 54.2 licensed practical nurses per 10,000 population (OPS 1988, 62, 96).

The remaining 50,000 nurses, in roughly equal numbers of auxiliaries and *empíricos*, have no comparable categories in the United States. The auxiliaries complete primary school (through seventh grade) and a nine- to twelve-month course of study in a hospital. About 1,000 auxiliaries graduate each year; currently about 22,000 to 25,000 are working (PAHO 1990*b*, 23). In 1984, Argentina had 5.6 auxiliary (post–primary school trained) nurses for every 10,000 inhabitants, whereas Chile had 23.8 and Paraguay 8.5 per 10,000 population (OPS 1988, 80).

The 25,000 nurses working in public and private hospitals as *empíricos*, or empirically trained nurses, generally have not completed the seven years of primary school. They were hired as cleaning personnel and learned nursing on the job (OPS 1989, 129). The *empíricos* constitute 39 percent of the nursing staff nationwide, but in many public hospitals they account for as much as 80 percent (PAHO 1990*b*, 22–23).

Empíricos and auxiliaries together are about three-fourths of the nursing work force, and it is they who have direct contact with the patients. In many public hospitals, they also are the nursing directors, due to the dearth of professional nurses (OPS 1989, 121–122). It is illegal to employ empirically trained nurses at all, much less in supervisory positions, but necessity compels public and private hospitals to break the law. At night, on weekends, and on holidays, it is the nurses without formal training or with the least training who are in charge (Wainerman and Geldstein 1990, 14, 22–23).

The development of professional nurses is thwarted by the lack of ongoing training opportunities as well as the lack of distinction in functions and remuneration between categories of nurses. The pay difference between professional and auxiliary nurses is only about 20 percent (Wainerman and Geldstein 1990, 33). "Little social prestige, low wages, and the training level associated with nursing make hiring very difficult and prevent raising hiring requirements" (PAHO 1990*b*, 23).

Nurses also are burdened with difficult tasks, extreme tension, long hours, and night work. The lack of oversight allows even public hospitals to violate rules regarding maximum workload, measured in number of patients or beds per nurse, hours, rest periods, tasks, rank, and promotion. The extremely low salaries compel nurses to have double and triple employment, exhausting and demoralizing them (Wainerman and Geldstein 1990, 3, 132).

Nurses train in the public hospitals and leave as soon as they can for jobs in private hospitals. Public hospitals continually bear the cost of training nurses for the private sector. The lack of information on the nursing profession, on nursing school enrollments, and on staffing makes it more difficult to address the nursing shortage (Wainerman and Geldstein 1990, 6).

Distribution of Nurses in the Hospital. Certain types of hospitals and certain wards have greater need for nurses. At the special Hospital for Burn Victims of the City of Buenos Aires, the job of nursing is particularly stressful. Nurses either leave after their first day or stay a long time. Their thirty-six-hour week includes a twenty-four-hour shift every second week. They make $500 a month and so must work two jobs or double shifts. Because of their special skills, the city makes a special allowance for double full-time appointments at the Burn Hospital. Each patient takes ten hours of nursing time every day. Unlike in other hospitals, there are more nurses on the weekends and at night because no doctors are available then. The nurses' care determines if the patient lives or dies.

The neonatology department of the provincial Diego Paroissien Hospital (La Matanza) has thirty beds and forty nurses on all shifts, including one of two university-trained nurses in the entire hospital, eight professional nurses, and about thirty empirically trained nurses, five to seven on each shift (Dr. Alberto Schwarcz, August 21, 1992). In other parts of Diego Parossien Hospital, the nurse-patient ratio is one to twenty or one to thirty. In the clinical wards (that is, everything but pediatrics, surgery, and maternity), twenty nurses are spread over three shifts. The absentee rate is 40 percent, because nurses work shifts in private hospitals to make money (Dr. Lucía Saracco, August 21, 1992).

The clinical ward has sixty beds, but because of structural defects in the building, only forty are usable. Six beds are for intensive care, ten for intermediate care, and twenty-four for standard care. On a typical day, five or six nurses are on the schedule, but the ward ends up with only two or three because the surgery ward takes priority. Surgery nurses have even greater incentive to be absent because the private sector pays much better for their specialized training (Dr. Lucía Saracco, August 21, 1992).

Ricardo Gutiérrez Children's Hospital has a staff of 1,000 doctors, of which 700 are fully trained and 300 are residents. There are 10 university-trained nurses and 300 other nurses, of which 25 percent are high school graduates (professionals). The remaining 75 percent are *empíricos*. In Gutiérrez, each ward has twenty beds. At night and on the weekend, one nurse has full care of two wards, forty children (visit, September 12, 1991).

Effects of the Shortage of Nurses on Quality of Care. The shortage of nurses affects medical practice, as well as the safety of patients. In pediatrics in Clínicas Hospital, the hospital's infection-control specialist instructs the residents to tailor their prescriptions to accommodate the lack of nurses, by increasing the dosing intervals and using general doses rather than a specific dose appropriate to each child's weight and condition. She explains that the nurses are too busy for more precision or frequency and that it does no good for her to fight for more nurses for pediatrics in the hospital hierarchy, because theirs is a very low status department (September 29, 1992, and October 19, 1992). In June, July, and August of 1992, there were no nurses at night in pediatrics. There were thirty children, two first-year residents, one third-year resident, and a telephone that did not always work.[2]

The lack of nurses has a direct impact on the infant mortality rate. The new Garrahan National Children's Hospital has all the facilities to make infant and child survival possible for those who are admitted. The doctors there have equipment, medicine, better salaries, and seventy intensive-care nurses in neonatology (Dr. Pedro de Sarasqueta, September 25, 1991). Seventy-five percent of the babies who are admitted to intensive care at Garrahan live (Dr. Isabel Kurlat, August 26, 1993). Eighty percent of those in respiratory intensive care survive (Dr. Pedro de Sarasqueta, September 25, 1991). But Garrahan accepts only one of five patients who need its level of care. Those who do not make it to Garrahan do not survive (Dr. Isabel Kurlat, August 26, 1993).

As medicine becomes more technologically advanced, it is nurses who keep patients alive by their attention in intensive-care units. Doctors diagnose, prescribe, and sometimes save lives by brilliant insight, but it is the nurses who give constant care. The doctor-nurse ratio in Argentina is inverted for advanced medical care. There is a solution to the nursing shortage. Students coming out of the medical schools in droves really are not well prepared as doctors. They could, however, be trained as nurses for intensive-care units and for primary care, screening, and referral. Even sophisticated facilities cannot fill the gap between a few competent doctors who leave at noon and nurses who have not finished primary school.

Cleaning Personnel

The safety and efficiency of a hospital depend to a large degree on the cleaning personnel. In the pediatric wards of Buenos Aires municipal hospitals, there was a clear inverse relationship between the number of cleaners in a ward and the rate of infection. Wards with one cleaner had five times the rate of infection of those with four cleaners (Manterola et al. 1989, 23).

The government has let hospital cleaning suffer both from the fiscal crisis and from corruption within the city administration. Hospital Muñiz, which specializes in infectious disease and AIDS in particular, and Hospital Penna were without cleaning or maintenance crews for weeks because the city failed to pay the contractor (*Clarín*, October 3, 1992, p. 36). When the provincial government imposed a new board of directors on Diego Paroissien Hospital, the board contracted out cleaning to a company that sends new people every day. The staff cannot explain every day how to wash down a room for surgery or deliveries, and so the nurses have to do it. The staff also cannot let the cleaning crew take charge of the linens because there would be nothing left; the linens would all be stolen (Dr. Alberto Schwarcz, August 21, 1992).

Physical Plant, Equipment, Supplies, Maintenance

The practice of medicine at the secondary and tertiary levels in Argentina is hampered by obsolescence of the physical plant, maldistribution of hospitals beds, shortages of equipment and supplies, poor maintenance of technically advanced equipment, and lack of normal janitorial services. The two periods of expansion of the public hospital system were in the late 1800s and during the first Perón administration (1946 to 1955) under Health Minister Ramón Carrillo. The physical infrastructure in place by the end of the 1950s allowed medical education to flourish briefly in Buenos Aires in the 1960s. Most of the provinces and most of Greater Buenos Aires went without significant investment in medical infrastructure. The economic crisis of the 1970s to the present has eroded the quality of hospital facilities to the point that many of these hospitals once famous across South America are now material for a modern horror movie.

Physical Plant

Although the data would suggest that Argentina has adequate, even excessive, hospital facilities, a number of factors contribute to a severe shortage of hospital space, at least in certain types of facilities and in certain regions. In the city of Buenos Aires and in La Plata, there are sufficient beds per person. In the counties surrounding those two cities, however, hospital space, even for routine needs such as maternity, is scarce.

The dilapidated condition of much of the hospital infrastructure limits the availability of bed space. Facilities that are not in disrepair are limited by the antiquated design of the wards. Lack of staff and lack of equipment create bottlenecks in services that extend patient stays, thereby causing bed shortages. "With five beds per thousand population the present hospital capacity would be more than sufficient, but the hospitals are obsolete, poorly maintained and have outdated equipment. The public hospital infrastructure is rapidly becoming unusable: 25 percent of the registered short-term capacity is dilapidated beyond repair and another 25 percent requires extensive upgrading. Long-term hospitals are even older and 50 percent of their capacity is totally obsolete. Outdated equipment and poor management contribute to the underutilization of capacity" (World Bank 1988, 16). The situation has worsened since the World Bank's report because of another decade of neglect and increasing demands placed on the public sector by higher unemployment.

The large, open wards of the older hospitals cannot be partitioned because of the shortage of funds and the lack of nursing staff, even though they contribute to high rates of intrahospital infection. In all pediatric wards of Buenos Aires municipal hospitals, the rate of intrahospital infection for children in separate rooms or partitioned wards was 7.4 percent; for patients in general wards, the rate was 12 percent (Manterola et al. 1989, 22). For respiratory and skin infections, both of which are passed directly from child to child, intrahospitally acquired infections were four times as prevalent in the general wards as in separate rooms. Infections passed through invasive procedures were distributed more evenly among locations (Manterola et al. 1989, 24).

Countries like Argentina, which have some advanced facilities in an essentially backward medical environment, face a special kind of problem. They have the equipment and the expertise to keep seriously ill patients alive, but they lack the hygiene practices and procedural norms that protect those patients and their ward mates from intrahospital infection. Immunocompromised patients with leukemia or lymphoma can survive a long time in Argentina, but only with large doses of antibiotics to overcome the lack of hygiene and the exposure to children with common infectious diseases. That overuse of antibiotics encourages the development of drug-resistant microbes, which threatens the very usefulness of the drugs (Manterola et al. 1989, 20).

Ricardo Gutiérrez Children's Hospital in Buenos Aires was built over 100 years ago. The pavillions surround a pleasant courtyard with a little bit of grass and some play equipment. The wings are open to the air and sunlight in the courtyards but also to the stray cats that wander from garbage dumpsters to wards and back again. The older wards in Gutiérrez have huge holes in the interior walls and are poorly equipped (visits, September–December 1991).

In those old structures, the staff tries to modify the facilities to fit modern medicine. At the old children's hospital in Mendoza (Emilio Civit), neonatal intensive care could not be provided within the old framework and in 1991 was housed in a tiny prefab bungalow of four rooms some distance from the main building. One room had bunks for the staff, a second room was for meetings, and the other two rooms were full of incubators with tiny babies hooked up to tubes and monitors (visit, October 31, 1991).

Outside Buenos Aires, it is an absolute lack of beds, rather than obsolescence, that is the problem. In the suburban county of General Sarmiento, which has one million mostly poor inhabitants, in-patient facilities have a total of 220 beds, approximately 1 bed per 4,500 people. In General Sarmiento, there are three patients for every bed: one in the bed, one on a cot, and one sitting and waiting. The staff have to rush patients out to make room for new patients, although they know that when they send a new mother and baby home they are sending them to dens of infection, with dirt floors and contaminated wells.[3] The patients soon will be back with respiratory infections and diarrheas. And they will be back again and again (Jorge Sparvoli, September 3, 1992).

Other hospitals have serious design flaws that lead to the condemnation of a large proportion of installed capacity. "The maternity hospital of San Francisco Solano was closed and evacuated by a judicial order due to neglect of the cesspool, which was causing water and waste to flow out of the drainage grates in the floors of the consultation rooms, wards and delivery rooms" (Kreplak 1991, 32).

Patients and their companions (mothers, children, siblings) at the emergency room of San Justo (La Matanza) maternal-child hospital stand by the hundreds in the bitter cold inside the hospital because a wall is missing. The hospital is not under construction or reconstruction; it is just missing one huge exterior wall in the waiting area. So the patients stand inside in the cold (there are no benches) and fight off aggressive, barking stray dogs that wander at will in the hospital hallways (visit, September 9, 1992).

Physical plant is also a problem at Diego Paroissien Hospital (La Matanza), in which only 120 of the planned 300 beds normally are in use, because of structural problems, including repeated flooding and serious roof leakage.

Equipment

The lack of staff is exacerbated by the lack of equipment or the lack of reliable equipment in public hospitals. Professionals use an enormous amount of time attempting to accomplish relatively simple diagnostic tasks, leaving less time for attention to patients. The lack of or poor condition of diagnostic equipment or the electrical or phone hookups to support equipment also jeopardizes the lives and health of patients, as well as complicating profoundly the organization of hospital attention and the use of beds.

From the simplest emergency equipment, such as oxygen, to the latest CAT scanners, serious deficiencies are found across the spectrum of hospitals. Although the public sector has twice as many beds as the private sector and four times as many in chronic care, the private sector has 75 percent of the equipment for sonograms, 72 percent for dialysis, 77 percent for mammograms, and 93 percent for CAT scans. The equipment in the public sector is older and not maintained. The gap between the two sectors has grown throughout the 1980s and 1990s. Information from importers and vendors indicates that in 1980–1981 the private sector added forty computer tomography units and no fewer than eighty gamma cameras, electrocardiographs, and other machines of the latest vintage (Katz and Muñoz 1988, 110–111). The public sector, meanwhile, added virtually nothing.

Even apart from sophisticated technology, the public hospitals are seriously deficient. In Gutiérrez Children's Hospital (MCBA) in 1991, the old wards had none of the basic equipment, including oxygen systems (visit, September 12, 1991). The doctors' association of Gutiérrez Hospital filed suit against the city because of conditions in the hospital. The doctors charged that many patients had died or suffered complications over the two weeks prior to the filing of the suit due to lack of nurses, lack of an oxygen system in working order, and the lack of essential medicines. Dr. Luis Becú, a former director of the hospital and, at the time of the lawsuit, a ward head, said that some of the deaths had occurred because children could not be transferred from the clinical wards to intensive-care units, due to lack of beds. In 1991, there were ten fewer beds in intensive care than two years earlier (*Buenos Aires Herald*, August 17, 1991, p. 11).

Newer public hospitals, even in poorer areas, such as Diego Paroissien Hospital in La Matanza, are equipped with oxygen in all wards, but only one of the ten EKG machines there was working when I visited. When the rains leak through the roof and ruin an x-ray machine, it is not replaced. The hospital has no CAT scanners, now a medical commonplace, and none of the even more advanced computerized tomography (Dr. Lucía Saracco, August 21, 1992).

Trying to practice modern medicine without equipment produces Kafkaesque complications. When a patient needs a CAT scan, doctors have to make an appointment at a private hospital. The appointments offered generally are at three in the morning. It usually takes two weeks to get the appointment, so the patient stays in the hospital, without any cure, taking up the bed of someone who needs to get in but cannot. The doctors also have to make an appointment for an ambulance to take the person. If there is no ambulance available, the patient cannot take that appointment. Or the appointed day (or night) comes, but the ambulance does not show up—perhaps it broke down or found a more remunerative fare—and the patient loses the appointment. The patient fills a bed for another two weeks waiting for another appointment (Dr. Lucía Saracco, August 21, 1992).

Delivery and Neonatology. Ninety-six percent of the babies in Argentina are born in hospitals, and yet they are very badly received. The delivery rooms in most of the hospitals in the country are cold and the conditions primitive, with the result that many infants do not survive a complicated birth, although they could and would have been saved in a hospital with minimal equipment, including suction or resuscitation equipment. The delivery rooms, including the one in Clínicas Hospital (University of Buenos Aires), could not pass inspection by the rules that are in effect now, due to the lack of basic equipment (Dr. Isabel Kurlat, August 26, 1993).

At Clínicas, if a delivery has to be changed to a Caesarean section, the mother has to be transferred from the second to the twelfth floor. The elevators in Clínicas are notorious for never working; their failure is even mentioned in professional journals (Arce and Roncoroni 1987, 36). In fact, the elevators do work, but they are kept out of service by personnel on the twelfth floor so patients cannot be referred to them. Pushing the button does no good. If a patient is in extreme danger, doctors on the second floor bang on the elevator doors and shout up the shaft that they have a critical emergency, and the elevator is sent to take the patient up to surgery (Dr. Isabel Kurlat and the residents, August 26, 1993).

The conditions to which the newborns are subjected also are primitive. Clínicas is an extremely important hospital. As the teaching hospital of the University of Buenos Aires, located in the Federal Capital, its facilities are superior to those of most hospitals in the country. The neonatology ward serves a designated population of high-risk mothers. That is, mothers who are seriously ill are referred to deliver at this important hospital. The babies of these sick mothers are themselves often in jeopardy. The neonatology ward serves 1,000 high-risk births per year, and yet until mid-1993, it had no special equipment or even a plan to acquire such facilities. The high-risk and often impaired babies were kept in old, unsophisticated incubators. There is no ventilating system; when the ward needs fresh air, the windows are opened, letting in the foul air of central Buenos Aires (Dr. Isabel Kurlat, August 26, 1993). (Since the time of my visit, Dr. Isabel Kurlat has become chief of neonatology and many of these deficiencies have been corrected.)

Neonatal wards in the newer hospitals are much more appropriately outfitted. In Garrahan National Children's Hospital, the equipment is up to date, as it is in the new Florencio Varela municipal hospital, called *Mi Pueblo*. These two examples are exceptions to the rule that hospitals lack the most basic equipment for a growing population of high-risk births. The prevention of premature or other high-risk births has been virtually abandoned at the primary-care level, which makes the equipping of intensive-care nurseries of critical importance for the survival and development of the infants so compromised.

Even basic furnishings are lacking in public hospitals, including facilities in the wards for washing hands. The absence of a sink for hand washing is associated with a much higher rate of intrahospital infection. Wards with no facilities or with only one sink have three times the rate of infection (16.3 percent of patients) as wards with two or three sinks. The use of disposable soap and the availability of hand-drying machines or throw-away towels also are associated with lower rates of infection, but the differences are not as dramatic as for the simple practice of washing the hands with whatever kind of soap (Manterola et al. 1989, 23). Given the inadequate consciousness on the part of doctors, nurses, and cleaning personnel of the importance of hand washing in preventing the spread of infection, the lack of equipment is all the more critical.

Electrical outlets are another obstacle. Sometimes in a whole ward there are no working outlets to plug in an EKG machine. Doctors ask for repairs, and the janitor tells them to fill out a form. Still nothing is done, wasting the doctors' time and making medical attention if not impossible, then certainly more laborious. Weeks pass and, by begging special favors, finally a doctor can get the janitor to fix the outlets so an attempt can be made to take care of patients (Dr. Lucía Saracco, August 21, 1992).

Another basic link in the provision of services—one that is taken for granted in more affluent countries—is the telephone. The phone system in Argentina is extremely primitive. In a hospital like Diego Paroissien, which lacks modern facilities, the phone is the link to modern medicine, to appointments for advanced equipment, and for patient referrals to better-equipped and better-staffed hospitals. But as often as not the phone does not work. A tremendous amount of the doctors' time is spent calling other hospitals. Even if the phone works that day at Diego Paroissien, it may not at any of the hospitals being called, so a doctor could spend all day just getting one patient placed. That creates a staff nightmare.

The province justifies the fact that none of the resigning staff has been replaced in three years, calculating that each patient gets fifteen minutes of a doctor's time. The fifteen-minute allowance does not take into account all the time wasted in equipment failure, referrals, and administrative hassles (Dr. Lucía Saracco, August 21, 1992).

Laboratories. Hospital labs have varied tasks, complicated by the fact that people come to the hospital for all kinds of reasons. Since there is no primary health care in most of the country, people go to the emergency room or outpatient clinic of the hospital for regular health care. So the hospital lab has very common work, such as pregnancy tests, as well as the more sophisticated diagnostic work (Rosana García, August 21, 1992).

The critical lack of staff is made more serious by the antiquity of the equipment. Nothing is automated in the lab. If seventy test tubes, all for the same test, need a drop or two of something and then to be shaken, each one has to be done individually and by hand. Diego Paroissien does not have the machines to do that automatically, so the lack of personnel is exacerbated. The technology also exists to do several tests simultaneously on one test tube of blood, but Diego Paroissien does not have the equipment to do it (Rosana García, August 21, 1992).

The Diego Paroissien lab has to send many tests to other hospitals, including anything that involves radioactive elements. For uncommon or complicated tests, such as immunofluorescence, the lab has to save them up and do them all together once a week. The tests themselves take several days, so there is a delay of as much as fifteen to twenty days in testing, keeping people waiting and beds occupied. The hospital has no computers and sometimes no disinfectants for washing the equipment or gloves for protection. The gloves are around the hospital somewhere, but an hour looking for them is an hour not working. So, in frustration, lab staff just go ahead and do the job without protection (Rosana García, August 21, 1992).

The hospital administrator at Diego Paroissien says that the new financial rules requiring hospitals to be self-financing mean they cannot get any new equipment (Carlos Ménguez, August 21, 1992). In Hospital Muñiz, the main hospital for AIDS cases, there also were no funds, and the hospital was left without the chemicals needed to test for AIDS. Charges flew back and forth between the hospital and the city, but somewhere along the line bad management left the hospital with no way to test (*Clarín*, October 3, 1992, p. 36).

The operation of the hospital as a whole is compromised, as is the health and safety not only of patients but of staff as well, by the combined crises of staff, equipment, and bed space in a large at-risk community. Workers in the emergency room are in danger from patients' companions who become aggressive. Seeing their sick or injured loved one denied a bed in the wards, they become desperate and beat up the doctor. They know that, when there are no beds, the patient just stays in the emergency room, where the doctors change every day. Nobody follows the case, and after ten or fifteen days in the emergency room, the patient may just die. Meanwhile, scores of patients take up beds waiting twenty days or more for tests or waiting for a diagnostic appointment outside (Dr. Lucía Saracco, August 21, 1992).

The doctors working in outpatient care also play a role in the overcrowding. Because there is a forty-day wait for lab tests for outpatients and the wait may be much less for admitted patients, some doctors will admit patients who do not actually need to be admitted just to get the tests done. The staff tries desperately to attend to their patients, but the conflicting and overlapping needs cause much infighting and bitterness among the staff (Dr. Lucía Saracco, August 21, 1992).

Over the past few years, the situation has worsened. In 1992, the doctors and residents in pediatrics at Hospital de Clínicas did not complain about lack of equipment. By 1993, after the new austerity imposed by the University of Buenos Aires, they reported having to fight for equipment and medicine. Other departments of the hospital, such as cardiology and other prestige specialties that treat those who can pay, were not as affected (August 23, 1993).

The equipment crisis certainly is not reserved to Buenos Aires. In fact, the situation in the interior is, in almost all cases, worse than in the capital. Doctors at the public hospital "4 de junio" in Sáenz Peña, Chaco, protested to the hospital director about the lack of respirators, monitors, endotracheal tubes, and other equipment. Due to lack of norms for surgery or out of sheer frustration, doctors plan surgery without making sure an anesthetist is available or discussing with the anesthetist the medication of the patient. Seventy percent of surgery is carried out without an assistant, which by itself lengthens the time a patient has to be under anesthesia. If any problem is encountered, the surgeon has to wait until someone arrives to help, while the patient is kept asleep. The prolonged anesthesia greatly increases the risk of the surgery. The doctors, at times, bring anesthesia apparatus from private hospitals to avoid having to transport the patients to the equipment in the private hospitals (*Norte*, April 15, 1992, p. 14).

An equipment problem that affects the health of the population at large is that fewer than half the hospitals in the country have incinerators for pathogenic waste. Those that do not have incinerators send untreated waste to open-air dumps (*Buenos Aires Herald*, August 29, 1993, p. 14). (See Chapter 5.)

Supplies

The availability of supplies, including gloves and medicines, varies among hospitals and among wards. In Gutiérrez Children's Hospital, due to lack of funds, no medicines were available in 1991 in this hospital of 1,000 doctors. Doctors gave family members a prescription to be filled at a private pharmacy outside the hospital. The availability of other supplies depended on the energy exercised by the ward chief.

At Diego Paroissien Hospital, doctors differ in their interpretations of the availability of supplies. Some say the items are not available, whereas others say that, with organization and persistence, the items can be located. In neonatology in La Matanza, the chief of the ward uses his personal computer and funds from an award he received to employ a computer specialist to keep track of the needed supplies. His is the only computerized ward in the hospital (Dr. Alberto Schwarcz, August 21, 1992).

The director of Hospital de Quemados (Burn Victims' Hospital), Dr. María Coruja, stretches her budget by maintaining stocks for only a few days, never more than a week. That way, she reduces the possibility of theft and keeps her funds available for what she needs, but it requires constant attention. She has to order medicine every day to keep up with the need. (Dr. Coruja calls this system "feminine management.") Quemados has everything the staff needs: disposables, medicines, equipment, electricity, gloves, and the equipment necessary to protect themselves from infection. The critical condition of their patients requires that everything function well, or people die. The emergency nature of their work keeps staff morale high and engenders a very giving spirit. Everyone in the hospital, from orderlies to surgeons, knows every patient and contributes ideas for the patients' care (Dr. María Coruja, September 16, 1992).[4]

In other hospitals, sometimes people just do not bother to have the right supplies. Equipment with dirty, broken tubes that could pass infection is used for births. Often the supplies are in the hospital, but one has to search for them. Having something in the wrong place is almost like not having it at all. Whether supplies are available in a department depends very much on the department chief. Some chiefs say they are doctors, not administrators or supply supervisors. But to do the job, the supplies have to be there when the staff is ready to work with the patients (Dr. Alberto Schwarcz, August 21, 1992).

All the doctors with whom I spoke agreed that what really is lacking are gowns and sheets. Technically there might be enough sets of surgical clothes and sheets, but nobody bothers to keep them going through the system. There is fabric and there are seamstresses; but the new sets do not get ordered from the sewing department. The maids roll up the used sheets from surgery and sometimes the linens are thrown out with the disposables. If there are twenty deliveries in a weekend, every set of sheets gets pulled off and thrown in a corner of the floor. Monday morning comes, and there are no sheets because for the whole weekend they have been piling up in a corner of the delivery room. If the sheets are left on the delivery beds and go back to recovery with them, some mothers take the sheets. The people who work in the hospital also take sheets home (Dr. Alberto Schwarcz, August 21, 1992).

Maintenance

Maintenance of the facilities is of two kinds: structural and cleaning. Structural maintenance varies greatly among hospitals; some hospitals are allotted more funds. Fernández Hospital (MCBA), for example, is in very good condition and is said to be the best public hospital in Buenos Aires for acute care. Fernández receives more money from the city because it just would not do to have a pestilential disaster in the middle of the affluent neighborhood of Barrio Norte. Although it is drab and dated in comparison with modern hospitals in the United States, it is well maintained. Even within Fernández, however, there are variations. The best-furnished areas are those with high prestige in the medical community, such as surgery and cardiology. Obstetrics and pediatrics get the hand-me-downs of equipment and furnishings from their more esteemed colleagues. Even Fernández has a doctor-nurse ratio of four to one (visit, interviews, September 9, 1992).

San Justo Municipal Maternity Hospital has no working toilets for the hundreds of patients waiting in the emergency room and the outpatient clinic. The room is there, with the broken shards of a toilet bowl stuck in the floor. But no comfort is afforded the pregnant women who have traveled by bus to wait hours for a prenatal checkup, nor for a mother with a young child with explosive diarrhea who comes to the emergency room because they have no other doctor and no primary-care facilities. In Gutiérrez Children's Hospital, there are only two stalls to accomodate the needs of the scores of women and children waiting for attention in the emergency room or for outpatient services.

Most of the hospitals are cleaned, which is not the same as clean. In San Justo, although the janitor swept the hall several times in one morning, it stayed dirty because the area surrounding the hospital was filthy and muddy, there was no wall, and dogs and people tracked in mud. In the hospitals that do have toilets for patients waiting for emergency or outpatient care, the toilets almost never work, flooding the floors. That means people walk in standing water and sewage.

At least in most places, there is an effort to maintain some dignity. In Gutiérrez Hospital, however, the workplace of a thousand doctors, every time I visited the public bathroom in the waiting area for emergency and outpatient services, it was disgustingly filthy. The floor was flooded and the toilets broken. It was not uncommon to see piles of human feces, at times as much as a foot high (thirty centimeters, estimated by sight only), on the bathroom floor. Mothers tried to bathe their children in the sinks, but there was no place to hang anything. The countertops were full of children and their muddy shoes, and the faucets yielded only a trickle of water.

Quality of Care

The lack of norms and the role of personality determine to a large extent the quality of care in the public hospital, as they do in primary care facilities, although perhaps to a lesser degree. The role of the hospital director is important, but even a good director can be undermined by subordinates whose leadership is lacking in their individual units.

Ricardo Gutiérrez Children's Hospital (MCBA)

At Gutiérrez Children's Hospital, I was told that some wards are good and some are bad, and the quality of service all depends on the chief of the ward. If the chief comes in early and expects the staff to arrive on time, work hard, do their jobs well, keep the ward clean, then the ward works well. The individual efforts of the ward chief even determine what financing the ward can get, from the hospital itself or from outside sources. Where the chief does not make the extra effort, the ward works poorly. Some wards are disasters: the chief arrives late, as does the staff; the staff is undisciplined; and the place is a filthy mess (Names withheld, September 12, 1991).

La Plata

In the regional teaching hospital of La Plata, the chief set the tone for the ward. Relations among the doctors were not cooperative. To maintain their positions in the teaching hierarchy, the doctors never consulted with each other and always defended their own diagnoses. The doctors kept the patients' files for their research, making it difficult for others on duty to treat them (Crivos 1988, 132).

Relations in the hospital as a whole were almost entirely vertical. Consulting between specialties and moving patients from one ward to another were rare, even when patients needed treatment that could not be provided in the wards to which they were first confined. The tone in the ward also was unpleasant for the patients. The teaching staff and residents talked about patients in their presence but did not talk to them (Crivos 1988, 129, 134–135).

Hospital de Clínicas General San Martín

None of the conditions described for the preceding facilities were found in the pediatric ward of Clínicas Hospital, the teaching hospital of the University of Buenos Aires. From the First Chair in Pediatrics, Dr. Carlos Ray, down through all the echelons of teaching staff, residents, and nurses, respect for the patients, for their families, and for each other was paramount. There was no divorce of teaching and curative functions. The faculty taught the residents how to cure. Consultation among the pediatric staff and the residents and between them and specialized departments of the hospital was constant and ongoing. Each week, specialists from outside the ward participated in the Tuesday *pasa de sala* (rounds) and in the Thursday *athenéo* (presentation of scientific findings).

On each daily visit to the ward, Dr. Ray spoke with each mother and with each child. He held the children and joked with the young children and teenagers. He evidenced a personal interest in each child, which was not lost on the patients or their families. Dr. Ray asked each parent if he or she was well treated by the staff. What is taught in this ward is not just the highest level of technical pediatric care but also the importance of each of these patients, who came from the most disadvantaged class. When I interviewed the mothers of children in this ward, they confirmed my observations. They told me how well they were treated by all the staff—their questions were answered, and their needs were met by doctors, residents, and nurses.

The seriousness of purpose and compassion exhibited by the faculty of the ward were carried on by the residents and the nurses. The chief resident in 1992, Dr. Ana Bernard, was extremely competent. Her medical knowledge was encyclopedic, and she conveyed it to the residents effectively. She was also a heroic motivator for the residents when they lost hope for a patient. The problem for the public hospital is that, in another year, the chief of residents or the First Chair might not be a person who embodies all those important attributes.

Children's Hospital of San Justo

San Justo Children's Hospital is one of the hospitals in Greater Buenos Aires that refers patients to the pediatric ward at Clínicas. In my interviews with the mothers, they volunteered the information that the pediatric ward at Clínicas stood in stark contrast to their experience when their children were patients at the Children's Hospital of San Justo. At San Justo, they told me they "were treated like animals." That also confirmed my observations at San Justo. I saw staff who treated each other badly, who were hostile to patients, and who generally created an environment that was extremely unpleasant. I observed this in my experience with the director of the hospital, with his office staff, and with all the doctors and other staff I encountered, with one exception, a woman who worked in the central office (September 9, 1992).[5]

Lack of Norms and Intrahospital Infection

Argentine hospitals frequently fail to meet world hygiene standards. "Saving money by minimizing hygiene is actually a false economy; treatment becomes far more expensive with constant infection while sterilizing dirty items is futile" (*Buenos Aires Herald*, August 29, 1993, p. 14).

In Diego Paroissien Hospital, the infection-control specialist has tried to educate the staff about AIDS, hepatitis, and other infectious disease transmission, but they do not have a consciousness of prevention. Sometimes they just go from one patient to another with the same dirty equipment. The auxiliary nursing staff come from the same population as the patients and also have little consciousness of cleanliness. They do not use water at home—why should they act any differently in the hospital? In fact, the nurses resent doing for the patient what they would not do at home (Dr. Lucía Saracco, August 21, 1992).

The lack of norms and standards of procedure that is endemic in the Argentine system has serious, even fatal, consequences for patients. Doctors at the children's hospital in San Miguel de Tucumán investigated the causes and the effects of the very high rate of intrahospital infection there. With their findings, the instituted corrective procedures, greatly reducing intrahospital infection and mortality. The results of the study are instructive because the conditions in Tucumán prior to the investigation reflect the lack of norms in most hospitals.

In Tucumán, 25 percent of patients contracted infections after being admitted to the hospital, resulting in mortality rates among children ten times those of children who were not infected in the hospital. Some of the children were infected two and three times, and the mortality rate among those with three episodes was fifteen times that of children who did not become infected. The outbreaks had been attributed to the low socioeconomic status of the area, with the malnutrition and lack of knowledge that implied. When the rates of infection reached 25 percent (in the United States, the rate is between 1 and 1.4 percent), lack of hygiene in the hospital and careless use of antibiotics became more plausible explanations. Salmonella, the agent in 70 percent of the gastroenteric infections, was found in the supplies of antiseptics and water vessels shared among the patients. Ten percent of the nurses, kitchen staff, and those who prepared infant formula were infected with salmonella. The infection spread further by the lack of sterilization, crowding, and the improper handling of diapers. Implementation of proper procedures was blocked by lack of funds, lack of information, and lack of consciousness of cleanliness on the part of doctors and nurses (Torres et al. 1990, 38–43).

The various procedures implemented during the second phase of the study made it clear that the staff essentially were starting from zero in safe hospital practice. They instituted hand washing before and after procedures and disinfection and proper handling of tubes, syringes, and other invasive equipment. Beds were redistributed to reduce crowding and to vary ages to reduce vulnerability. More careful handling of diapers, checkups for personnel, and the elimination of common water and antiseptic vessels were initiated.

The study investigated twenty cases of sepsis (systemic infection), all fatal. The doctors decided that intravenous and other invasive techniques were used much too frequently and without clean procedure. For infection acquired by surgical patients, the hospital instituted hygienic methods in the preparation and movement of the patients, in the cleaning and airing of incisions, and in surgical techniques. For respiratory infections, the disinfection of respirators between patients was implemented. For each type of infection, the most basic hygiene was introduced (Torres et al. 1990, 41).

The other major problem found by investigators was in the use of antibiotics. Eighty-four percent of patients were being treated with antibiotics, 68 percent for therapeutic reasons, the remaining 16 percent for prophylaxis. Twenty percent of the therapeutic prescriptions were not indicated by the pathology present. Thirty percent of all children had received antibiotics for more than the proper length of time. Forty percent of the patients were given the wrong type or dose of antibiotic for the wrong duration or at improper intervals. Only 3 percent of those treated with antibiotics had been tested for bacterial infection.[6] Fifty-one percent of the ampicillin, 70 percent of the trimetoprima, and 100 percent of the penicillin were improperly used. The hospital had not purhased the types of antibiotics that were needed (Torres et al. 1990, 41).

The result of the anarchic use of antibiotics was an extremely high level of resistance to drugs. In the burn unit, the resistance to rifampicin had gone from 10 percent to 80 percent over a short period of time in 1984. With the implementation of norms of prescription and administration during 1985–1986, the resistant strains were eliminated. By 1987, it was found that the proportion of patients treated with antibiotics was reduced from 84 percent to 15.8 percent (14.3 percent for therapy and 1.5 percent for prophylaxis). Of those, 99 percent were found in the audit to have been properly indicated. The average length of stay was reduced from 12 days to 5–8 days between 1983 and 1986. As a result of all the changes instituted in hygiene, use of antibiotics, and length of stay, intrahospital infection fell from 25 percent to 4 percent by the end of the first year. In the two subsequent years (up to the time of the report), the rate ranged from 1.2 percent to 3.5 percent. Mortality fell from 30 percent of those infected to 10 percent (Torres et al. 1990, 42–43).

The overall conclusions of the study at the children's hospital in Tucumán are good news for public health in Argentina. A significant reduction in costs resulted from the large reduction in purchases of antibiotics, from the reduced complications from intrahospital infection, and from the lower use of hospital bed-days. The cost reduction was achieved with greatly reduced levels of mortality and morbidity among the patients (Torres et al. 1990, 44).

Similar success was achieved in the neonatal intensive care unit at the Emilio Civit Hospital in Mendoza. The rate of intrahospital infection there was zero, by virtue of the simple practice enforced in that unit that nurses wash their hands after each contact with an infant (Dr. Adriana Obilla, October 31, 1991). This kind of success is not unique, but the results are isolated and not widely publicized.

While the success in Tucumán and at Emilio Civit is encouraging, what it highlights is the lack of generally accepted norms, which is the cause of much avoidable suffering. In Tucumán, doctors attributed high rates of intrahospital infection to the population characteristics of the patients rather than to their own procedures, until the rates were twenty-five times U.S. norms. Procedures they instituted were as basic as hand washing and washing tubes for invasive procedures. Hand washing was sufficiently uncommon that at Emilio Civit a doctor volunteered the information that in neonatology they washed their hands. In many doctors' bathrooms in hospitals I visited, there was no paper and no soap.

Throughout Argentina, doctors and nurses attempt to practice medicine in dilapidated buildings, without basic equipment, without medicines, without supplies. They work, most of them valiantly, in dirty buildings, accompanied by dogs, cats, and lice, with no sink to wash in, no soap, no gloves. If they eat the hospital food, they may get hepatitis A. If they turn away a patient, they may be attacked by the relatives. If they still care how it all turns out, they could get a bit discouraged.

The worsening conditions in most of the public hospitals produce grim results for the poor. Part IV looks at the outcome of poor living conditions, national indifference, and inadequate or even dangerous medical care. Chapter 10 covers infant and child mortality; Chapter 11 deals with child and adolescent development; and Chapter 12 discusses adult health.

Part IV
The Human Toll

Ten

Infant and Child Mortality

When the *Titanic* sank in 1912, three percent of the passengers in first class lost their lives, 16 percent of those in second class and 45 percent of those in third class. In an imaginary boat, representative of Latin America, there would be 345 million passengers on board, subject to different risks, by social class, as cruel or even more cruel than those of the *Titanic*. Annually almost one million bodies of children under five years old are thrown overboard, the majority of them coming from "third class" who, for the most part, should not have perished.

Dr. Hugo Behm[1]

Previous chapters examined housing deficiencies, the lack of clean water, inadequate disposal of human wastes and garbage, the hazards of a weak state and backward civic culture, and the inadequacies of public medicine. This chapter evaluates the effect that those factors have on infant and child mortality, the most widely used indicator of a nation's health. As a first approximation, infant and child mortality rates indicate the standard of living of a group of people or a country as a whole because children under five years of age are most sensitive to differences in housing, sanitary facilities, nutrition, and access to medical intervention.

The rate of infant and child deaths shows great variation between and within countries, by region, by province, by urban and rural setting, by personal characteristics, such as age of the mother, and especially by economic class. The extent of mortality of infants and young children, its variation among various regions and groups in the country, and its causes are the subject of this chapter.

Infant and Child Mortality Worldwide

In general, the level of economic development is an important determinant of a nation's health, and infant mortality rates tend to have an inverse relationship with GDP per capita. Government policy, however, is crucial in affecting mortality outcomes for infants and children. The commitment of a government to sanitation, nutrition, and the success of targeted medical interventions shows itself most in infant and young child mortality rates. Public health measures can have a significant impact in lowering infant and child mortality below what would be expected from GDP data alone. Table 10.1 shows selected countries, ranked by GDP per capita (by purchasing power parity), and the rate of infant mortality in those countries in 1965, 1985, and 1993.

It is clear that distribution of income and the extent of public health services alter the inverse relationship between GDP and health. The United States has the least equal distribution of income of the industrial countries and is the only one without a national health system. Its infant mortality rate of 9 per 1,000 is more than twice that of Japan, higher than Ireland's (which has about half the GDP per capita), and equal to that of the Czech Republic (where GDP per capita is one-third that of the United States).

Among developing countries, the structure of the economy and the commitment to public health also are reflected in infant mortality rates. In the Americas, Chile, Costa Rica, and Cuba have been the most successful in lowering infant mortality. Argentina has more than twice the GDP per capita of Cuba and reports twice the infant mortality. In Asia, Sri Lanka, working with a GDP per capita one-eighth that of the United Arab Emirates, has a slightly lower infant mortality rate. In Africa, Tanzania has a GDP per capita only 70 percent that of Sierra Leone but has an infant mortality rate about half that of Sierra Leone.

Mortality rates fell dramatically in the 1970s all over the world. Although mortality continued to fall during the 1980s, the rate of decrease in Argentina was slower. While it is true that rates of infant mortality tend to fall more slowly when the rate itself is lower, Argentina is not yet in the group of countries with very low rates for which that slowing of improvement is expected. In comparison, from 1985 to 1993, rates continued to fall in Costa Rica and Chile, where the level in 1985 was already below that of Argentina in 1993. For the entire period 1950–1987, the rate of decrease in infant mortality rates was greater in other countries in Latin America, including Costa Rica, where the under-five mortality rate fell at 5 per year, and Mexico, where it fell at 3 per year throughout the thirty-seven years. In Argentina, the rate of decrease was 2.2 per year (Werthein 1989, 309). Some of the countries with already low rates that had notable success in the period 1985–1993 were Japan (33 percent decrease), Ireland (30 percent), Greece (38 percent), and the Czech Republic, during a period of significant economic adjustment (40 percent).

_____ *Table 10.1* _____

Infant and Child Mortality Rates, Selected Countries

Country	1992 Real GDP per Capita (PPP$)	Infant Mortality Rate (per 1,000)		
		1965	*1985*	*1993*
United States	23,760	22	11	9
United Arab Emirates	21,830	100	35	18
Canada	20,520	23	8	7
Japan	20,520	18	6	4
Ireland	12,830	25	10	7
Argentina	**8,860**	**58**	**34**	**24**
Chile	8,410	107	22	16
Greece	8,310	34	16	10
Czech Republic[a]	7,690	26	15	9
Costa Rica	5,480	72	19	14
South Africa	3,799	124	78	52
Cuba	3,412	38	16	12[b]
Sri Lanka	2,850	63	36	17
Sierra Leone	880	220	175	164
Tanzania	620	138	110	84

_____

Sources: World Bank 1995, Table 27; World Bank 1987*b*, Table 29; UNDP 1995, Tables 1, 4.

[a] Data for 1965 and 1985 are for Czechoslovakia.

[b] 1992.

Among Third World countries, Argentina has a relatively low rate of infant and child death. Still, mortality is much higher than can be justified by its GDP per capita, its level of education, the number of doctors, the degree of urbanization, or its self-concept of modernity. Sixty to seventy percent of the 20,000 infant and child deaths per year are avoidable (Vinocur 1991, 269; also James Grant, executive director of UNICEF, quoted in *Buenos Aires Herald*, April 5, 1992, p. 18). The vast majority of unnecessary deaths are among the poor, and they die because they are poor in a country that has abandoned them.

Variations in Argentine Infant and Child Mortality

The distribution of infant and child mortality in Argentina corresponds closely to the distribution of poverty by province. Because of the large number of births in the Greater Buenos Aires area, the number of deaths also is great. One-third of infant and child deaths occur in the Buenos Aires area, but more than one-third of the births. The rate of mortality is much higher in the provinces of the Northeast and the Northwest, but the highest rates are in the poor settlements of Greater Buenos Aires, where doctors report death rates of over 100 per

_____ Table 10.2 _____

Infant and Child Mortality and Poverty, by Jurisdiction

Jurisdisction	1990 Percentage of Preschoolers in Poverty	1987–1988 (per 1,000) Mortality Rate <1	Mortality Rate <5
Formosa	64.4	40.5	49.1
Chaco	63.6	38.0	45.7
Jujuy	56.7	36.5	44.0
Salta	55.9	32.6	41.3
San Luis	41.2	32.9	37.3
Misiones	55.0	29.9	36.1
La Rioja	43.4	32.6	35.6
Corrientes	58.0	27.8	32.9
Catamarca	51.2	26.5	32.6
Río Negro	50.0	28.3	32.4
Tucumán	53.5	28.8	32.3
Santiago del Estero	60.4	27.6	31.2
Argentina	**40.2**	**26.6**	**30.4**
Santa Fe	37.5	27.0	29.6
Buenos Aires (province)	36.5	25.9	28.6
San Juan	40.8	25.3	28.5
Mendoza	33.2	24.3	28.5
Córdoba	31.3	24.7	27.8
Chubut	45.3	23.4	27.1
Entre Ríos	43.4	24.4	27.0
La Pampa	29.8	24.3	26.3
Neuquén	49.1	22.1	25.5
Santa Cruz	31.9	23.4	24.9
Tierra del Fuego	29.4	20.0	23.9
Federal Capital	11.6	15.9	19.9

_____

Source: Derived from UNICEF n.d., Tables 3, 6.

_____

1,000 (Dr. Pedro de Sarasqueta, September 25, 1992; Dr. Mario Rípoli, November 27, 1991).

Table 10.2 lists the provinces in descending order of rate of mortality for children under five (last column). The data also show which provinces are above the national average and which are below. The table also shows the percentage of young children in each province living in homes with unsatisfied basic needs and the provincial average mortality for children under one year of age. The ranking by mortality rates conforms fairly closely to ranking by percentage of children living in poverty.[2] The most prominent exception is the province of Neuquén, where half the children live in poverty, but mortality rates are among the lowest. Neuquén instituted an aggressive public health program in the 1970s.

Formosa, Chaco, Jujuy, and Salta all take their expected rankings by poverty level and mortality rates. All are in the impoverished Northeast and Northwest, in the Chagas' endemic zone, with large indigenous populations in isolated settlements, large numbers of migrant farm workers, very low levels of water and sanitary service, and shortages of medical facilities and personnel. Provinces whose reported mortality rates are unexpectedly low are Santiago del Estero and Catamarca, poor interior provinces in the Chagas' endemic zone, and Misiones and Corrientes, in the humid Northeast.

Just as the pattern of mortality rates between provinces shows clearly the effects of poverty and of health policy, so too do the differential rates of decline over time. Argentina benefited from the decreases in mortality brought about worldwide by the introduction of oral rehydration therapy and vaccinations. In the mid-1970s, the poor were hit with both the collapse of the economy, in which their sources of income disappeared and cycles of high inflation eroded purchasing power, and the assault of the military *Proceso* on the public health system. Income distribution became much more unequal, and the public health sector was sacked. The changing pattern of mortality from 1976 to the present vividly illustrates the impact of economic and health policies on an already vulnerable poor population.

Between 1970 and 1987, there was considerable improvement in infant and child mortality nationally and a narrowing of the gap among the provinces, although large differences still exist. Improvement slowed down and then reversed from the 1980s on. Table 10.3 gives the rates of infant mortality (under one year) for each jurisdiction for 1970, 1981, and 1987. (Tierra del Fuego is not included because it was not yet a province.)

In absolute terms, the range between the highest and the lowest jurisdictions (Jujuy and the Federal Capital), which had been 116.1 in 1970, closed to 33.7 between Salta and the Federal Capital in 1981, and decreased further to 20.2 between Formosa and the Federal Capital in 1987. In relative terms, too, the gap closed. In 1970, Jujuy's rate was 2.4 times the national average and 4.7 times that of the Federal Capital. In 1981, Salta had a rate that was 1.5 times the national rate and almost three times that of the Federal Capital. In 1987, Formosa's rate was 1.4 times the national rate and 2.3 times that of the Federal Capital.

In spite of improvements, the poorer provinces still are more than two decades behind the Federal Capital. By 1987, Chaco, Formosa, and Jujuy had not yet reached the level that the capital had reached in 1970; Catamarca, La Rioja, and Salta barely had done so. In fact, the infant mortality rate in Formosa in 1987 was equal to that of the capital in 1954. There has been some catching up, however; Jujuy's infant mortality rate in 1970 was equal to that of the capital in 1892 (Mercer 1990, 124).

Between 1964 and 1988, infant mortality fell noticeably in Argentina, but at

_____ Table 10.3 _____
Infant Mortality, by Jurisdiction, for Selected Years

Jurisdiction	Infant Mortality Rate (per 1,000)		
	1970	*1981*	*1987*
Argentina	**62.0**	**33.6**	**26.0**
Federal Capital	31.3	17.7	15.5
Buenos Aires (province)	56.8	33.1	24.8
Catamarca	70.9	43.9	30.9
Córdoba	50.4	24.9	25.5
Corrientes	78.9	44.7	27.7
Chaco	97.4	48.0	33.0
Chubut	83.1	36.9	22.9
Entre Ríos	59.1	31.1	22.7
Formosa	57.2	40.1	35.7
Jujuy	147.4	47.5	35.3
La Pampa	40.6	37.4	21.3
La Rioja	85.5	42.5	31.0
Mendoza	55.1	25.9	22.3
Misiones	76.7	47.9	23.5
Neuquén	106.5	29.5	23.6
Río Negro	92.6	37.6	25.6
Salta	109.0	51.4	30.8
San Juan	80.0	32.4	24.6
San Luis	74.0	36.5	24.9
Santa Cruz	54.7	32.8	21.6
Santa Fe	56.2	32.2	28.0
Santiago del Estero	76.4	31.2	24.5
Tucumán	73.8	37.2	27.8

_____
Source: OPS 1989, 27, from Argentine Ministry of Health and Social Action.

very different rates in the different provinces. While in the country as a whole the rate of decrease was 58 percent, in nine jurisdictions the decrease was more than 60 percent, including Neuquén's dramatic 81 percent improvement. In seven provinces, the decrease was between 50 percent and 60 percent, and in six provinces the decrease was less than 50 percent, including Formosa where the decrease in infant mortality was only 34.5 percent over the twenty-four year period.[3] In Córdoba, the annual rate of decrease in infant mortality between 1964 and 1988 was about 1 percent, but for the 1980s the rate of decrease was 0.1 percent per year (Battellino and Bennun 1991, 50).

In the period 1976–1981, the pattern for the 1980s, that of slowing improvements, was beginning to be in evidence. Although the rate fell continuously throughout the period 1976–1981, its descent slowed. Two-thirds of the decrease for the years 1976–1981 occurred in the first half of that period. In fact, one-third of the decrease was recorded between 1977 and 1978. In spite of the deceleration, the improvement over the period was important. The change in the rate from 1976 to 1981 meant that 35,000 lives were saved. In 1981 alone, 10,500 children who would have died by 1976 rates survived. The Federal Capital was among the jurisdictions that showed the most improvement. If all the jurisdictions had rates as low as the capital, 45 percent of infant deaths nationwide would have been averted (Mychaszula and Acosta 1990, 3–8).

The improvements came about by bringing down the highest rates and also by lowering the lowest rates. Although the range overall did not increase, the spread between the bottom and the median increased. By 1981, all the provinces except Salta were below the median for 1976. The median stopped falling in 1980, and the upper quarter stopped falling in 1981. In 1981, the median began to increase, indicating a worsening in the worse provinces (Mychaszula and Acosta 1990, 15).

Official infant and child mortality rates are potent political tools. Consequently, the numbers reported by the government continued to show declines even after increases were definitely occurring in many parts of the country. The government chooses the data that are supplied to international organizations. Data for the 1990s from primary sources, from doctors working in the provinces, show increases in infant and child mortality. Often the very existence of disease outbreaks is not reported by the government. The deterioration in the collection of vital statistics is also a causal factor. For events to be recorded, health workers have to be working in the area. The collapse of the public health system meant the cessation of data collection and delivery of data to national agencies.

In Salta, infant mortality increased from 30 per 1,000 in 1987 to 36 per 1,000 in 1990. Of the infants who died, 38 percent had no medical attention in the illness that led to their death (Villa 1991, 85). In Salta, some areas have the highest infant mortality rates in the country. In Iruya, Salta, the rate was reported to have increased from 46 per 1,000 in 1988 to 126 per 1,000 in 1990. In another isolated area of Salta, in Santa Victoria Oeste, the infant mortality rate increased from 58 per 1,000 in 1988 to 76 per 1,000 in 1990. (All these higher figures predate the cholera outbreak in Salta that began in 1991.) Even parts of the country with much lower rates were reporting increases (even in official data). In the province of Buenos Aires, the rate increased from 22.6 to 23.4 from 1989 to 1990, a significant increase for such a large sample over such a short period of time (Cravino 1992, 2). The rate continued to climb, according Congressional delegate Miguel Angel Blazze, to 28 per 1,000 in 1992 (*Buenos Aires Herald*, August 22, 1992, p. 11).

The reasons that the rate of improvement slowed in the 1980s and actually turned upward again in some provinces are the worsening crisis in the Argentine economy and the neglect of health programs for vulnerable groups. The next section discusses the differences in infant mortality within provinces, differences that derive from economic and social class.

Intraprovincial Differences in Infant Mortality

Not only do interprovincial differences show the link between poverty and mortality, differences in infants' chances of survival within a province also correspond to differences in socioeconomic conditions of their families. It is not surprising that children in homes that provide little shelter from the elements, who drink contaminated water, who play in toxic waste dumps, whose homes expose them to risks of burns and punctures, who spend their days unattended by an adult, who are unvaccinated, and whose visits to a clinic are arduous and cold and offer little attention and high risk of iatrogenic illness would run a higher risk of illness and death than children who are sheltered in all the ways that affluence permits. This section presents various studies that examine the differential mortality risk within provinces for children of different social groups.

Córdoba

In the province of Córdoba for the period 1987–1989, the highest infant mortality rate (33.6 per 1,000 live births) was in the resource-poor northwestern zone. Not only is the region poorer, it also has less medical attention available. The area with the lowest rate (15.9) was in the southeast of the province, a fertile agricultural area with more regular sources of employment and better accessibility and better quality of medical care (Battellino and Bennun 1991, 51, 55).

Differences among socioeconomic classes were even greater than regional differentials. The rate of infant deaths increased significantly as economic status decreased. The rate for children of agricultural and industrial workers was 5.5 times that for children of employers, directors, and high-level managers (Battellino and Bennun 1991, 53). The mortality rate for children of the highest economic level is approximately what is possible in Córdoba with the current state of the art in environment and medical attention. Deaths in excess of that rate among children of the other three classes (professional and commercial, technicians and service workers, and agricultural and industrial workers) can be considered deaths attributable to differential access to goods and services that maintain health. In the period 1987–1989 in the province of Córdoba alone, 1,000 deaths of children under one year of age would not have occurred had the children been of the top income class (Battellino and Bennun 1991, 52).

Chaco and San Juan

The Pan American Health Organization conducted a study of infant and young child mortality in fifteen sites throughout the Americas, including two in Argentina, San Juan and Chaco. The incidence of mortality in children under the age of five was examined, with the data disaggregated by social, economic, and biological characteristics. The findings with regard to mortality in homes without piped water, without toilets, by number of rooms, and by crowding were discussed in Chapters 3 and 5. Father's occupation and mother's education, as direct indicators of economic class, are considered here. In all study sites in the Americas, death rates were higher among children of unskilled workers than among skilled workers or professionals. In Argentina, the death rate of children of unskilled workers was three times that of children of professional and clerical workers in both San Juan and Chaco (Burke 1979, 37).

Mother's education is an important factor in infant and child mortality, as a proxy for economic class and for the independent role it plays in promoting child survival. In the PAHO study, the incidence of death was found to vary negatively with mother's education, although not monotonically in all study sites. In Chaco and San Juan, however, there was a precisely inverse relationship. In Chaco, children of mothers with no education were seven times as likely to die as children whose mothers had been to secondary school. Children whose mothers had one to two years of primary school had six times the chances of dying as children of mothers with secondary or better education. In San Juan, the death rate among children of mothers with one to two years education was four times that of children with secondary school–educated mothers and nine times that of children whose mothers had been to university (Burke 1979, 36).

Misiones

A study of infant mortality and social inequality in Misiones compared deaths among children according to place of residence, father's occuption, and mother's education. While even the official mortality rates used in the study show enormous differences, they understate the gap between rural and urban areas and between social classes, because there are more unreported deaths in rural areas than in urban and at the lower end of the economic scale than at the upper. Rural people have to go to urban areas for hospital services. Registration of death occurs at the site of service, not at the habitual place of residence of mother. That overstates deaths of urban residents and understates deaths of rural residents. The infant mortality rate for all rural areas was 73.4 percent higher than for urban areas. Between the largest urban areas and the smallest rural settlements, the difference was 114 percent (Müller 1984, 63–67).

Infant mortality in the highest economic class, measured by father's occupation, was 27.3 per 1,000 and 86.1 per 1,000 for the lowest economic class. Since the overall rate for the largest urban areas was 50.9 per 1,000, clearly class plays an even stronger role than location as a risk factor in infant deaths. Mothers with secondary or more education had infant mortality rates of 39.2 per 1,000 and illiterate mothers 96.5 per 1,000 (Müller 1984, 69–70).

_____ Table 10.4 _____

Misiones Infant Mortality Rate, by Occupation, Education, and Region

| Father's Occupational Level | Mortality Rate (per 1,000 Live Births) | | | | |
| | Mother's Educational Level | | | | |
	12+ years	*7+ years*	*<7 years*	*Illiterate*	*Total*
Large Urban Areas					
High	27.8	42.6	40.7*	—	33.0
Medium	32.0	52.0	55.6	71.1	50.9
Low	55.0	25.6	76.1	91.7	67.2
Rural Towns					
High	117.7*	39.0*	38.5*	125.0*	64.9
Medium	26.7*	88.1	67.5	54.0	68.2
Low	130.4*	37.6*	85.8	109.1	84.0
Rural Villages and Settlements					
High	50.0*	27.0*	73.2*	—	48.8*
Medium	47.6*	85.0	88.0	112.2	89.8
Low	333.3*	113.6	145.5	212.7	156.1

_____

* Fewer than 10 deaths.

Source: Adapted from Müller 1984, 79.

Combining mother's educational level with location, the study found that the rate for children of rural illiterate mothers was five times that of children of educated urban mothers. Although mother's education is a help to child survival, the data from Misiones show that when sanitary and health services are unavailable in the rural areas, the beneficial effects of maternal education are weakened. In the same educational class, death rates in rural areas and small cities were more than 2.5 times that for large cities (Müller 1984, 75, 77).

Combining location with socioeconomic class by father's occupation and mother's education shows the enormous gulf that exists in child survival by socioeconomic class and by region. An eightfold difference was recorded between the extremes of the social spectrum.[4] Infant mortality among households in large urban areas with mothers of secondary or more education and fathers of the two highest socio-occupational classes was 27.8 per 1,000 live births. The rate for households in rural areas with illiterate mothers and with fathers in the lowest socio-occupational class was 212.7 per 1,000, or more than one out of every five children born in rural poverty to uneducated mothers (Müller 1984, 79).

Table 10.4 details the rates of infant mortality by subgroup.

Distribution and Causes of Infant and Child Deaths

The distribution of infant and child deaths by age group reflects to some degree the causes of death. We divide the age groups into neonates (infants under 28 days), postneonates (one month to one year), and young children (one to four years).[5] This section discusses the chief factors that contribute to infant and child deaths for each age group. Generally, countries or regions with high infant mortality rates have higher proportions of deaths in postneonatal and child groups. As mortality rates fall, it is the postneonatal rate that falls first, reflecting improvements in environmental factors. In low-rate countries, neonatal rates predominate since they reflect a preponderance of congenital problems. We shall see, however, that assumptions based on the experience of low-rate countries about the causes of death for poor children do not apply in moderate- to high-rate countries, including Argentina.[6]

Table 10.5 shows the distribution of deaths by age among the various jurisdictions. In the areas of higher overall rates, the neonatal threshhold is but one of many hurdles to cross before a child makes it to the fifth birthday. The postneonatal and postinfant periods are as dangerous for children in poverty and in isolated areas as is the neonatal period. The pattern for jurisdictions with relatively low rates of under-five mortality is that, having survived the critical neonatal period, children have a greater likelihood of surviving.

Argentina has not entered the phase where postneonatal rates are insignificant compared to neonatal rates. In half the provinces and in the country overall, postneonatal and child mortality is equal or almost equal to neonatal mortality, and in recent years, postneonatal mortality is increasing. Because Argentina has relatively low infant mortality among Third World countries, some analysts look at the rates for the Federal Capital and consider neonatal deaths to be the outstanding challenge for Argentine pediatrics (Moscona et al. 1985, 307). Argentina should not be confused with a low-rate country with First World problems. Even the "easy" solutions, those for postneonatal survival, have not yet been implemented. The still-high rates of neonatal mortality reflect the degree to which Argentina's neonatal mortality is due to avoidable causes rather than congenital defects.

A small proportion of neonatal deaths is irreducible regardless of medical access, and some neonatal deaths are caused by the state of medical art in a region, regardless of class. Thus, there is greater variation among economic classes in postneonatal rates than in neonatal rates. In the Córdoba study, for the two highest economic classes, neonatal deaths were well more than half of total infant deaths, but for the lower-income groups postneonatal deaths predominated. Postneonatal deaths in the highest socioeconomic class were 1.8 per 1,000, but for the lowest socioeconomic class they were eleven times that.

_____ Table 10.5 _____

Mortality Rates by Age and Jurisdiction, 1987–1988

	Mortality Rate, per 1,000			
Jurisdiction	Neonatal <28 days	Postneonatal 1–11 months	<Young Child 11 months–5 years	Total <5 years
Formosa	24.4	15.9	8.8	49.1
Chaco	21.4	16.4	7.9	45.7
Jujuy	17.7	16.8	9.5	44.0
Salta	16.9	15.5	8.9	41.3
San Luis	19.5	12.7	5.1	37.3
Misiones	17.9	11.7	6.5	36.1
La Rioja	21.5	10.9	3.2	35.6
Corrientes	17.0	10.6	5.3	32.9
Catamarca	13.9	10.6	8.1	32.6
Río Negro	16.7	10.3	5.4	32.4
Tucumán	16.9	9.8	5.6	32.3
Santiago del Estero	14.8	11.1	5.3	31.2
Argentina	**16.5**	**9.5**	**4.4**	**30.4**
Santa Fe	18.2	8.7	2.7	29.6
Buenos Aires (province)	16.2	9.0	3.4	28.6
San Juan	16.2	9.1	3.2	28.5
Mendoza	17.0	7.3	4.2	28.5
Córdoba	16.4	7.9	3.5	27.8
Chubut	13.4	9.8	3.9	27.1
Entre Ríos	17.2	7.0	2.8	27.0
La Pampa	17.0	7.3	2.0	26.3
Neuquén	16.4	7.8	1.3	25.5
Santa Cruz	18.2	5.2	1.5	24.9
Tierra del Fuego	16.6	3.4	3.9	23.9
Federal Capital	11.7	3.9	4.3	19.9

_____

Source: Derived from UNICEF n.d., Table 6.

Neonatal deaths among the lowest economic class were more than three times those of the highest class, demonstrating that Argentina is nowhere near the current irreducible biological minimum in neonatal deaths, which may have been achieved in a country like Japan and which would be invariant with respect to class (Battellino and Bennun 1991, 53).

Neonatal Deaths and Stillbirths

In developed countries with good health coverage, most neonatal and perinatal deaths are caused by congenital and largely inevitable factors.[7] In poor countries, as seen in the preceding section, neonatal rates are much higher and exhibit large variations among classes and regions. Factors in the physical and social environment are responsible for most neonatal deaths among the poor. Maternal malnutrition contributes to low birth weight, even in full-term infants. Lack of prenatal care is strongly associated with prematurity and, consequently, low birth weight, which greatly prejudice a newborn's chance of survival. In Argentina, the main cause of neonatal death is low birth weight, due chiefly to prematurity. Thirteen percent of births in Greater Buenos Aires are low-birth-weight infants (less than 2,500 grams, or 5.5 pounds), and 1.5 percent of births are very low birth weight (less than 1,500 grams, or 3.3 pounds) (Clivaggio 1991, 131). Low-birth-weight infants account for two-thirds of neonatal deaths. Very low birth weights constitute two-fifths of all neonatal deaths (Moscona et al. 1985, 311, 312). The Inter-American study had similar findings for all sites: 65.3 percent of neonatal deaths were of infants with low birth weight, whereas only 10 percent of sample births were low birth weight (Burke 1979, 42).

The incidence of low and very low birth weights varies with economic class. In Greater Buenos Aires, of 49,700 low-birth-weight children, the rate for the nonpoor was 8.5 percent of live births; for the impoverished, 12.2 percent; and for the structurally poor, 10.3 percent. For 3,400 very low birth weight infants, the incidence among the nonpoor was 0.1 percent; among the impoverished, 0.7 percent; and among the structurally poor, 1.6 percent (UNICEF 1990a, 94).[8] In Greater Buenos Aires, the incidence of low birth weight has increased since 1985 from 7 to 12 percent among the poor population served by the public hospitals, according to the only computer record of birth weights in the region (Dr. Alberto Schwarcz, August 21, 1992).

The extent of injury in the intrauterine period is important in determining a malnourished infant's chance of survival. Preterm infants who are small for their gestational age, that is, had suffered fetal growth retardation, have much greater mortality than premature infants whose weight is adequate for gestational age. Babies who are small in both weight and length (proportional growth retardation) have much higher mortality than babies who experienced greater retardation in weight in relation to length (disproportionate retardation). Because babies grow in length throughout the intrauterine period but put on most of their weight in the last several weeks of gestation, proportional growth retardation indicates deprivation throughout the intrauterine period. Disproportional growth retardation, that is, low weight for length, indicates deprivation at later, less vulnerable, stages of gestation. The death rate for premature infants undernourished throughout the interuterine period was 208.3 per 1,000 in a Mexican study (Balcazar and Haas 1991, 59–60).

At the Durand Hospital (MCBA), premature infants most likely to present pathologies or to die were those of lowest birth weight. Even among full-term infants, low birth weight by itself correlated with pathology and death, so that low weight, by itself, was seen to be an injury (Digregorio et al. 1988, 20).

Poor maternal nutrition and smoking are responsible for much of the fetal growth retardation and low birth weight. The other factor that is responsible for much of the low birth weight is prematurity. In the mid-1980s, doctors at Diego Paroissien Hospital (La Matanza, Greater Buenos Aires) investigated the causes for the high levels of neonatal death. At Paroissien, the rate was 24 per 1,000 live births, whereas at Sardá Maternity Hospital (MCBA) at the time, it was 15 per 1,000 and in developed countries, about 8 per 1,000. The high infant death rate in La Matanza did not correlate with many of the expected variables, including education, parity (number of previous pregnancies), age of mother, or type of birth (C-section or other). The factor that was most significant in determining neonatal death was the lack of prenatal checkups. The death rate for infants of mothers without any prenatal care was 60 per 1,000. For 81 percent of the children who died, there was severe maternal pathology that was almost entirely preventable or treatable (Schwarcz 1987, 545).

When the doctors at Paroissien participated in the organization of a local clinic to attend to pregnancies, they found none of the expected variables to explain the women's prior lack of prenatal care, such as lack of education. What they did find was that the very poor quality of attention they received at the public clinics had driven the women away (de Sarasqueta 1987, 549).

There is much evidence, in La Matanza and internationally, that prematurity is strongly connected with both maternal and amniotic infections. The La Matanza study found that in stillbirths of less than 3.3 pounds, there were infections in 75 percent of the placentas. Almost 90 percent of the placentas of premature infants had some pathology (de Sarasqueta 1990, 724). Another alarming finding of the La Matanza study illustrates the inability of doctors to fully counter the destructive force of falling living standards with high-tech facilities. After the initiation of the intensive-care unit at Diego Paroissien Hospital, doctors brought the neonatal death rate for the hospital down from 24 per 1,000 to 15 per 1,000 in three years (1984 to 1987). The fetal death rate (stillbirths), however, increased. In fact, the number of stillbirths exceeded the number of liveborn children who subsequently died in the perinatal period (de Sarasqueta et al. 1988, 194, 196).

Doctors cannot do anything about placenta previa after the child is long asphyxiated. They cannot repair a ruptured amniotic sac when an infection has invaded. If there is no prenatal care, the mothers come to them when it is already too late. It is an enormous waste of resources, maternal as well as medical, in addition to a tragic loss of life or impairment of ability, to allow simple, preventable, or treatable diseases, such as vaginal or urinary infections, to destroy a child or bring it to birth when it is not sufficiently mature.

We can express this health dilemma in economic terms: there is an intertemporal trade-off between preventive care and reparatory care in which the functioning of the price system does not assign adequate resources to prevention

(Katz and Maceira 1990, 175). The cost of preventive care is an out-of-pocket expense for the public system now. The benefits of prenatal care are personal and economic. The surviving infants and their better quality of life from healthy birth and the health and happiness of their mothers are reason enough. But society, too, benefits. It is a waste of human resources to squander so many people who could survive, who could live productive lives. It is also a waste of human resource to put mothers through pregnancy after pregnancy to achieve the number of children they want. It is an enormous expense to build neonatal intensive care units to accommodate all the casualties of a neglected population. In human terms, it is irrational to deny treatment until the newborn is asphyxiated and thus born severely retarded. There is an economic rationale: under the pricing system that currently exists, sophisticated equipment generates private profits, while preventive care does not. Competent prenatal care rarely requires more than a speculum and an attentive ear, but it is not profitable in the private sector. The government has abandoned the role that only it can perform.

Even for the babies who do make it to an intensive-care nursery, there is a difference in survival rates for very low birth weight infants in public and private hospitals because of the differences in equipment and nursing staffs (Moscona et al. 1985, 310). In Buenos Aires, babies weighing 850 to 1,000 grams (1.9 to 2.2 pounds) had a 50 percent survival rate in public hospitals and a 90 percent survival rate in private hospitals. With an in-house neonatal nursing program, in one year public hospitals could decrease infant mortality by half, according to the chief of neonatology at Sardá Maternity Hospital (MCBA) (Clivaggio 1991, 131). The problem is probably more intractable than that, but not without solution. There is little elasticity of substitution between labor and capital in neonatology. A nurse or a doctor cannot take the place of sophisticated equipment or drugs. And no amount of technology can substitute for the almost constant attention that is required from trained personnel. The public hospitals lack both. In both private and public, there is a dearth of neonatal specialists, doctors and nurses. Consequently, at night and on weekends, when inexperienced residents are in charge, there is a much higher rate of neonatal death. The critical importance of experience is also seen in the fact that there is no difference in the neonatal mortality rate between hospitals with and without intensive-care nurseries. What does make a difference is whether the hospital has fewer than or more than 2,000 births per year. With fewer births, personnel cannot advance their learning, even with advanced equipment (Katz and Maceira 1990, 180–192).

Postneonatal Mortality

Some critically ill newborns, especially in an intensive-care unit, may survive the neonatal period of twenty-eight days but die later. Such postneonatal deaths are due directly to prenatal and perinatal causes, such as maternal malnutrition, lack of prenatal care, incompetent delivery, or congenital problems. Many other infants who were injured in the prenatal or perinatal phase and who survived due to costly intervention succumb to infections in the postneonatal period due to continuing malnutrition and lack of adequate primary health care. Healthy infants, too, fall ill and die, weaned early to diluted formula and exposed to contaminated water and dirt floors in cold, damp, crowded houses with virulent cases of tuberculosis and noxious fumes from gas or charcoal burners. Because of the protection afforded by maternal antibodies through breastfeeding, fewer infants of one to six months become ill than older infants (six to twelve months), who may be weaned and who also are more mobile. But the case fatality rate is higher for the younger, more vulnerable infants (Waterlow 1987, 48).

In a study of postneonatal deaths in 1987 in the city of Buenos Aires, 50 percent of deaths were from infections and 24 percent from congenital heart disease. The distribution of deaths by cause profiles a relatively advantaged population, since the Federal Capital has nearly universal water service (except for the *villas*) and more access to medical facilities than the rest of the country. There were relatively few deaths from immunopreventable diseases, such as whooping cough, measles, and tuberculosis, and fewer deaths from diarrhea, compared to the country as a whole (de Sarasqueta and Basso 1988, 328).

Postneonatal mortality rates for infants from the Greater Buenos Aires suburbs are closer to national postneonatal rates, but they still reflect a relatively privileged population compared to the interior provinces. Infants under three months were 47 percent of the deaths, and 78 percent of infants who died were under six months of age. In 32 percent of the deaths due to infections and congenital heart defects, malnutrition was a contributory factor. More than half the postneonatal deaths had some problem in gestation or delivery that caused malformation, chromosome damage, low birth weight, or neonatal asphyxia (de Sarasqueta and Basso 1988, 331).

There were fewer deaths from acute respiratory infection compared with national averages because these babies have some access, although not ideal, to medical attention. Also notable was the high incidence of deaths from congenital defects that are correctable. Certain risk factors that occur in 10 to 15 percent of births, including low birth weight, asphyxia, and malformations, were present in 60 percent of postneonatal deaths (de Sarasqueta and Basso 1988, 332).

The fact that the Federal Capital has been relatively successful in lowering postneonatal deaths from the causes common elsewhere in Argentina and the Third World (acute respiratory infections, diarrhea, immunopreventable diseases) highlights the long-term impact of inadequate prenatal attention. Most of the postneonatal deaths in the Federal Capital have some prenatal or perinatal risk factor. That is, babies with prenatal injury who were low-weight and asphyxiated newborns survive into the postneonatal period but die from subsequent injury. Better prenatal care would lower postneonatal as well as neonatal death rates. These clearly high-risk babies are not being followed up adequately (de Sarasqueta and Basso 1988, 332). What happens is that the babies are seen again and again for this problem or that but always by a different doctor. They become weaker; no one is looking at their overall health problem, which perhaps originated in the prenatal or perinatal environment, and one day they die (Dr. Pedro de Sarasqueta, September 25, 1991).

The lethal effect of inattentive medical care is seen in many of these avoidable deaths. Doctors at Garrahan Children's Hospital studied sixty postneonatal deaths, in which three-fourths of the babies died of respiratory infections and one-fourth from enteric infections. More than half of those who died of respiratory infections had been sick for ten days when they came to the hospital, and almost all died within two to three days of arriving. These were not cases of powerful infection overwhelming a child rapidly. Almost all the children had been taken to a doctor for a minor respiratory infection and had been given medication. The medication did not help; at some point, they could not breathe, were taken to the hospital already in very bad shape, and died. Of the fifteen children who died of diarrhea, twelve had been sick more than ten days, and all had been taken to a doctor and rehydrated using oral solution. These were children who were malnourished but were treated as though they were eutrophic (of proper weight and size) (de Sarasqueta 1990, 726–727).

There are many more studies of neonatal deaths in Argentina than of postneonatal, although 1 percent of liveborn children die in the postneonatal period from avoidable causes (compared to 1.7 percent neonatal). The bias in medicine toward high-tech solutions influences researchers' interests. Neonatal problems are treated with sophisticated tools and drugs. Postneonates need more breast-feeding and warmer shanties, neither of which has been awarded a Nobel prize in medicine nor generated much private profit.

Mortality of the Young Child

Deaths of young children, like those of infants, reflect changing conditions in the Argentine economy, society, and medicine. Table 10.6 shows the ranking of causes of death for 1970, 1981, and 1982–1983. Measles was the second leading cause of death in young children in Argentina in 1970. Regular vaccination for measles was introduced in Argentina in 1971, and data for 1981 and 1982–1983 show the effect of coverage. (When vaccination was neglected, there were serious epidemics in 1984 and 1991.)

In the midst of the *Proceso*'s Dirty War, accidents and violence jumped to first place as cause of death. Most of the children were not killed by the military, but the data give us a glimpse of a society falling apart. By 1982–1983, accidents and violence had become the leading cause of death for both sexes, but for boys not

_____ *Table 10.6* _____

Five Principal Causes of Death of Children 1 to 4 Years of Age

Cause	1970		1981		1982–1983	
	Percentage	*Rank*	*Percentage*	*Rank*	*Percentage*	*Rank*
Flu, pneumonia	13.3	1	9.5	2	8.1	3
Measles	12.3	2	1.8	—	—	—
Diarrheas	11.5	3	7.9	3	15.1	2
Accidents, violence	10.4	4	17.8	1	23.1	1
Nutritional deficit	4.2	5	5.8	5	7.6	4
Congenital anomaly	—	—	6.0	4	5.9	5
Heart conditions	—	—	—	—	5.9	5

Source: Mercer 1990, 135. Reprinted with permission of UNICEF.

only had claimed the number one spot but also had exceeded the next two causes combined, which traditionally had been the most important (infections and parasites; and influenza and pneumonia) (OPS 1989, 35). Also noteworthy is the increasing percentage of deaths directly due to nutritional deficit and the near doubling of the percentage due to diarrheas, both signals of the deteriorating economic situation.

A very high proportion of infant and child deaths are associated with nutritional deficiency. Even in Argentina, believed by many to be a country without malnutrition, there is a clear correlation between malnutrition and avoidable infant and child deaths. The correlation is not just a product of the crisis of the Argentine economy in the 1980s and 1990s. The Inter-American study of mortality in childhood for the years 1968–1969 demonstrated the role played by malnutrition in all causes of death and, in particular, as a contributory factor in deaths from diarrheal diseases, measles, and acute respiratory infections.

In the provincial capital of Resistencia, Chaco, 57 percent of all postneonatal and child deaths were associated with nutritional deficiency. Of fifteen sites in the Americas studied by PAHO, only two showed higher rates of malnutrition-associated deaths, Recife and Ribeirão Preto, both in Brazil.[9] For deaths from specific diseases, the percentages associated with malnutrition for Resistencia were diarrheal diseases, 67.3 percent; measles, 66.7 percent; and respiratory infections, 50 percent. Only the two Brazilian cities had higher rates of malnutrition-associated deaths for each of the specific diseases. The same pattern was found in rural Chaco and Resistencia and in suburban and rural areas of San Juan (Sai 1984, 64).

Excess Female Mortality Due to Malnutrition

Another aspect of malnutrition emerges rather dramatically when the data on mortality are disaggregated by sex. Genetically, females are stronger than males and, consequently, at every age, mortality rates tend to be higher for males than for females. The far greater prenatal and infant mortality for males is due to biological, not environmental, factors. Clearly, social and environmental factors influence the greater male mortality in later life, especially in the significantly higher rates of mortality due to accidents and violence.

The significant reduction or even reversal of the mortality rate differential between the sexes is an indication that social and cultural factors in the environment are causing excess female mortality (PAHO 1990*a*, 114). In many countries, the low status of women and girls is dramatically manifest. In India, bride burning because of inadequate dowry is a serious problem. The use of amniocentesis to identify girl babies for destruction is widespread. In India, it has reached genocidal proportions. There are villages in India that boast of having no girls (Dr. Raj Arole, March 18, 1996). In China, the abandonment of girl infants still is practiced. In a broad belt of countries from Asia across North Africa, female mortality is abnormally high in several age groups.

The results of Pan American Health Organization and World Health Organization studies of differentials in male-female mortality show the effect of the low value placed on girl children in numerous countries. Malnutrition is the lethal tool that raises female mortality. For all countries in the Americas, except the United States and Costa Rica, the ratio between male and female mortality drops to its lowest level in the age group one to four years. In that age group, the causes of excess female mortality are all preventable and strongly related to nutrition, including deaths directly attributed to nutritional deficiencies, as well as those influenced by malnutrition, such as measles and intestinal infections.

Malnutrition is directly linked to excess female mortality in eight Latin American countries, including Argentina. "The reasons for this disparity must be sought in the distribution of food within the family, particularly when resources are scarce. . . . as reflected in the proverb: 'Cuando la comida es poca, a la niña no le toca' (When food is scarce, young girls get none)" (PAHO 1990*a*, 116–117).

Age of Mother as a Factor in Infant and Child Mortality

The Misiones study mentioned earlier also examined infant mortality rates by age of mother. In both urban and rural areas, the graph of infant mortality by age of mother showed the U-shape that reflects the higher rates of mortality to children of teenagers and of older mothers (Müller 1984, 84).

In 1991, 30 percent of births in Greater Buenos Aires and 18 percent of births in the Federal Capital were to adolescent mothers (under nineteen years old).

——— *Table 10.7* ———————————————————————
Young Mothers and Child Survival

Location	Age of Mother	Percentage in Age Group with Liveborn Children	Mortality Rate (per 1,000)
National	14–24	24.9	47.0
	14–16	3.4	107.0
	17–19	16.9	50.0
	20–24	43.3	43.0
Urban	14–24	23.3	43.0
	14–16	2.9	117.0
	17–19	15.1	46.0
	20–24	40.5	39.0
Rural	14–24	33.7	59.0
	14–16	5.2	81.0
	17–19	26.9	62.0
	20–24	59.7	56.0

Source: INDEC 1985, 48.

The proportion is growing every year, as is the proportion of births to mothers under fifteen years old. From 1985 to 1989, births to girls under fifteen years old in Buenos Aires Province increased by 25 percent.

While adolescent motherhood is increasingly common in Greater Buenos Aires, doctors in the interior told me that it had always been a problem there (Las Heras Health Center, Mendoza, November 1, 1991). As shown in Table 10.7, the percentage of women in all three age groups with liveborn children is higher for rural women than for urban women. The prevalence of young adolescent motherhood (fourteen to sixteen years old) and among seventeen- to nineteen-year-olds is 80 percent higher in rural areas than in urban areas.

Young adolescent motherhood entails high risk in any setting, but it is particularly unsuccessful in urban areas where the mortality rate is 117 per 1,000. It is not clear whether the lower mortality for the youngest mothers in rural areas is the result of the greater support structure of the extended family, the greater acceptance of adolescent and single motherhood, or the underreporting of deaths in rural areas.

Some of the higher mortality rate among children of young mothers is a reflection of their lower economic class. Like their older sisters, young mothers lack access to prenatal care. However, much of the higher mortality is due specifically to the physical and emotional immaturity of the child-mothers. Their bodies are not fully developed, so the malnutrition they suffer is exacerbated by the increased demands of motherhood. Their pelvic structure is insufficiently mature, which leads to higher rates of both perinatal and maternal mortality. Many other complications are more common in adolescents, including eclampsia, which generally is fatal for both mother and child.

The girls' lack of maternal experience and their immaturity are a double hazard. First-time mothers of all ages make more mistakes, which, while usually minor, are sometimes fatal. Combined with the sometimes juvenile thinking of a teenager, lack of experience is more dangerous still. A great emotional burden for the girls and a serious danger for their infants is the fact that these mothers often have difficulty bonding with their children if they are the products of rape or incest, which is common among the younger girls (interviews in Florencio Varela and Gregorio La Ferrere, both in Greater Buenos Aires, and in Las Heras, Mendoza).

Distribution of Avoidable Deaths of Infants and Children

The Córdoba study found that a majority of the infant deaths related to conditions of the pregnancy and delivery were avoidable with the technology now available in Argentina. An additional 20 percent of deaths were caused by other avoidable infections, pneumonias, accidents, and nutritional deficiencies. There was a large increase in deaths from nutritional deficiencies over the period 1987–1989, from 26.7 deaths per 100,000 births in 1987 to 93.7 in 1989. In 1990, 4.3 percent of infant deaths were directly attributed to malnutrition, up from 1 percent in 1987 (Battellino and Bennun 1991, 52). Avoidable deaths amounted to 82 percent of neonatal deaths for the lowest socioeconomic class, but only 22 percent for the highest class. Avoidable deaths for postneonates were 82 percent of deaths for the lowest income class, but 14 percent of deaths in the highest class (Battellino and Bennun 1991, 54).

Not only does socioeconomic class assign different rates of infant mortality, it also produces different profiles of sicknesses and deaths. Those of the lower strata suffer from sicknesses and die from conditions that are preventable with the current level of medical knowledge. Added to the chronic poverty of a large segment of Argentine society are the additional burdens of the latest economic crisis that, at the family level, include "worsening of the quality and quantity of food, lessening of the medical care received by the mother and/or the child during the pregnancy, delivery and postnatal period, increase in the affective instability and emotional deterioration of the family group, reduction in access to social infrastructure and essential services," which lead to health problems and sometimes to death (Battellino and Bennun 1991, 56). It is not surprising that the infant mortality rate slowed its descent in the 1980s and climbed again in the 1990s.

In the Misiones study, for the province as a whole, 70 percent of deaths were avoidable using known health or sanitary methods. Deaths from sanitary conditions and from accidents are the two categories most closely connected with living conditions and constituted more than 50 percent of postneonatal deaths for both urban and rural infants. While illiterate rural mothers had three times as many deaths as urban educated mothers, postneonatal mortality specifically from sanitary conditions and accidents was nine times as common for rural illiterate mothers as for educated urban mothers (Müller 1984, 92).

In a 1985 study of Greater Buenos Aires, in all but one county, more than half of neonatal deaths were associated with unfavorable living conditions. In fifteen of the nineteen counties of Greater Buenos Aires, more than 40 percent of young child deaths were from causes related to poor living conditions (Marconi et al. 1990, 47).

According to data for all of Argentina for 1981 and 1985, while the number of deaths declined, the proportion of deaths from avoidable causes increased from 51.4 percent of the total to 66.4 percent of the total. The proportion from undefined causes also increased from 5.4 percent to 12.4 percent (Mercer 1990, 134).

Sixty children die every day in Argentina from avoidable causes:

- because it took a two-hour ride on a crowded, dangerous bus to wait in line from four in the morning in a cold, dirty hospital with no bathroom so the mother could have prenatal "care"
- because the unattended mother got a vaginal infection that could have been treated and forgotten
- because the mother did not get enough of the family's food supply
- because the mother did not have a tetanus shot or was untreated for Rh incompatibility
- because the baby did not have a BCG shot at birth and caught TB from a family member, and it took the form of tubercular meningitis
- because somebody sold vials of contaminated water to the hospital on the pretense that it was medicine.

But the overriding reason is that they are poor.

Eleven

Stunted Development in Children and Adolescents

In spite of maternal malnutrition, low birth weight, contaminated and ill-equipped delivery rooms, cold and dirty houses, parasites, and lack of vaccines, most babies survive, even in the poorest countries. How well do these survivors live when they go home to shanties, tenements, and *ranchos*? The growth and development of the child and the adolescent in conditions of poverty are the topic of this chapter. In most poor countries, more than half of the population is under the age of fifteen. Most of those children and the ones born in the next decade will stay in the work force until the middle of the twenty-first century. How well those children grow—physically, neurologically, and emotionally—indicates the health and wealth of the nation and predicts its future development.

Infant and child mortality rates generally are the indicators used to measure the health of a nation. The advantages of vital statistics are that births and deaths are well defined statistically, and they are more likely to be registered than are other variables, such as illnesses or disabilities. But even vital statistics are only rough approximations in most poor countries.

There are shortcomings to measuring health with its opposite. Clearly, mortality rates do not reveal the damage done to surviving children. Morbidity rates would give a better approximation of national health, but they are difficult to gather, particularly among those of lower income levels who have poor access to health care. Furthermore, health is more than an absence of disease. It includes normal growth and development of physical capacity, strength, endurance, resistance to disease, energy, sense of well-being, intellectual capacity, and appropriate behavior.

The Elements of Growth

Three groups of factors contribute to proper growth and development: sufficient and balanced nutrition, good health, and a positive social environment. A good diet is the factor we most often associate with growth. Diet is certainly a key factor, but the physical and mental development of a child or adult is more complex than mere food intake. Essentially, nutrition, health, and the social environment of the home and the neighborhood act independently and in concert to propel a person toward normal, healthy growth or to stunt his or her development. Malnutrition, although we tend to think of it as lack of food, is actually the result of all three forces. The role of each of these elements is discussed and then the effect of malnutrition on development.

Food Intake

Undernutrition and the lack of specific nutrients are widespread throughout the Third World.[1] Protein-calorie malnutrition affects perhaps as many as 1.2 billion people; 6 million people have been blinded due to Vitamin A deficiency; goiter due to iodine deficiency affects 150 million people (Chen 1987, 65). Twenty million children are born every year underweight; more than 200 million children under five are stunted; more than 650 million people, many of them pregnant and lactating women, are anemic due to iron deficiency (Maxwell 1992, 4).

One in five people cannot get enough to eat each day, and yet there is no shortage in world food supplies. Inadequate food intake is caused by both supply and demand factors. Supply disruption by drought, blight, plagues of locusts, floods, and infertile soil—all are easily visualized. In fact, however, in the modern world, those factors are rarely the cause, or at least the sole cause, of famine. Wars disrupt transportation links and make it impossible to distribute the available food. Sometimes the belligerants use the food supply as a weapon. Famines in Somalia and Ethiopia are recent examples of war-induced starvation.

Even more common is the supply disruption caused by the operation of and interferences in the market. Forty percent of world grain supplies are fed to livestock, contributing to higher prices and reduced stocks for human consumption. Many developing countries continued the colonial practice of commodity-marketing boards buying an entire national crop at prices below world market price. Farmers smuggle their crop outside the country for free market prices; or they cannot afford to invest in quality seeds and fertilizer because of small returns; or they give up production of a cash crop entirely and produce for their own subsistence. Since 1960, food production per capita has dropped in sub-Saharan Africa.

Demand factors probably are even more significant sources of undernutrition for the poor. Low incomes and high prices add up to inadequate effective demand. The market recognizes only wants that are backed up by purchasing power. The market can clear at prices that create famine. In the Bangladesh famine of 1974, there were adequate supplies of food, more than in the years before or after. Flooding interfered with rice planting, which caused unemployment among rural laborers. At the same time, anticipating shortages the following season, the more affluent hoarded food supplies. Food prices rose dramatically, as did hunger deaths. The Bengal famine of 1943, the Ethiopian famine of 1973, and Irish famine of the 1840s were all the result of inadequate purchasing power, not inadequate supply. Food was exported from Ireland to England during the years that at least 1 million Irish died of starvation (Sen 1993, 41–42).

The amount that the poor spend on food out of their total household budget is very high. Studies of household expenditures in Latin America show a range of 47 percent in Venezuela to 68 percent in Colombia going to food purchases (Mellor 1987, 32). Because food takes up such a large share of the household income, price increases in food can have a serious impact on family survival. This is analogous to the Irish situation, when the increase in the price of potatoes was disastrous.

Another factor that affects nutrition is the quality of food. Lack of storage facilities leads not only to losses from rodents but also to mold. Mold is not just distasteful; it is also unhealthy. Scientists are now considering that the devastating nutritional disease kwashiorkor might be provoked by aflatoxin mold, because it often occurs in children even when adequate supplies of food are available (Nowikowski 1992, 9). In Argentina, the response of food producers to rising input prices in the 1990s was to lower the quality of foods. Even in moderately affluent neighborhoods, it was increasingly difficult after 1991 to find pastas that were not adulterated. (The adulteration of foods and beverages in poor neighborhoods was documented in Chapter 6.)

The modern diet has a great impact on migrants to urban areas. "When rural inhabitants move to the cities, their eating changes drastically. The adoption of an urban style of life signifies that they tend to use foods of quick preparation which the body can absorb quickly. Travelling to and from work and cooking constitute conflicting needs. Mothers who work outside the home have trouble breastfeeding their children, and advertising induces them to buy processed foods of little nutritive value" (Lunven 1987, 84).

Cycle of Illness and Malnutrition

Food intake is only one factor in the child's growth environment. In fact, most child malnutrition is recorded in homes that have enough food (UNICEF 1991, 10). Health is another important key. Serious or prolonged illness can set back a child's growth. Of course, health and nutrition, or the lack of both, interact. The sick child cannot benefit from food that is available. "Efficient biological utilization of food in large measure depends on a person's health status, which, in turn, is conditioned by access to water supply and waste disposal systems and to health services. The high prevalence of infectious diseases among children, particularly diarrheal diseases, acute respiratory infections, and diseases preventable by immunization, increases nutritional requirements and interferes with the biological utilization of nutrients" (PAHO 1990*a*, 186). Diarrhea, measles, respiratory infections, and malaria are among the main diseases that provoke anorexia (loss of appetite), burn up calories in fever, and inhibit the absorption of nutrients. Frequent or prolonged illnesses result in malnutrition (UNICEF 1991, 10).

Children do not have to be starved to the extremes found in Biafra or Ethiopia to be at significantly greater risk from even minor diseases. Malnutrition and disease become enmeshed in a vicious circle that undermines a child's (or an adult's) health. The undernourished child succumbs more readily to sickness, and the sickness takes a much more serious course. The illness worsens the malnutrition, thereby making the child more vulnerable to other infections. Measles, diarrhea, and upper respiratory infections generally are not life threatening to a well-fed child, but they are potential killers to one who is malnourished (Mahler 1987, 11). Immunization prevents some of the infectious diseases that unleash malnutrition, but it is precisely those children most at risk of infectious disease who do not have access to primary health care and immunizations.

Children in their first year, whether they are from affluent backgrounds or poor, tend to experience numerous periods of illness. The difference between the two groups is in the outcome of the episodes. A study of sickness and health in infants in Rosario substantiated what had been observed in other studies as well, that "[t]he relative frequency of episodes of sicknesses suffered did not show any difference between both groups of children (extreme poverty—not extreme poverty), on the other hand the total number of days of sickness during the year is substantially greater among the children of extreme poverty" (Enria 1991, 67). Some of the children were sick almost every day of the year.

Social Environment

The final elements that contribute to growth and development are social characteristics and stress factors, such as family stability, crowding in the home, family size, birth order, and a condition that may be difficult to specify statistically, pleasantness of the environment, which could include the amount of filth, garbage, violence, personal insult, or indifference that a person must confront every day. All these factors influence not only the amount of food a child gets but also how usefully it can be converted into healthy energy. Obviously, too, factors in the physical environment, such as water supply and waste disposal, have an immediate pathogenic impact that interacts with lack of resistance to produce wasting diarrheal diseases, hepatitis, and other infections.

The environmental factors may be extreme. "[M]any of the severely malnourished children live in homes that could be considered in a state of disaster. The mother has problems; she could be abandoned, sick or unemployed or be too young—whichever of these it is, it deals with greater problems than the simple need for food or medical attention. . . . If the food distribution center or health center were right next door, the mother could not take the sick child there, simply because she is incapable of functioning" (Chafkin 1987, 80).

The Hunger Cycle

The cycle of deprivation begins before birth. If the mother is chronically malnourished, lack of nutrients over the long term have slowed her physical development and her intellectual growth. If she is acutely malnourished, she is not receiving enough nutrients to maintain her health. If the mother is a teenager, she has double demands for her own growth and that of her child. If the mother is older, she already may be exhausted by numerous pregnancies with only short intervals between them to recuperate. Old or young, she continues her usual work, which uses up all the calories she consumes. If the mother's malnutrition continues through the pregnancy, the baby will suffer intrauterine growth retardation. Proportional growth retardation (weight and length) indicates inadequate nourishment throughout gestation. Disproportional growth retardation (low weight, normal length) may indicate only late deprivation, which is less injurious because the baby's organs are well formed and the brain has had better nourishment early on (Balcazar and Haas 1991, 60).

The nourishment of the child *in utero* is key to reaching the child's full genetic potential. Placental growth is important for brain-cell development (Shneour 1974, 38). The capacity of the placenta to transfer nutrients is determined by maternal nutrition. Studies of placental weight of mothers in various socioeconomic classes found differences of up to 50 percent between women of high and low economic class. Low socioeconomic class also correlated with numerous pathologies of the placenta (Nuñez 1988, 56–57).

The low-birth-weight baby will be born with 40 percent fewer brain cells than the full-term baby (Berg 1973, 9). Longitudinal studies of low and very low birth weight infants in the United States show a high prevalence of neurological and developmental problems. IQs below seventy were recorded for 21 percent of the children, 9 percent had cerebral palsy, 25 percent had very poor vision, and 45 percent required special education in school (Kolata 1994, A25). In poor countries, these tiny babies are much more likely to continue to suffer malnutrition both because of the environment in which they live and because of their own weaker immune systems and absorptive capacity. This astounding waste of human potential results mostly from avoidable causes.

In middle and high socioeconomic levels, birth weights above 2,500 grams (5.5 pounds) are considered not at biological risk, but for poor populations the minimum nonrisk weight should be at least 3,000 grams (6.6 pounds) since, in adverse environmental conditions, there are fewer opportunities later to increase to adequate weight. In the UNICEF study of Greater La Plata/Greater Buenos Aires *villas*, there was a marked correspondence of lower birth weights and more severe degrees of malnutrition later in childhood (UNICEF 1990*b*, 82).

In the Rosario study of health and illness in infants, 45 percent of women belonging to the group characterized as extreme poverty did not gain the minimum amount of weight suggested by obstetric norms (15 pounds), and some women even lost weight over the pregnancy. The average weight of poor infants was 300 grams (eleven ounces) less than that of the total infant population. The lowest birth weights (1,000–2,000 grams, or 2.2 to 3.3 pounds) were recorded among poor infants, and the poor also showed a relatively greater incidence of prematurity (8.9 percent, compared to 5.6 percent). The injuries suffered by poor newborns include intrauterine growth retardation (9 percent of newborns in poverty), infections and parasites (5 percent), respiratory infections (4.5 percent), congenital anomalies (4 percent), clotting defects (2.5 percent), infections resulting from problems of the mother, the pregnancy, or the birth (1.5 percent), and depression at birth (0.5 percent) (Enria 1991, 64–65). The greater number of premature births and of fetal malnutrition and the greater percentage of children who at birth had deficient physical-functional conditions were found in all four categories of fathers with working class jobs but especially workers in unstable positions (Torrado 1986, 332).

Breastfeeding

For babies of low birth weight or normal weight, breastfeeding is a nutritional imperative. The advantages of breastfeeding cannot be replicated with any other feeding method. Breast milk provides maternal antibodies to disease that protect the child for six months to a year, the most vulnerable period of life. Breast milk is pure, uncontaminated, cheap, plentiful, and provides the proper nutrients for human growth and development, in particular brain development.[2] Premature infants given breast milk scored significantly higher on intelligence tests than babies given formula, even controlling for differences in affective behavior on the part of mothers by tubal feeding (*Boletín de la Oficina Sanitaria Panamericana* 113(3) 1992, p. 254).

Breastfeeding also protects against intestinal infections from contaminants in the environment. Mixing the formula with contaminated water exposes the baby to all the pathogens in the water supply. Keeping the bottle and the nipple clean in a house with dirt floors and without a spigot is next to impossible. Formula feeding also increases the risk of malnutrition because the mother may be illiterate and mix formula and water in the wrong proportions, giving the baby too little sustenance. To stretch her food budget, the mother may dilute the formula.

An Argentine study found that only 35 percent of mothers prepared the formula in the proper proportions (Anigstein et al. 1987). In fully breastfed infants, the diarrheal diseases generally do not appear until weaning. Shortened breastfeeding brings diarrheas and malnutrition to an earlier and more vulnerable stage of infancy (UNICEF 1990*b*, 49).

A study of growth and development of the young child conducted under the auspices of UNICEF between 1986 and 1989 surveyed 920 families with 1,520 children under the age of six who lived in the squatter areas of Greater La Plata and the southeast region of Greater Buenos Aires. Almost all the children in the survey (97 percent) were breastfed initially. The average duration for exclusive breastfeeding was 2.4 months, compared to the recommendation of the Argentine Society of Pediatrics for five to six months of exclusive breastfeeding and UNICEF's recommendation of a lower limit of at least four months. By UNICEF's standards, only 7.8 percent of the children were satisfactorily breastfed.

The mothers reported insufficient milk supply as their reason for giving up breastfeeding. Even allowing for misinformation among the mothers about how to maintain successful breastfeeding or recognize signs of insufficiency, the fact that 60 percent of the sample attributed the need to suspend feeding to lack of milk suggests that maternal malnutrition could be widespread. In the UNICEF study, only two-thirds of the infants who ingested cow's milk received a quantity sufficient to supply their needs (UNICEF 1990*b*, 52).

The diet of children older than twelve months also was inadequate in quantity and variety, with only half the children eating fruits or vegetables. Only 60 percent of the children had three meals and a snack. The rest did not eat dinner but rather had *maté* (tea), in some cases accompanied by bread (UNICEF 1990*b*, 54). In populations with high-starch diets around the world, weaning the infant between six months and a year leads to malnutrition.

Results of the Malnutrition Forces

The most profound impact of the interaction of inadequate food, impaired utilization, and other hostile environmental factors is the excessive and preventable mortality in the population at risk. But mortality is not the only outcome. Fortunately, most children do not die of disease, even aggravated by malnutrition. But hundreds of thousands more children each year recover from the immediate illness to live impaired lives from the interaction of malnutrition and disease.

The connection between nutrition and physical growth is fairly obvious. It may be less obvious that sufficient quantities of good-quality food and the body's ability to utilize it are also of critical importance for normal development of mental capacity, good behavior, and social adjustment. The angry or frustrated child, of any economic class, may be only badly fed, in quality terms if not in quantity.

Malnutrition also has been shown to make people depressed and, in particular, fatalistic. The prospects for success are slim when people give up. That is true not only in an individual's life but also for a developing nation, when a significant proportion of the population has lost hope. Fatalism produced by chronic malnutrition is an enormous obstacle to a country's development.

The effect of malnutrition on a child's growth and normal development will be influenced by how early in life the deprivation occurred and the gravity and duration of episodes of undernutrition. The younger the child, the more severe the deprivation, and the more extended the period of time suffered, the greater will be the retarding effect on the malnourished child.

Height, weight, and head circumference are the measures used to evaluate physical growth. These measurements are easy and inexpensive to obtain. Developmental progress is observed in the infant and the toddler and compared to standards of what most children the same age can do. Weight-for-height is not an adequate measure of a child's development because it cannot discriminate past and present malnutrition. If, in the past, the child has been deprived for a sufficient period of time, he or she will be short-for-age or stunted (chronically malnourished). Children of normal height for their age but of low weight for their height are experiencing current or acute malnutrition and are said to be wasted, or emaciated.[3]

Variations in weight and height are important not so much in themselves, but as indicators of other important health factors. The failure to grow and develop affects all of a child's or young adult's body. The child is less strong, with less brute strength, less endurance, less resistance to disease, less energy and enthusiasm, and less mental capacity, and is less able to behave correctly or respond rationally to situations. The apathy and low responsivity of the severely malnourished child means that the child receives fewer stimuli from the environment and less attention from the mother, thus aggravating developmental retardation (Thomson and Pollitt 1977, 33).

All three groups of contributory factors—quantity and quality of nutrition, diseases, and social factors—are related to the socioeconomic level of the family. There is no one-for-one correspondence of income to weight, height, and mental capacity. But in studies of large populations, there are significant correlations between the growth and development of children and the economic level of the population.[4]

The subject of variations in mental capacity among groups is a sensitive one. Allegations of natural differences in intelligence have been used to justify racist and class-biased social systems. Because of the vicious nature of those theories, scholars have avoided or handled too delicately information about the damage to poor children of the effects of their environment. Two clarifications need to be made. First, it is not necessary to accept or reject the existence of innate differences in intelligence in individuals. Whether all children are innately equally gifted or there are innate differences between individuals is not at issue here. Second, to say that malnutrition, neglect, or emotional injury cause lower physical and mental capacity in the poor does not say that the poor are, as a group, as a race, or as a class, innately less capable. On the contrary, it is environmental factors that determine capacity. Because of distortions that have maliciously used data about the damage to poor children, not enough is said about this enormous waste of potential.

Malnutrition in Argentina

Argentines are accustomed to thinking of their country as a place of bounty, without malnourished children. That generally was true in the past, and a higher proportion of Argentine children are well fed than in many other developing countries. For many Argentine children and adults today, however, there is not only a serious lack of specific nutrients but also an absolute lack of food for the poor in urban and even in rural areas.

The Ministry of Health and Social Action estimates the proportion of children under five suffering from malnutrition to be 30 percent. PAHO considers that figure to be a little high, although it concedes that in the rural areas of the northern provinces it is probably accurate (PAHO 1990*b*, 15). The 1980 census found that 12 percent of children under five years of age had a critically low level of subsistence (OPS 1989, 58). In numerous interviews with pediatricians, however, 35 percent was their estimate of child malnutrition. Doctors working in the poorest *villas* estimated adolescent malnutrition to be even higher (Dr. Mario Rípoli, November 27, 1991).

Argentina is a major food-producing and food-exporting country. Overall, the country still enjoys access to plentiful food. Per capita food intake in 1984–1986 was almost 1,000 calories more than international standards for daily consumption, although that was a decrease from earlier years.[5] Protein consumption traditionally has been high, primarily of animal origin. In 1978–1980, per capita daily intake of protein was 111.9 grams, well above the recommended minimum (PAHO 1990*a*, 185, and 1990*b*, 15).

The crisis of Argentine production affected agriculture, and food supply fell from 1979–1981 to 1987 by 4 percent. Nevertheless, the problem with Argentine food is not essentially one of supply but rather of demand. Real incomes for the majority of the population fell throughout the 1980s, and effective demand for food has been curtailed. The more-than-adequate figures for per capita calorie and protein consumption are averages that mask the variations among income levels. While the rich still have steaks of *lomo* and *bife de chorizo* every night, the poor have a dinner of *maté* and perhaps white bread. Argentina's former middle class is going hungry, too.[6]

Evaluating the developmental state of the nation is complicated by the lack of adequate and comparable data. Doctors do not routinely evaluate a child's development during health visits. When they do, the evaluation is not routinely recorded. If it is recorded, the information is not aggregated for the national population (Morasso and Lejarraga 1984, 1). Consequently, nationwide studies of child development are few in Argentina. Regional and national studies are summarized next.

Rosario is an industrial city in Santa Fe hard hit by the economic crisis of the 1980s and 1990s. Poor children there were hit hard by their environment even before the latest crisis. (The results of the growth monitoring carried out by the medical association of Rosario were reported in Chapter 1.) The children from families in extreme poverty suffered physical and psychomotor retardation (Enria 1991, 66, 68).

In the UNICEF study of more than 1,500 squatter children in the Greater La Plata/Greater Buenos Aires area, one-fourth were malnourished on the basis of weight for age. UNICEF was critical of underregistration of malnutrition in official data and reported numerous other studies of children in the squatter settlements that also show one-fourth of the children malnourished (UNICEF 1990*b*, 82). Forty percent of the children were below normal height for their age, twice the rate for the population at large. Disaggregating by sex and age indicates that boys (in squatter families) begin to show higher prevalence of lower stature between six and eleven months of age, whereas the girls begin to show the effects at twelve months of age. Females show a greater genetic resistence to alterations of growth (UNICEF 1990*b*, 85).[7]

Although 56 percent of families had children whose physical growth was normal, and 66 percent of families had children with normal psychological development, only 41 percent of families had children who were growing and developing adequately by both measures (UNICEF 1990*b*, 87).

The UNICEF study included standardized tests for psychomotor development among children from birth to two years and from two to five years. Among the squatter children, two-thirds appeared to have normal development, one-fourth were at risk, based on their scores, and 9 percent showed retardation or developmental lag. Among the poor children, three times as many had developmental delay and twice as many were at risk as in a control group from the general population (UNICEF 1990*b*, 69).

In the group under two years of age, disaggregated by half-years, the degree of retardation increased dramatically from younger to older groups. In the first half-year, there were no cases of slowness, but in subsequent half-year periods, the proportion of children with delayed development increased from 6.5 percent to 8.2 percent to 18.9 percent. The percentage of apparently normal children, those not at risk, fell from 74.8 percent among the youngest to 55.6 percent among the 18- to 23-month-olds. The gap between children of different social classes widens at the point when language emerges. The degree of retardation is greatest in the area of language and smallest in the area of movement. Gross motor skills were more developed than small motor skills, which were more developed than language.

The UNICEF study attempted to evaluate if there was a cultural bias to the psychomotor testing. Bias would be expected to affect all children of the same socioeconomic class similarly. The great variation among poor children confirms what had been the suspicion of many researchers and the source of some hope, that some children actually do survive and develop normally, even under the most adverse circumstances. The variation also seemed to disallow the testing bias. Furthermore, the differences in development appear early, and the skills tested involved behaviors that seem bias free, such as pointing to their shoes or feet, walking backward for a few steps, naming an object, or saying at least a few words (UNICEF 1990*b*, 75).

The effects of going to school hungry show. The falling IQ scores of Argentine children as they go through school that were reported by Gino Germani in 1955 certainly raise interesting questions about the quality and type of education offered (Germani 1955, 241). However, the combined effects of poor nutrition, poor health, and environmental factors are sufficient cause to render Argentine children, on average, increasingly unable to cope physically and mentally, even if the curriculum were stimulating.

The problems of nutrition, environment, and health are compounded as years go by. Although it would seem that a tiny infant is most at risk in a situation of retarded growth and development (and if the only risk considered is mortality, that is so), in fact, prolonged exposure to poor nutrition, poor home environment, and poor health takes its toll on primary-school children and adolescents.

Doctors working in medical centers in the *villas miseria* in Greater Buenos Aires estimate that one-fourth of patients under five years of age are undernourished, but the proportion of patients under fourteen years old who are undernourished is an even more alarming 40 percent (Dr. Mario Rípoli, November 27, 1991). The consistency of the results in changing economic circumstances is interesting. A 1975 study in Salta found roughly the same proportions. In children under five years of age, 29 percent were significantly below the standard of weight-for-age. Of those aged five to fourteen, 42 percent were seriously underweight for their age. Within the province of Salta, the distribution of malnutrition was marked, with 46 percent of the younger children studied in remote Orán underweight for their age, and in the older group 51 percent had low weight-for-age. Half the children of Orán under fourteen years of age suffered chronic and current malnutrition (Morasso and Lejarraga 1984, 4).

In 1980, the Salta Institute of Nutritional Research surveyed children under fourteen years of age in the provinces of Salta, Santiago del Estero, Tucumán, and Jujuy. Prevalence of malnutrition was 22 percent among those under one year of age, 35 percent among two-year-olds, more than 50 percent among seven-year-olds, and 42 percent among eleven-year-olds by the standard of weight-for-age. Malnutrition was first degree for 32 percent of the children, and second and third degree for 10 percent of the children. (An example of third-degree malnutrition is kwashiorkor.) Weight-for-height measurements showed that between 10 and 20 percent of the sampled children had signs of recent malnutrition (emaciation).

In Catamarca in 1982, 56 percent of schoolchildren in the west of the province were stunted, and 22 percent were emaciated. In comparison, in the east, the prevalence of stunting was 36 percent, of wasting (emaciation), 3 percent. In the western zone, 34 percent of children in urban areas were stunted. In rural areas of western Catamarca, 84 percent of children were stunted.

In a 1979 study of Santiago del Estero, 20 percent of the children in both age groups were emaciated, while 34 percent of the under-fives and 54 percent of the older group were stunted. Again, in a province already severely affected by malnutrition, it is possible to observe even higher rates in certain departments. In Tacañitas, among children five to fourteen years, 59 percent were stunted and 45 percent were currently malnourished, or emaciated (Morasso and Lejarraga 1984, 5). These are children who go to school hungry, not feeling well and not learning.

Malnutrition is also a problem in more affluent regions. In Buenos Aires, a 1985 household survey of 485 children under two years of age found that 17 percent of males and 15 percent of females were emaciated and that 27 percent of the males and 20 percent of the females were stunted (PAHO 1990*b*, 15). The Pan American Health Organization surveyed the nutritional status of 40,000 schoolchildren from all the provinces, beginning in 1985, and found that 10 percent of the children were stunted (OPS 1989, 59).

Nationally, the distribution of growth retardation matches the distribution of poverty. A 1983 study by the Argentine Society of Pediatrics with anthropometric data from eleven provinces found malnutrition to range from 12 percent to 39 percent in children under two years of age (Calvo et al. 1989, 134).

The same correlations between poverty and growth retardation among provinces were demonstrated in a study of over 15,000 high school students in 1986. There were significant differences in weight and height between students in public and private schools, even though the entire sample showed a strong bias in favor of middle and upper classes simply because it was a study of secondary students. That was confirmed by data on the job classification of the parents of sample children (Lejarraga et al. 1986). Another finding of this study was the small but significant difference in height in favor of children from smaller cities and rural areas compared with the largest cities in each province. That would seem to indicate the role of pleasantness of the environment.

In a study of army conscripts in Argentina in 1987, there was a significant correspondence between provinces with a high percentage of homes with unsatisfied basic needs and the proportion of young men of lower weight and height. Young men in Jujuy attain an average height three inches shorter than those in the Federal Capital. Their average weight is eight kilograms (almost eighteen pounds) less than that of young men in the Capital (Lejarraga et al. 1991).

Combining averages for weight and height by province with other indicators of health and economic status shows striking correlations, especially with infant and child mortality. Low weight, the indicator of acute malnutrition, shows higher correlation with infant and child mortality than stunted height. Chronic malnutrition (stunting) was less likely to produce death than the combination of chronic and acute malnutrition, as evidenced in low weight-for-age (Lejarraga et al. 1991).

Lack of Specific Nutrients

In addition to the devastating effects from generally inadequate diet combined with illness and environmental stress, the poor suffer from a disabling lack of specific nutrients, including vitamin A, iron, iodine, calcium, and vitamins B and C. These nutritional deficiencies are widespread and can have serious, even fatal, consequences.

Vitamin A

Vitamin A is necessary for cell metabolism, healthy skin and eyes, and development of immune mechanisms. Deficiency in vitamin A generally occurs in population groups with low-calorie diets and is particularly lethal for preschoolers (PAHO 1990*a*, 194). Vitamin A deficiency is the major cause of blindness in developing countries, blinding at least 250,000 children per year (Horwitz 1987, 2). Because blindness hampers a person's chances of survival, the number of blind survivors understates the extent of the problem. In addition, visual disability affects a significant proportion of the population. Xerophthalmia (vitamin A–deficiency blindness) can be prevented with vitamin A supplements at a cost of 25 cents per person per year (Foster 1992, 15). The productivity loss of vitamin A deficiency, year after year, is staggering but avoidable.

Vitamin D

Another avoidable deficiency disease in some parts of the developing world is rickets. Girls in *purdah* (completely covered in robes) have so little sun exposure that they suffer from vitamin D deficiency, which affects the development of bones and joints (Berg 1973, 15). There would be no monetary cost in allowing the girls to play in the sunshine.

Iodine

Iodine deficiency leads to thyroid problems, including goiter (endemic in the Andean region and in parts of Asia), deaf-mutism, and cretinism. At least 3 percent of people who live in the Andes become cretins, that is, with profound mental retardation (Horwitz 1987, 2). In poorer communities, the percentages are much higher, with estimates of goiter of 50 to 60 percent in some Bolivian communities, with 5 to 10 percent cretins. The iodization of table salt, at a cost of one-sixth of a cent per person per year, eliminates goiter and cretinism (Berg 1973, 26).

The injury to populations with endemic goiter goes far beyond overt cretinism and deaf-mutism. Other children in the endemic areas are affected to a less obvious degree. In one area of endemic goiter, 19 percent of the children, while not overt cretins, were below the tenth percentile in national standards of intellectual achievement, compared to only 6.6 percent of children in a control village (Stanbury 1977, 50).

In an investigation of highland Ecuador, 7 percent of adults were identified as cretins, but an additional 23 percent of adults were retarded to some degree. The Ecuador study attempted to evaluate the extent to which a society and an economy are limited by the presence of such a large proportion of the adult population who are mentally deficient and unable to pass on "the full informational content and behavioral repertoire of the culture" (Greene 1977, 57, 88). Not only cretins and near-cretins raise this dilemma. Any society in which a significant proportion of the population are not able to function near their intellectual or physical potential will be held back.

China recently has recognized the enormity of the problem of iodine deficiency in the country. More than ten million cases of mental retardation, including hundreds of thousands of cretins, are attributed by the Public Health Ministry to lack of iodine. Probably tens of millions of people have lowered intelligence due to milder iodine deficiency. In 1995, 35 to 65 percent of newborns surveyed in every provincial capital exhibited iodine deficiency. As many as 25 percent of children surveyed in the 1980s had IQs between fifty and sixty-nine (Tyler 1996, A1, A10).

In Argentina, the endemic goiter zone encompasses all the western provinces along the foothills and *altiplano* of the Andes. Mendoza Province began iodization of salt in 1953, and it was required nationwide between 1967 and 1970. Since 1970, the official national rate of goiter has dropped from 44 percent to 5 percent. Apparently the law is evaded by clandestine mining, smuggling, or improper production of salt. In 1981, prevalence of goiter among schoolchildren in the province of Salta exceeded 30 percent. Fourteen percent of families in the province were found to consume noniodized salt. The population at risk of goiter in the province of Salta alone reaches 25,000 (PAHO 1990*b*, 16). Even in Buenos Aires, well outside the supposed endemic zone, goiter prevalence among schoolchildren was 8.5 percent in 1986, eighteen years after iodization was begun (Salvaneschi et al. 1991, 99–105).

Calcium

Calcium is important not only for bone and tooth development but also for healthy pregnancy. Deficiency of calcium is implicated in hypertension of pregnancy, with its resulting toxemia and eclampsia, which often are fatal to both mother and baby. In the Ecuadorian Andes, a high rate of maternal and perinatal death was shown to be caused by calcium deficiency in pregnancy-induced hypertension (*Boletín de la Oficina Sanitaria Panamericana* 110(2) 1991, p. 135). In a national study of Argentine students, the prevalence of calcium deficiency was estimated to be 26 percent (OPS 1989, 58). In Greater Buenos Aires, 49 percent of children surveyed were found deficient in calcium (Calvo et al. 1989, 144). In Salta, 80 percent of families sampled randomly from the population were deficient in calcium. In Catamarca, only 10 percent of seventh graders were found to get enough calcium from food available at home (Morasso and Lejarraga 1984, 2, 7).

Iron

Iron deficiency is the most widespread nutritional deficiency in the world. Anemia during pregnancy is associated with low birth weight. Infants and children are at high risk because of elevated requirements of iron for growth, especially if they are of low birth weight, are weaned early, or suffer repeated infections. The result of iron deficiency in advanced cases is anemia, but other functions affected are muscular metabolism, work capacity, cognitive function, resistence to infections, and regulation of body temperature, all of which can occur without anemia being evident (Calvo et al. 1989, 131–132).

Among children in Greater Buenos Aires, only 2 percent got enough iron in their diet. The ingestion of iron was associated strongly with the socioeconomic level, not the age, of the children. Ascorbic acid ingestion, important for the absorption of iron, was below the recommended level for 61 percent of the children. In Argentina, the only foods supplemented with iron are baby formulas. Only 25 percent of infants receive formula (rather than just milk) and usually only before four months of age, when supplementation is of little effect, at least for the full-term baby, who still has prenatal reserves of iron (Calvo et al. 1989, 144–145, 153).

Iron deficiency is a public health problem of significant proportions in Argentina. In no region of the country is prevalence of anemia less than 22 percent among children up to two years of age (PAHO 1990a, 192–194). In Salta, the prevalence is 35 percent; in Greater Buenos Aires, the prevalence of iron-deficiency anemia is 47 percent; and in Misiones, the prevalence is 55 percent.

Teen Pregnancies and Growth

These stunted children are also the adolescent mothers and fathers whose babies, not surprisingly, suffer from emaciation while still in the womb and, born at very low weight, begin another cycle of retarded growth, disease, and underdevelopment. Girls of twelve, thirteen, and fourteen have not finished developing physically, and certainly not mentally or emotionally. As of the 1980 census, 13 percent of births in Argentina were to adolescents (INDEC 1985, 49). The pregnancies strain their developing bodies, and the responsibility of feeding another person takes away from the food the woman-child and man-child can obtain. The highest rates of infant mortality and maternal mortality are among adolescent mothers. Malnourished teens are lethargic, depressed, and inattentive mothers who provide inadequate stimulus to their babies, who are themselves too listless to demand attention anyway.

Again it is the low economic level and social factors that have launched the epidemic of child-pregnancies—the lack of incentive for staying in school and extremely high rates of youth unemployment (60 percent) make having a baby a pleasant option. Crowding, promiscuity (in both senses), poor education (sometimes lack of sex education), low status of women relative to their partners, lack of money for contraceptives or lack of power vis-à-vis men, and incest also are reasons for the very high rate of child pregnancies.

The Stunted Nation

A nation of children with retarded mental and physical development is very costly. Thirty-five percent of the children admitted to the Garrahan National Children's Hospital and to Gutiérrez Children's Hospital (MCBA) are malnourished (Dr. Pedro de Sarasqueta, September 25, 1991). At San Isidro Children's Hospital, 70 percent of the children come from poor households, 36 percent are malnourished, and 40 percent are not properly immunized (Waserstreguer et al. 1987, 192). Add to that the cost of hospitalizing malnourished children in all the provincial hospitals, and we have only a glimpse of the monumental direct cost of malnutrition and retarded growth. The indirect costs of a retarded work force are unmeasured.

All these children, who simply need food or good water and sewers, are being treated with hospitals of high complexity. Worse yet, the children are not cured, because they must go back to the same homes, with the same lack of food, contaminated water, and crowding from which they came. And they go right back on the track of retarded growth and stunted development.

Fortunately, the situation is not hopeless. Provided with the right growth environment at an early enough stage in their lives, children can recover. A child whose development is retarded because of lack of proper nutrition, illness, or other factors, when those problems are overcome, will return to a growth path similar to that of a child not impaired. But without an improvement in the growth environment, that child is condemned to a stunted life, physically and mentally.

Clearly, this is not a medical problem. The most brilliant and dedicated doctors, with which Argentina is well endowed, can only treat the illnesses of the children brought to them. They cannot feed all the children of the country. Some have a hard enough time feeding their own. The solution to retarded growth and development of Argentina's young people is better nutrition, safe water supplies, clean disposal of waste and garbage, better housing, cleaner environment—all in the realm of economists and politicians to correct. Rather than improving, however, living conditions are worsening for the poor.

Throughout the life cycle of the poor, multiple factors conspire to inhibit proper physical growth and mental development. The baby is starved in the womb because the mother is ill fed. Placental insufficiency thwarts the proper development of brain cells. Infection interrupts the pregnancy, and the child is born prematurely, at very low weight, and vulnerable. The mother gives up breastfeeding, from either malnutrition or lack of information, or because she is at work for long hours away from the child. The child is deprived of the protection afforded by the mother's antibodies, the proper nutrition of human milk, and the wholesomeness of uncontaminated food. Frequent infections, especially diarrheal diseases, and acute respiratory infections or immunopreventable diseases, such as measles, rob the child's appetite. Inadequate feeding, deficient in specific nutrients and in overall protein and energy content, stunts the growth of the child and diminishes the opportunity for mental development (Martorell 1987, 53).

Many infants die in the process; many more are permanently maimed, physically and mentally. Even having survived the most difficult years of early childhood, the hungry child is a listless student and an indifferent worker. Girls of small stature tend to have underdeveloped bone structure, especially of the pelvic area, and are at greater risk in childbirth, especially when prenatal care is lacking and delivery services are inadequate. Parents of the next generation, workers for the next century—what kind of macabre experiment in human development is being carried out in Argentina, in the Third World, between regions, between classes, between the sexes? A better formula for undermining national development could not be devised.

Twelve

The Debilitated Work Force

The industrialized world experienced an epidemiological transition from a predominance of infectious and parasitic diseases to a preponderance of chronic, degenerative diseases. Cancers, cardiovascular diseases, and metabolic disorders are the most important causes of morbidity and mortality for populations spared an early death. Death and disease in the developing world reflect an epidemiological accumulation rather than a transition: poor populations continue to suffer from the ancient plagues, but they also have higher rates of degenerative diseases. Poor people are not spared the degenerative diseases, nor are those disorders as inevitable as was once thought. These chronic illnesses often result from poor diet, environmental and occupational exposure to toxins, stress, and lack of preventive care, all of which are more prevalent among the poor.

This chapter focuses on the adult illnesses and disabilities produced or aggravated by poverty and underdevelopment and on the impact of disabling conditions on productivity and national wealth. First, some of the causes of adult ill health are discussed. Then, three areas of adult health greatly influenced by poverty but not treated in depth elsewhere in this work are considered: mental health, women's reproductive health, and occupational safety. Some of the ways that poor health and disability affect national development are suggested at the conclusion of the chapter.

Causes of Adult Ill Health

Poor adults face the same infectious and parasitic diseases due to poor housing and contaminated water and food as children and also suffer the cumulative effect of a life of deprivation. Other conditions, however, are specifically related to adult occupational or sexual activity. Occupational and procreative hazards affect the poor almost exclusively. Sexually transmitted and chronic non-communicable diseases affect the population at large but impose the greatest burden on the poor, who have the least access to preventive and therapeutic care. Adult illness and disability that result from a legacy of childhood deprivation and ongoing malnutrition are addressed first. The obstacles, both objective and subjective, to adult access to medical care are considered next.

The Effects of Childhood and Adult Deprivation

The impact of poverty on children and adolescents was addressed in Chapter 11. The malnourished child is small and weak and does poorly in school. In addition to the general effects of protein-calorie malnutrition and recurring illnesses, there are specific retarding effects of deficiency of iodine, iron, calcium, and other nutrients, and blindness due to vitamin A deficiency. The burden of disease and disability from childhood deprivation does not lighten with age, and for the adult (and adolescent) work force, productivity on the job suffers. Although they are still children developmentally, poor youth play an adult economic role. Entry into the work force increases the strain of malnutrition. Among the chronically poor in all Argentine cities surveyed, more than half began working as children. In Buenos Aires, 18 percent of adults who are now poor were working by the time they were nine, another 52 percent by age fourteen (INDEC 1990, 133).

Adult health is affected by a lifetime of poor nutrition. Recent research indicates that heart disease and diabetes are highly correlated with low birth weight in full-term infants (Brody 1996, C1, C6). Fetal malnutrition has a long reach in shortchanging the adult of a full, healthy life. Poor diet affects health not only in the prenatal age but throughout life, contributing to degenerative disease and its consequent disability and loss of productive years of life. While the affluent population also suffers from chronic degenerative diseases, rates of morbidity and mortality are higher in all age groups (except the oldest) for the poor. The reasons are clear. The poor eat cheaper, lower-quality food, have less information about health-promoting behavior, and have less access to health care that would provide an early warning signal for diabetes, heart disease, and cancer.

As in the United States, obesity in developing countries is much more common among the poor and is increasing, as fast food and low-quality starches and fats replace traditional foods. Migration to cities disrupts traditional sources of food supply and eating habits. The urban lifestyle includes foods of quick preparation and quick absorption. Urban workers trade commuting for the cooking they would have done in rural areas, where they would work closer to home (Lunven 1987, 84). Indigenous people in the United States experienced high rates of diabetes, heart disease, and obesity when they adopted the standard diet of the poor. Fifty percent of Native Americans in Southwest United States have diabetes by age thirty-five, fifteen times the national average (Brody 1991, C21). In

Argentina, 17 percent of young people in the Federal Capital are obese, but in Jujuy, one of the poorest and most traditional provinces, only 3 percent are obese (Lejarraga et al. 1991, 185).

Cardiovascular diseases are the leading killers in Argentina, causing 46 percent of deaths, one of the highest rates in the world. About half of the population between fifty and sixty years of age has some coronary defect, as do about 80 percent of persons over seventy years (*Buenos Aires Herald*, November 28, 1993, p. 4). Smoking, stress, Chagas' disease, and a diet high in animal content and salt are all contributing factors. More than eight million Argentines, 26 percent of the population, suffer from hypertension, half of them unknowingly and so not receiving treatment (Clivaggio 1993*b*, 43). These serious health problems in Argentina are not specific to the poor. President Menem lost two economy ministers to heart attacks in two years. Treatment, however, is less accessible for the poor.

Tobacco use also is not specific to the poor, nor is it a result of childhood deprivation. It is such an important killer, however (and interacts with other causes of degenerative diseases), that it must be mentioned here. Of the 5.5 billion people now alive, as many as half a billion will die from tobacco use if current trends in the developed countries continue. Half the people who begin smoking as teenagers die from it, twenty to twenty-five years earlier than life expectancy would suggest (Peto et al. 1994). Because tobacco use generally increases as national income increases, improvements in developing country incomes will mean more deaths from tobacco use. A study by the Pan American Health Organization found that cigarette smoking caused 13,000 deaths in Argentina in 1981 from heart attack and lung cancer alone. Other tobacco-induced conditions, such as emphysema, fetal growth retardation, and infant pneumonia, were not included in the study (PAHO 1990*a*, 98).

Smoking during pregnancy is the most frequent cause of fetal growth retardation in developed countries. Smoking in pregnancy affects the amount of adipose tissue in babies and also the development of vital organs, including the brain (OPS 1992*b*, 255). As women in Third World countries adopt First World habits, smoking is taking a higher toll in female and infant mortality. One of the disadvantages of a country like Argentina, at an intermediate stage of development, is that it has some of the customs of developed countries, especially those that are heavily advertised, without having the consciousness of health prevention that affluence eventually produces. Women use their freedom to smoke in Argentina, as in the United States, to keep from gaining weight. In Latin America, smoking is an extreme hazard for women, increasing ten times the risk of cardiovascular accident for those taking oral contraceptives, the most common form of birth control in the region (PAHO 1990*a*, 126).

In Chile, smoking causes 11 percent of all deaths and 11 percent of infant mortality. The presence of smokers in the home increases acute respiratory infections in infants by 30 percent. For infants of smoking mothers, the increase in acute respiratory infections is 700 percent. Smoking doubles the incidence of miscarriage and premature births and leads to lower birth weights, even for full-term infants (Medina and Kaempffer 1991, 112–121). There are few studies of the effects of smoking in Argentina because of the generalized lack of preventive consciousness, even among doctors. A 1985 article in the *World Health Statistical Quarterly* reported tobacco use by young people in a number of countries. Argentine data in the report was over a decade old (1971–1972), although other countries reported data from the early 1980s. Among Argentines, fifteen to twenty-four years old, 31 percent of women and 57 percent of men smoked at that time (Friedman 1985, 259). In spite of the decrease in national income and real wages from 1970 to 1985, per capita cigarette consumption increased in Argentina 3 percent over that period (PAHO 1990*a*, 98).

Infectious and parasitic diseases of childhood also leave a legacy of disability, although some of the damage is not apparent until young adulthood. Chronic Chagas' disease, contracted in infancy, is evidenced in cardiac and digestive anomalies in the adult. Repeated infection with guinea worm or schistosomiasis or an enlarged spleen from recurrent malaria disables the young worker. In parts of the developing world, the prevalence of river blindness has been a deterrent to development. Years after first entering the body, the larvae of onchocerca worms cause blindness by working their way to the optic nerves or cause disfigurement by erupting on the skin.

Poor nutrition combined with recurrent infectious and parasitic illnesses also affect the next generation. Safe motherhood is undermined by past and present deprivation. The development of the pelvis in the growing girl can mean life or death in childbirth, especially in home births where Caesarean sections are not possible. Anemia also predisposes the mother to problems in pregnancy, and calcium deficiency can cause eclampsia, which is often fatal.

Adult Access to Medical Attention

Medical intervention can moderate the effects of chronic degenerative diseases and permit longer, more productive, more comfortable lives. Lack of medical attention aggravates adult illness. It is difficult and costly to get medical care for poor people of any age. Poor adults, however, often get less attention than poor children. Parents are more likely to bring their children for care, overcoming obstacles that appear insurmountable. When their own health is at stake, financial barriers, the need to continue working, and subjective factors interfere with seeking care.

Lack of primary health care facilities and the financial hurdle of user fees are not the only barriers that people face. Even getting to the clinic is too expensive for some. As bus fares increase in Argentina, doctors say that patients come to them in worse condition. Doctors have adapted the practice of medicine to what they can accomplish in one visit because they know that is the only contact they will have with most patients (Llovet 1984, 46–48). Inflexible work schedules and scarcity of clinics in poor and industrial areas keep workers from attending to health problems in the early stages.

When a poor person does go to a doctor, the communication is less satisfactory than for patients of the middle and upper classes, with whom doctors feel a similarity of interests (Llovet 1984, 31). Surveys of waiting time in five cities indicate that seeing a doctor is more onerous for the poor. Waiting more than four hours for medical attention was two to four times as common for poor people as for the nonpoor, depending on the city (INDEC 1990, 203).

Given their inflexible schedules and their discomfort in medical settings, poor people instead rely on networks of family and friends more than on public or private medical care, but those networks offer diagnoses that are not always accurate (Llovet 1984, 38). For a routine birth, an untrained attendant is sufficient. But for more complicated cases, informal networks can lead to tragedy. Such was the case for the mother of twins in Florencio Varela who was attended in birth by her mother and who hemorrhaged to death when the second baby was not delivered (see Chapter 8).

Finally, the imposition of fees in the public hospitals under the military government in Argentina posed more than an objective financial hurdle. People who were unable to pay could have the fees waived, but the fee system made seeking medical care much more bureaucratic. Paying bills on a monthly basis, keeping receipts, and applying for reimbursement are complicated tasks for people who do not manage their daily lives that way (Llovet 1984, 124). When people keep all their financial assets in a little plastic bag, insurance forms and copayments can be insurmountable barriers. Throughout the world, countries trying to reorganize public services are instituting fee-for-service plans. Such plans may well be necessary, but administrators should recognize the barriers that literacy and recordkeeping pose for the poor.

The institution of fees and rules also can produce results that appear irrational (Llovet 1984, 137). Because outpatient clinics charge fees, people wait until clinics close at noon and then go to a hospital emergency room, which is free. In Argentina, in all the census cities surveyed, a much higher percentage of poor people used emergency rooms, ranging from two to ten times as high as for nonpoor (INDEC 1990, 201). Overuse of emergency rooms requires patients to wait longer and ties up more costly infrastructure than if people used neighborhood clinics. Poor people are responding rationally to the fee structure by going to emergency rooms, but doing so further strains the public system.

Subjective and Cultural Factors in Health

Most of this work has been concerned with the objective circumstances of people's lives that make them more vulnerable to a long list of diseases and other health hazards. The physical deficiencies of their houses and water supply are due chiefly to poverty. Lack of preventive or therapeutic medical care facilities, the high price of medicine and medical services, bus fares, and inflexible work schedules keep people from seeking medical attention. Nevertheless, there are opportunities that people allow to slip by. Given the inadequacy of health care facilities and the horror stories described in previous chapters, it is not surprising that the poor find it difficult to deliver themselves up to the medical establishments. But the home environment of the poor and the dereliction of the state present so many health hazards that one is compelled to ask why poor people do not seek to protect their health in whatever way possible. Although the main obstacles to health are objective, many subjective, cultural, and political factors, conditioned by poverty, add to the complex web of discouragement that prevents poor people from protecting their health. Failure to perceive disease, refusal to submit to symptoms, fatalism, and superstition are among the factors that impede public health, as well as the process of democracy and development.

Poor adults tend to recognize illness in themselves less frequently than do nonpoor adults. When babies and children are sick, generally they cry, break out in fever or a rash, are irritable, vomit, or will not eat. Adult illnesses are both more subtle and more complex and require some education to envision maladies, through the greater use of scientific vocabulary and abstraction. The perception of symptoms depends on the learned ability to memorize and categorize sensations and their associated disorders (Prece and Schufer de Paikin 1991, 28). The use of abstraction is an acquired skill that gives the educated person the ability to identify symptoms independent of discomfort or incapacity (Llovet 1984, 36). Self-perceived morbidity is greater in the United States than in India (Murray et al. 1992*a*, 114), although life expectancy in the United States is fifteen years greater. The comparison of perceptions of poor and nonpoor in five cities in Argentina shows this disparity as well. In all but one of the locations studied, a significantly smaller percentage of poor people perceived themselves as ill than did nonpoor people. In Neuquén, in contrast, which is the only province with a serious public primary health care system, a slightly larger percentage of poor people perceived illness (INDEC 1990, 197).

There are even greater differences in the proportion of people who went for a health visit without having perceived symptoms of disease. In each location, between two and three times as many nonpoor went for a health checkup as did poor people. In Santiago del Estero, only 1 percent of poor, and in GBA fewer than 5 percent, had gone for a checkup without having symptoms of disease (INDEC 1990, 198).

There are differences between the health behaviors of the poor and the middle and upper classes even when symptoms are present. The more physical a person's work, the more the body is viewed as a tool. The imperative of making a living eclipses long-term health concerns. The intensive use of the body increases the threshold of noticing symptoms and makes it easier to deny problems (Llovet 1984, 27).[1] What doctors told me in the public hospitals and what is reported in the literature are that poor adults do not go to the doctor until their condition prevents them from carrying out their daily tasks, which may well be when the condition is already terminal (Dr. Lucía Saracco, August 21, 1992). The place that poor people seek attention indicates both the lack of public primary care and the stage at which they submit to symptoms. In the five-city census, for those poor people who did seek attention, a very high proportion went directly to the hospital compared to the nonpoor. The proportion of poor people who went to a doctor's office for medical care was about one-fourth the rate for the nonpoor (INDEC 1990, 201).

Fatalism causes people to resign themselves to illnesses and disabilities that are preventable or curable. Malnutrition and the inuring effects of an environment of suffering produce fatalism. People also become fatalistic and passive when they live under repressive political and social systems. Fatalism also has subjective and cultural roots. Chapter 2 addressed the economic role that belief in fate or luck has in dampening effort and of the perception of a hostile supernatural environment in generating a fear and loathing of strangers. Chapter 6 examined the combined impact of a hostile social environment and a weak state apparatus on public health. Those cultural factors affect adult health in other ways as well.

When people view nature as essentially malevolent and see themselves as pawns of fate, their own actions seem unimportant. Their experience of hunger, pain, and repressive governments seems to confirm the belief in a malevolent world. That passivity can infect persons of any stratum of the population because it is part of their common beliefs and experience. Affluence, however, affords a preventive approach to health because people have money, time, flexibility of schedule, and access to information. Affluence also offers confidence in lieu of fatalism, a sense of the usefulness of planning for the long run, and the knowledge that certain risks can be minimized. For the poor, discouragement, fatalism, and the banality of suffering compound the objective conditions of their unhealthy environment.

Fatalism takes on a more sinister character when other people are considered part of a hostile natural and supernatural environment. Superstition and the belief in magic play an important role for many in Argentina and elsewhere.[2] Magical notions and the distrust of strangers contribute to the belief in *mal de ojo* (the evil eye), the idea that a person can make others sick simply by looking at them.

It is a source of great concern in some societies if a stranger smiles at a baby, since it is assumed that any stranger would wish ill on the child. Not only does that belief contribute to the continuation of a mentally unhealthy environment (distrust of all strangers, hatred, in fact, of those outside the circle of intimates), it also discourages seeking a cure. If the family believes a relative has been cursed, solutions like correcting the contaminated water or other source of infection, as modern medicine would see it, are irrelevant.

Maladies are seen as a curse, either through magic or as a punishment from God. Consequently, disabilities are a source of shame and fear, and negative attitudes toward the disabled develop as a result. The disabled population in Argentina includes persons born with congenital conditions and those injured in birth, in the home, in the workplace, and at war. Although disability is at least as common in Argentina as in the United States, it is unusual to see mentally and physically challenged persons on outings with their families.The disabled are hidden at home, children are not mainstreamed at school, and adults are not given rehabilitation and occupational therapy.

The abhorrence of the disabled, combined with the wounded pride of losing the war in the Malvinas, has meant an abandonment of Argentina's wounded war veterans. In a society without a spirit of occupational therapy, they are the unwanted, legless reminders of a humiliating war who lift themselves around the streets and sidewalks of downtown Buenos Aires at other people's knees, begging for coins.

Adult Medical Problems

Mental health, women's reproductive health, and occupational safety and health—all predominantly adult health issues—are profoundly influenced by income, class, and access to medical care. Some of the problems in these areas are due to deprivation in childhood, whereas others result from hazards experienced as adults. They are the three most important areas in which poor adults face risks that are distinct from those of nonpoor people.

Mental Health

The World Health Organization lists depressive disorders and violence fifth among causes of mortality and disability burden in the developing world (Bobadilla et al. 1994, 174). In Argentina, as in many developing countries, there is little primary care for mental health problems. Sufferers either receive no attention or go directly to asylums (*Buenos Aires Herald*, July 8, 1990, p. 4). Considering that the prognosis is poor for those confined to state asylums, the "penalty" for mental illness is high. Only in the province of Río Negro has there been a serious effort at treating mental patients on an outpatient basis (Cohen 1987, 357–364; Sainz 1992*b*, 10–11).

Mental health problems are aggravated during economic crisis. For most people, being unemployed significantly impairs mental health. Even for people who still have their jobs, an increase in the local unemployment rate has been shown to increase the level of anxiety in the community over potential job loss, contributing to mental distress (Warr 1987, 59, 201–202).

Suicide from economic causes increased in Argentina in the crisis of the 1990s. In 1994, Argentina reported suicide as the fifth leading cause of death among fifteen- to forty-nine-year-olds. Argentina has the highest suicide rate in Latin America and ranks eleventh in the world (*Buenos Aires Herald*, May 22, 1994, p. 4). In the first ten months of 1992, 520 people committed suicide in Greater Buenos Aires. Police reported that 25 percent of suicides were due to economic problems (*Buenos Aires Herald*, October 17, 1992, p. 11).

Suicides among people dependent on retirement pensions reached epidemic proportions in the second half of 1992. In the two-month period from late August to late October 1992, seventeen pensioners committed suicide, one every three days (Lamazares 1992, 42). The government refused to pay any pensions above the minimum level, which meant that people who had paid into voluntary plans for twenty-five years had to live on $150 to $200 per month, at a time when the cost of living in Argentina was equal to that of the United States. The government had kept no records of the $65 billion taken from the workers over the years, so there was no trace of what amounts the pensioned workers had contributed to their retirements (*Buenos Aires Herald*, February 21, 1992, p. 3). (In addition to suicides, deaths of persons over sixty years of age increased 70 percent in several districts of Buenos Aires in 1991 alone [*Buenos Aires Hearld*, March 12, 1992, p. 11].)

In times of structural adjustment in most developing countries, it is not surprising that indices of poor mental health, such as alcoholism and other substance abuse, are rising among workers and unemployed teenagers. The Argentine Health Secretariat reports three million alcoholics in a country of about thirty-three million people (*Buenos Aires Herald*, August 3, 1992, p. 7). The crisis years saw a large increase in on-the-job use of illegal drugs. In 1987, 3 percent of Argentine workers were reported to use drugs at work, including cocaine, marijuana, and illegal use of controlled pharmaceuticals. By 1991, 8 to 12 percent of workers, including surgeons, nurses, school bus drivers, journalists, and stockbrokers reported using drugs on the job, citing stress and competition as their reasons (*Clarín*, second section, March 1, 1992, p. 14). (See also Chapter 7, which describes the abuse of tranquilizers in Argentina.)

Teenage alcoholism is a health problem of increasing importance and is the second most serious endemic disease in Argentina, after Chagas' disease, and the third leading cause of death, after heart disease and cancer. The "drug" most used by young street children is glue. In the early 1990s, increased drug use and exposure to the summary use of violence by the police led to a disturbing trend of random killings by children in the *villas bravas* (Giubellino 1992, 32). Violent crimes are still less common in most developing countries than in the large cities of the United States, but the increase indicates a fragmenting social fabric.

The hatred of the "other" is even more capable of harm—both physical and mental—when combined with the authoritarian state. The deaths during the Dirty War are variously estimated between 20,000 and 30,000, although some venture even higher figures (Zwi and Ugalde 1991, 208). Individually recorded deaths acknowledged by the Argentine government commission after the return of democracy numbered about 9,000. In Argentina, very few of those imprisoned and tortured were released, so the most important morbidity effect of the repression is its impact on the psyche and the soul of the Argentine nation.

The tactics of the Argentine military in 1976 to 1983 were designed to paralyze political action by creating a mood of terror through the indiscriminate use of violence.[3] They killed children and old people, men and women, Argentines and foreigners, priests, nuns, doctors, and nurses. It was sufficient that a person could be in any way linked to a progressive, even to the extent of merely being in the same university class (Zwi and Ugalde 1991, 207; numerous personal accounts from Argentines).

Argentina is by no means alone in its perpetration or tolerance of torture and political killings. Amnesty International reports that one-third of the countries in the world practice or condone systematic torture and psychiatric abuse as means of political control (Stover and Nightingale 1985, 3). In countries where civil war involves the civilian population, torture can be widespread, as in Rwanda and Bosnia. The public health impact is staggering.

The effects of torture on those who survive are permanent. Scars, burns, fractures, deafness, and impaired vision are among the physical effects. Insomnia, headaches, depression, anxiety, withdrawal, sexual dysfunction, memory loss, and confusion are some of the other effects of torture (Allodi et al. 1985, 69).[4]

The legacy of the repression in the population at large in Argentina is said to be reflected in the lower level of public civility. "Public cruelty is replicated by everyday cruelty. . . . The brutal authoritarian regime unleashed brutality" on the street and in the family (Corradi 1987, 119). The threat of random disappearance led to a passion for ignorance, and the inuring effect of exposure to public cruelty eroded the sense of solidarity and mercy that once existed (Corradi 1987, 119). Certainly, the experience of those years and the fear instilled by the hyperinflation must be factors in the muted response to current, unprecedented levels of unemployment. The reports of fellow Argentines surviving on grubs, rats, and snakes in a country with fifty million head of cattle raise only a ripple of protest fifteen years after the repression and less than a decade after the hyperinflation.

Violence against women is a serious public health problem in most of the world, including the developing countries. In many countries, the government or the society at large does not take abuse of women seriously. As a result, women have little support or recourse. Although domestic violence is reported in all countries, there are variations both in the prevalence of abuse and in the accuracy of reporting. A national survey in Colombia concluded that one in five women is abused by her partner. In Papua New Guinea, 67 percent of rural women and 56 percent of urban women were found to be physically abused by their partners. Eighty percent of women in Chile reported having been abused, and 63 percent said they were in abusive relationships at the time interviewed (Heise 1993, 172–173).

Domestic violence leads to serious injury and death. It also causes depression and is the cause of a high proportion of female suicide. One-third of women seen in emergency rooms in Lima, Peru, were injured by their partners. Six percent of *all* serious injuries and deaths in Shanghai, China, were abused wives. Eighteen percent of all wives in Papua New Guinea have sought hospital treatment for injuries inflicted by their husbands (Heise 1993, 173).

Around the world, most women who are murdered are murdered by their partners, from 62 percent of women victims in Canada to 75 percent in Papua New Guinea. In Bangladesh, half of *all* murders are wives killed by their husbands. Of special concern in the 1980s and 1990s in India has been the epidemic of dowry deaths. Husbands and their families make increasing demands on the bride's family for dowry. If the extortion is not met, the bride is killed, often by dowsing her with kerosene and setting her on fire to make it appear a kitchen accident. Only a fraction of bride burnings have been acknowledged by police, but one-fifth of deaths to women in India from fifteen to forty-four years of age are due to "accidental" burns, and the death rate from burns has been increasing since 1979 (Heise 1993, 174–175). Other categories of violence against women that pose serious public health menaces are rape, which is extremely widespread, and genital mutilation, which is common in Africa and the Middle East. While violence against women is worldwide, isolation, the grip of tradition, and the lack of democratic rights for women make it an especially difficult public health problem in developing countries.

Women's Reproductive Health

While women suffer from all the nutritional, infectious, and parasitic diseases that men do—often to a greater extent because of their low status in the household and society—they also are vulnerable to other injuries because of their gender. Women are exposed to numerous health hazards through sexual activity and childbearing. Neither of those, of course, is hazardous to a healthy woman with a healthy partner. One woman in 3,300 in the United States and 1 woman in 7,300 in Canada die from complications of pregnancy and childbirth. In sub-Saharan Africa, 1 in 13 women dies from pregnancy or childbirth. In South Asia, 1 woman in 35 dies from obstetric causes. According to UNICEF, over half a million women each year die from reproductive causes, and 18 million are disabled. UNICEF's 1996 report, *The Progress of Nations*, estimates 75,000 deaths per year from abortions, 75,000 from eclampsia, 100,000 from blood poisoning, 40,000 from obstructed labor, and 140,000 from hemorrhage (UNICEF 1996). Almost all the carnage is avoidable with simple prenatal care and accessible delivery centers for complicated births. These are horrible, protracted deaths that are easy to prevent.

Instead of improving, the situation is worsening in some places. In the Argentine province of Salta, maternal mortality increased from 110 deaths per 100,000 in 1987 to 150 per 100,000 in 1990, a 27 percent increase in four years. One-fourth of births in Salta are in the home (Villa 1991, 85). The rate in Salta is said to be three times the national rate, but the latter is widely thought to be a gross underestimate. The measurement method attributes deaths to obstetric causes only during a limited period of time and fails to count deaths that are not immediate. A study in 1985 of deaths of all women between fifteen and forty-nine years of age in Buenos Aires and Córdoba found that, when death certificates were checked against medical histories, the actual rate for Buenos Aires should have been 79 deaths per 100,000 live births, not 50, and for Córdoba the rate should have been 76, not 32, per 100,000 live births (Pignotti 1992*b*, 17).

The causes of maternal mortality are strongly correlated with, if not strictly dictated by, poverty. Cephalopelvic disproportion results from inadequate pelvic development of the mother due to malnutrition and causes death when she does not have prenatal care and access to a life-saving Caesarean section. As a result, two lives are wasted in a gruesome ordeal. Eclampsia, too, results from nutritional deficiency and lack of prenatal care.[5]

A category of maternal mortality that is difficult to quantify is that of deaths due to induced abortion, certainly a grave problem in Argentina and elsewhere. In Argentina, where abortion is illegal, 10 percent of abortions lead to hemorrhage or infection. In the Federal Capital, 4 out of every 1,000 women who enter the hospital after an abortion die. Some estimates are as high as 1,000 abortions a day in Argentina and one maternal death every other day (*Clarín*, November 24, 1991, p. 38). That would mean that 5 percent of all women from fifteen to forty-nine years of age have an abortion every year, an estimate I find too high to be credible.[6] Twenty to 40 percent of the beds in gynecology wards in public hospitals are said to be occupied by women suffering complications from illegal abortions (Pignotti 1992*b*, 17). There are many reports on abortion in the Argentine press, but much of the data come from the same source, and the methodology in that source is seriously flawed.

Early research on induced abortion by Tietze and Murstein (1975) excluded data from Latin America because they concluded that women's reporting of pregnancy loss was unreliable in the region. Women would not report abortions, which were both illegal and socially sanctioned. A Pan American Health Organization report by Santiago Gaslonde (1975) initiated a methodology that counted all unsuccessful pregnancies as induced abortions. Key Argentine researchers, following that methodology, assume that all abortions are induced, that is, that there are no miscarriages or stillbirths (Llovet and Ramos 1988, 10–11). That approach ignores the most salient fact, that most unsuccessful pregnancies and most maternal deaths occur among poor women. Neither problem can be correctly addressed when bad epidemiology fails to identify the poverty-induced causes of child and maternal death.

Doctors who work with poor women and who have collected the only data on prenatal, perinatal, and neonatal death, find that stillbirths outnumber neonatal deaths and that stillbirths and miscarriages are generally the result of infection. (See Chapter 10.) Maternal death due to induced abortion is a hazard almost exclusively for the poor (because wealthier women can pay for safer abortions), but maternal mortality is not solely due to induced abortion. Poor women die in pregnancy because they are malnourished, because they lack prenatal care, because they get vaginal infections, because they are unattended or badly attended in birth, and because they hemorrhage or get infections from unnecessary Caesarean sections performed for the convenience of doctors and the profit of the hospital. Also, many die because they have illegal, induced abortions.

It is possible that a reason, conscious or unconscious, for adopting such a methodology was to provide a rationale for legalizing abortion. To focus health services for women on the provision of abortion, however, does not serve the needs that poor women face. As the Pan American Health Organization notes, "Rather than being an option itself, abortion reflects a lack of options" (PAHO 1990a, 123). Abortion is a poor response to sexual violence, lack of information, and the spread of misinformation. It does not answer women's needs for equality and respect in domestic relationships. It is not a good solution for women who wish to plan their families. If services to women are defined as access to abortion, they do nothing to reduce the mortality and morbidity from infection, malnutrition, and lack of prenatal care.

The problem is framed as though the difficulty of family planning resides in the refusal of health practitioners to help women rather than in the broader issue of gender relations. The World Bank reported in 1987 that "Public hospitals and health centers do not provide family planning care; physicians working in public services provide covert advice and prescriptions in exceptional cases only; and Social Security [obras sociales] pays for contraceptives in exceptional cases only" (World Bank 1987a, 6). That information is dated or offers a very limited view and does not accord with what is observed in the health centers. Although there are not enough primary health care centers, the ones there are provide information on fertility control. Every center I visited in Argentina provided contraceptive advice and counseling, privately or in classes. When the health center was far from the neighborhood, the gynecologist went to the soup kitchen to give classes in fertility control. It is estimated that half the 700,000 women who take the pill have self-prescribed it because in Argentina it is available over-the-counter (Pignotti 1992*b*, 17). The pill, however, is an unreliable method for many poor women because they cannot always be sure of having the money for it.

The biggest obstacle for women is not the lack of information or the lack of services. It is their unequal status in relationships, which is not a condition specific to the poor. Social workers told me that the women with whom they worked preferred to practice rhythm and attended classes at the health centers in natural family planning. If the husbands came home drunk, however, the women's planning was to no avail (Health Center Number 149, Godoy Cruz, Mendoza, November 1, 1991). Many women opt for sterilization, although they are not happy with it. In the context of their low status, they see it as the only workable solution (PAHO 1990*a*, 135). Inequality of responsibility and risk, of course, is not only an issue for poor women or those in the developing world. Information alone will not defend women who have no rights. What women need is for community organizations to make men's responsibility and women's equality a top priority. Social organizations, women's groups, church groups, governmental offices, and nongovernmental organizations would advance public health generally and overall development if they were to make a priority of women's rights and dignity within the family. The ability to plan healthy families follows from that status. Planning when to be pregnant seems pointless if nothing else in a woman's life is under her control and if even the pregnancies she plans fail because of infection or malnutrition.

Maternal mortality is one area of health that can improve with or without changes in income if the government decides to make it a priority. "Experiences in countries in the [Panamerican] Region and elsewhere have shown that reductions in maternal mortality do not parallel economic development. Maternal mortality can be reduced through well-provided and well-organized maternal care systems, even under those conditions where it is impossible to improve the overall living conditions of women of childbearing age" (PAHO 1990*a*, 122). Because childbearing is a discrete event, rather than the fabric of a person's life, it can be addressed in community campaigns for prenatal care and institutional births (where needed). The added advantage of prenatal care is the opportunity to educate women in other aspects of their own health and that of their families. The fact that maternal mortality can be reduced even without other changes in the environment of poverty does not contradict the assertion that health is an economic issue. For specific health conditions, such as childbearing or parasitic diseases, direct medical or sanitary intervention is effective. The decision to allocate national resources to such interventions is an economic choice.

Other health hazards with disproportionate impact on women are sexually transmitted diseases (STDs). For many women, STDs are occupational diseases, which they contract not only as sex workers but also in their occupational role as housewives. In Thailand, it is said that the greatest risk for women of contracting AIDS is in marriage (Wheeler 1996, A9). The unequal status of men and women in most countries means that women will be exposed to STDs by their husbands or boyfriends who also utilize prostitutes or have multiple partners. There is a bitter cycle for some women who contract STDs from their husbands, who have been infected by prostitutes. The reproductive tract infection renders the woman infertile, and she is then abandoned by her husband and his family. Her only means of survival may be to join the ranks of the prostitutes. It is estimated that 70 percent of infertility in developing countries is due to STDs. Another serious hazard for women is ectopic pregnancy. Eighty percent of ectopic pregnancies are thought to be caused by pelvic inflammatory disease from STDs. Ectopic pregnancy is an important cause of maternal mortality and, in survivors, of infertility. Papilloma virus is sexually transmitted and causes cervical cancer. About 350,000 women die of cervical cancer each year in developing countries (Jacobson 1992, 10–13). With an early Pap smear and treatment, women generally will survive cervical cancer. A study of cancer in Rosario, Argentina, showed a high correlation between cervical cancer and illiteracy, unskilled occupations, and poor housing (Poletto and Morini 1990, 201–205).

There are a number of reasons why it is difficult for women to protect themselves from STDs or to seek a cure. In unequal relationships, men have the say over birth control. The use of condoms would help to protect women from their partners' infections. In the developing world, the few clinics that treat STDs are used by men and prostitutes and, therefore, are avoided by women, who do not want to be ostracized. Sex education and diagnosis of STDs are not incorporated into primary health care, even where that is available (Jacobson 1992, 14, 16). A fundamental problem with control of STDs is the failure of health centers to educate the public. Husbands and their families blame the woman for the infection and the infertility. If the prevalence and etiology of the diseases were understood, it would be clear that the infected woman is suffering from a situation not of her own making and experienced by many of her sisters as well.

The extent of the epidemic in STDs is astounding. The rates vary among diseases and populations, but in many cases are extremely high. Up to 23 percent of women in some African regions are infected with chlamydia. In some rural areas of India, almost 50 percent of women have reproductive tract infections. In one study of rural Maharashtra State in India, 92 percent of women examined had at least one gynecological infection. The average number of infections per woman was 3.6 (Jacobson 1992, 12). Median estimate of gonorrhea prevalence in Africa, based on thirty-nine studies, was 10 percent. Up to 40 percent of women aged thirty to thirty-four in some central African cities were found to be infected with AIDS. Some estimates of the proportion of adults in sub-Saharan Africa and Southeast Asia infected with hepatitis B are as high as 95 percent, but I do not find that estimate credible. (McDermott et al. 1993, 92–93).[7]

For women working in the sex industry, rates of STDs, including AIDS, are even higher. In many countries, prostitution is common, and in some, the sex industry is a major source of foreign exchange. As AIDS has become both more widespread and more well known, STDs have become a pediatric concern as well. European and North American sex tourists have created a demand for younger and younger victims in the belief that a younger partner is less likely to be infected. In fact, children are more fragile and more likely to suffer abrasions or other injuries that invite the transmission of STDs. The prevalence of AIDS among prostitutes is extremely high and the widespread frequenting of prostitutes makes the disease a national health problem.[8] Other STDs are an important cofactor for AIDS, and sex workers, who are also poor and poorly attended in health care, have high rates of STDs. Prostitutes tend to aggregate on truck routes and in hub cities. In Argentina, in addition to the usual downtown locations for prostitutes, women stand out along the highways under the overpasses and wave down truckers (visit, Rosario, September 1993). Transport workers have been a key transmission factor in West Africa, Southeast Asia, and elsewhere that AIDS is extremely prevalent. They carry the infection to prostitutes around the country and also to their wives and girlfriends at home. Prison populations have very high rates of HIV, and conjugal visits carry the infection outside. In Argentina, it is estimated that one-third of prisoners are HIV positive, although the lack of broad screening could mean that is a serious underestimate. In Brazil, 20 percent of male prisoners and 35 percent of female prisoners are HIV positive (Sims 1996, A4).

In malnourished populations, HIV infection seems to spread faster, possibly accelerated by vitamin A deficiency. Studies in Malawi indicate that when mothers are vitamin A deficient, they pass on the infection to their newborns more readily (Altman 1995c, A17). Although HIV transmission appears to be slowing in the industrialized countries, that does not yet appear to be the case in the developing world. Because the disease takes up to a decade to manifest itself, deaths will continue to rise for years to come. The daily increase in new cases is estimated by the United Nations to be 7,500. In 1995, there were about 980,000 deaths from AIDS. The estimate for 1996 is over 1.1 million deaths (Simons 1996, A3).

Occupational Safety and Health

Occupational hazards are another form of physical and psychological abuse, but with ends that are economic instead of political. The need for survival compels workers to ignore the daily threat to their safety and psychological well-being. Employers are not required to protect the work force, because legislation either does not exist or is not enforced. In developing countries, danger on the job is also aggravated by informality, since work in the informal sector is not covered by safety regulations. When one-fourth or more of the labor force works in the informal sector, it is difficult to control the workplace (Novik 1988, 364). National policies contribute to the lack of prevention. Social security generally pays for occupational disabilities (for those in the formal, covered sector) but rarely for preventive expenses (OPS 1992*a*, 256).

The association between economic class and vulnerability to occupational hazards is clear. A collapsing earthen wall, an exploding gas canister, chronic exposure to lint, metal particles, and noxious fumes—such hazards are all more likely for farm, industrial, and construction workers than for executives and professionals. Occupational exposure exacerbates other factors, including crowding at home, lack of ventilation, malnutrition, and long workdays. Particulate damage to the lungs, for example, contributes to tuberculosis (Epelman 1988, 362–363).

In most poor countries, preventive measures for job safety are inadequate, and few data are gathered to obtain a good epidemiological profile of occupational risk. The nature and the magnitude of the problem of occupational health have not been subject to systematic inquiry. The symptoms of occupational diseases, risk factors, and preventive measures are neglected in medical training (OPS 1992*a*, 256). The practices of medical diagnosis do not foster accurate data collection, especially for chronic conditions. Clinical histories give scant attention to place of work as a factor in disease or disability (Epelman 1988, 362).

Unless the cause of an accident is immediately obvious, it may be assumed to have been "an act of God." Explosions in factories are considered a matter of fate or bad luck rather than the result of carelessness that could have been avoided (Piccinini 1988, 371). A half-hearted and unscientific investigation is abandoned without instituting measures to prevent the next explosion. Such injuries are not an act of God but rather an act of carelessness, not necessarily of the worker, but of the social context of their work. Lack of emergency and first aid facilities aggravates the burden of injury, leading to greater mortality and disability (Smith and Barss 1991, 256).

When the effects of toxic exposure are not immediately visible, recognition of chronic health effects depends on follow-up exams, which are less likely where workers have little access to health care. Workers just leave the job and suffer and die, not realizing that their condition was work related. They do not receive the appropriate therapy, and their occupational disease is unrecorded by epidemiologists.[9]

Studies of occupational safety and health suggest an enormous toll in mortality and morbidity throughout the developing world, with very high costs. PAHO reports that costs of accidents alone to amount to 10 percent of GNP for developing countries (OPS 1992*a*, 256). Based on data provided by national governments, the World Health Organization estimates that there are fifty million work accidents each year worldwide, of which 180,000 are fatal (Epelman 1988, 360). But those statistics appear to be gross understatements. The Pan American Health Organization estimates 50,000 deaths per year in the Americas. That is an improbably low estimate, since there are more than 6,000 deaths per year due to work accidents in the United States alone (Nordheimer 1996, F1), and PAHO estimates that the incidence of accidents and occupational illness is six to ten times greater in developing countries than in industrialized countries. In industrialized countries, about 10 percent of workers have a work accident each year. In Brazil, reported work accidents affect one in every five workers. In Argentina, epidemiological data of all kinds deteriorated under the military dictatorship, but occupational health and safety in particular was neglected (Epelman 1988, 360–361).

Although many of the hazards overlap, the following discussion is divided into rural work, industrial work, hospital work, work stress, and the particular hazards for women. The toll in morbidity and mortality is enormous. Millions of people go to work every day putting their lives on the line.

The extent of work injuries is least known in the rural areas because epidemiological research generally is conducted in city hospitals and because rural people often go to traditional healers. Rural workers either die from their injuries or recover, but neither event is recorded. An Indian study of occupational hazards in the countryside found that injuries constituted 14 percent of all morbidity. Agricultural machinery, such as threshers and fodder cutters, are the source of numerous injuries, including hand crushings and amputations. Extrapolating from the data collected in the sample region, researchers estimated serious injuries related to agriculture to amount to five million per year in India, with 500,000 deaths (Mohan 1993, 12–13). That suggests a large upward revision of WHO estimates for worldwide incidence.

An important occupational hazard of agricultural workers is exposure to pesticides, many of which are banned in the United States and other industrialized countries. Toxins enter the body through the skin, the respiratory system, and the digestive system. Sometimes multiple toxins have additive effects. The effects might neutralize each other, but more generally, they add together, increasing the toxicity of individual chemical exposures (British Medical Association 1991, 66–72). Agricultural workers, poorly clothed even for normal work, are not protected from skin contact with caustic chemicals they spray from foggers or that is sprayed on them from airplanes. Workers and often their children are used as field markers, to indicate to cropdusters the fields to be sprayed (Wright 1990, 20). Often they live in or at the edge of fields that are sprayed from the air. In addition to skin contact, particulate and gaseous poisons enter the lungs through breathing passages. Pesticides also settle on foods, cooking utensils, and eating areas of shacks in and near the fields. Pesticides also remain on the hands and clothes and are ingested. The workers wash in irrigation canals and get their drinking and cooking water from those same chemically contaminated sources (Michaels et al. 1985, 97). Agricultural workers are particularly at risk because they often are illiterate and cannot read the warnings on labels or the instructions for proper use.[10] The hazard to rural workers is exacerbated by their isolation. Workers who attempt to find out about pesticide hazards, farm union organizers who attempt to warn workers, and doctors who report pesticide poisonings have disappeared and have been tortured and killed (Faber 1993, 102).

One pound of pesticides for every person on the planet is used every year (Weber 1992, 20). Although 80 percent of pesticide use is in the industrialized world, 80 percent of reported pesticide deaths are in the developing world (Gardner 1996, 90). Of the one million pesticide poisonings per year, three-fourths result in chronic disability, including dermatitis, nervous disorders, and cancer. Estimates of deaths from accidental poisoning range from 4,000 to 19,000 per year (Weber 1992, 20). China recorded 10,000 deaths from pesticide poisoning in 1993 (Gardner 1996, 90), which makes 19,000 deaths for the entire world seem a very low estimate.

Poisonings that do not result in immediate death can still have serious consequences, including respiratory diseases, cancers, reproductive disorders, and birth defects. In 1993, the World Health Organization reported that 21 percent of Indonesian farmers exhibited three or more symptoms of poisoning during the spraying season. In Costa Rica, a pesticide banned in the United States for its toxicity caused sterility in 1,500 male banana plantation workers (*World Resources 1994–1995*, 115). In Mexico, field workers on tomato farms that export produce to the United States market suffer from nervous disorders from organophosphate poisoning. To prevent workers from going to local doctors, who are required to report the poisonings, foremen treat workers in the field with a temporary antidote, atropine (Wright 1990, 41).

Recognizing pesticide poisoning can be hampered by inadequate research on how work is actually performed. When researchers studied floriculture workers in Greater Buenos Aires, they expected that the pesticide sprayers would exhibit the greatest effects of poisoning. When they observed the work methods, it was clear that the sprayers were the least affected, since they passed through the greenhouses with the fog falling behind them. The women and children who entered the tightly sealed greenhouses afterward were immersed in the poisonous fog. In the floriculture of Florencio Varela (GBA), among symptomatic and asymptomatic workers, 43.5 percent had low white-cell counts consistent with chlorofluorocarbon pesticide poisoning, which causes leukemia and bone marrow cancer (Albiano 1991, 136). Another unexpected category of exposed workers was truck drivers because agricultural products often are sprayed in the truck. The poison control center for the city of Rosario, a major shipping point for agricultural products, handled 8,400 cases of pesticide poisoning, including 1,300 cases of acute poisoning, from 1976 to 1985 (Carbonara 1991, 84–85).

The hazards of pesticides extend beyond the workers to the consumers. Examples abound of accidental poisoning from careless storage or shipment of pesticides. In one case in 1985, a number of babies died in Salta because powdered milk was shipped in a truck used to carry parathion, a pesticide. Epidemiological monitoring of pesticide poisoning was abandoned in Argentina for lack of budget. In spite of illiteracy and low education levels, pesticide poisoning is not inevitable. Workers can be trained in the safe use of pesticides through audio-visual materials that could also teach people about personal hygiene and washing equipment and clothes (Higa de Landoni 1991, 165, 175).

The hazards of rural work defy complete enumeration but include bites by stray, possibly rabid dogs; goring by cattle, buffalo, and wild pigs; crocodile attacks; bites and stings by insects, arachnids, and reptiles; and drowning. Farm and forest workers are most affected by unconquered viruses, such as Argentine hemorrhagic fever (a hantavirus), and parasites, such as leishmaniasis, a disfiguring parasite for which there is neither prevention nor cure (*Diario de Cuyo*, November 5, 1991, p. 4). Farmers and fishermen in many developing countries also are more likely to contract schistosomiasis due to their greater contact with still water where the snails that carry the parasite reside. Migrant workers live in unhygienic shelters provided by farm owners. Four years after the cholera outbreak began in northern Argentina, northern migrants to Río Negro and Neuquén still were housed in "cramped, makeshift shelters with no running water or sanitary facilities" (*Buenos Aires Herald*, January 21, 1996, p. 4), threatening to bring the disease to the southern provinces.

The hazards of industry include explosions, burns, amputations and crushings from unguarded machinery, and exposure to noise, noxious fumes, and particulate pollution. The exposure is aggravated by the long work week in most developing countries. Safety standards established in the United States are based on a presumption of exposure in a five-day, forty-hour week. But in Argentina and other countries, the typical work week is six days, so the time of exposure is longer. Further, toxic effects can be increased by malnutrition. Anemia produced by lead exposure is aggravated by hookworm, for example (Michaels et al. 1985, 103–104). The list of disasters around the world involving mercury, arsenic, polyvinyl chlorides, manganese, lint (causing byssinosis, or brown lung), as-bestos, dioxins, chrome, and organophosphates is sickeningly long. The injuries are not isolated cases. A large proportion of the workers in each plant are af-fected. In one chloralkali plant in Nicaragua that had puddles of mercury on the floor, one-third of workers exhibited central nervous system damage (Ives 1985, 181). In battery factories in Medellín, Colombia, 71 percent of workers were found to have extremely high lead exposure. In other industries in Colombia, 28 percent of textile workers suffer from pulmonary disease; 15 percent of coal min-ers suffer from pneumoconiosis; and 70 percent of workers exposed to high noise levels suffer hearing loss. Forty percent of tin miners in Bolivia have sili-cosis or tuberculosilicosis. In São Paulo, Brazil, 87 percent of electroplaters had chromium-induced lesions, including people who had worked less than a year at the job (Michaels et al. 1985, 99–100).

Minimal safety equipment is not available. Workers get ulcers on their feet be-cause they stand in pools of acid wearing only sandals. When safety equipment is available, it often is inappropriate, such as gloves that are too short or easily punctured (Michaels et al. 1985, 101). It is commonplace to see workers in the streets of Buenos Aires using welding equipment without eye protection.

Even where health and safety legislation exists, lack of enforcement permits ongoing pollution and work hazards. Dock Sud is across the Riachuelo River from La Boca, in Avellaneda (province of Buenos Aires). Environmental control of Dock Sud was transferred to the province in 1993. Because the province does not enforce the federal hazardous waste law, municipal authorities have been hampered in attempts to clean up the area. Workers unload bulk sulphur, soda ash, and urea without protective clothing or breathing apparatus. Uncovered trucks with loads of toxic powders drive from the docks and into the city. Doctors in the surrounding neighborhoods report that skin and bronchial illnesses ac-count for 80 percent of doctor visits (Tucker 1995, 13).

The Argentine government not only ignores safety violations, it perpetrates them itself. In 1995, a government bomb factory exploded twice in the same month. The November 3 explosion at Río Tercero killed seven people and injured 330. The explosions hurled bombs into the neighborhood surrounding the plant, dropping live, two-foot-long mortar shells into a house nearly a half-mile from the factory. When warm weather set off a fire and further explosions at the plant on November 24, another person was killed. The Defense Minister admitted that the government knew there was risk of further explosions but kept people working at the plant. In spite of the government's assurances that the factory would be closed and the director fined, again in May of 1996 residents of Río Tercero had to be evacuated because of a nitric acid leak at the arms factory (*Buenos Aires Herald*, November 5, 1995, pp. 1, 4; November 26, 1995, p. 1; May 12, 1996, p. 4).

Disregard of safety is not restricted to farm and industrial workers. An Argentine Ministry of Labor study of nurses and surgery teams found that "absolutely no preventive norms were respected." They handled carcinogenic cleaning substances without protection. "[T]he concentration of anesthetic gases in the surgery theaters was as much as 100 times acceptable levels" (Rodríguez 1988, 386). The gases increase the risk of cancer 2.7 times, affect fertility, and provoke miscarriages and malformations. An expenditure of $50 could provide the protection required. The Labor Department investigators found a level of fatalism among the hospital workers that they expected to find only among factory or farm workers. Hospital workers who complain of the dangers are dealt with repressively. Hospital workers reacted dramatically to AIDS, although there have been many more deaths of medical workers from hepatitis B (Rodríguez 1988, 386–387).

Laundry workers are at high risk because they handle soiled linens. The staff often leave needles in the bedding, which results in numerous puncture wounds. In radiology, not one of the workers interviewed knew how many rems (units of radiation) he or she received per year, because there is no procedure for recording the exposure of each worker. The hazard is that much greater because most hospital workers in Argentina, whether doctors or nurses, have to work double shifts due to low pay (Rodríguez 1988, 387).[11]

There are many categories of job stress for workers, both blue collar and white. Insecurity of job tenure and the threat of lost income are among the most severe stresses, especially since the majority of workers have no savings. The stresses created by employers' attempts at cost cutting are costly in themselves. Stress leads to absenteeism, high turnover rates, and sabotage. Half of absenteeism is preventable, and 40 percent of turnover is due to stress (Karasek and Theorell 1990, 168). To the stress of insecurity is added the daily insult of the bad manners of supervisors, deprecating remarks, physical discomfort of badly designed work spaces, noise, odors, filth, lack of chairs, poor lighting, dirty windows, poor ventilation, drafts, extremes of temperature, lack of water fountains, ill-maintained and unattractive bathrooms, low-quality food in the cafeteria, and the daily trudge through an unpleasant neighborhood to get to the job site (Shostak 1980, 27). For women, the stresses are aggravated by remarks and behavior of male coworkers and supervisors that threaten and demean women sexually.

Women workers face additional risk at work because of the fatigue induced by their double work loads. A study of women in Guadalajara, Mexico, confirmed what so many others have shown, that even women employed full-time outside the home work thirty-four to forty-two hours per week in domestic tasks (Uribe Vásquez et al. 1991, 104). Women are used in work requiring speed, mental and visual acuity, concentration, and manual dexterity, all of which have particular injuries, such as carpal tunnel syndrome, loss of sight, and headaches. Piecework, which is common for women in textile work, is stressful and causes higher rates of stomach ulcers and tranquilizer use. In the health sector, women tend to work in the lower-status and more dangerous jobs and are exposed to radiation and biologically and chemically toxic substances (Paltiel 1989, 147, 151, 153).

One out of every five women working in cities in Latin America in 1985 was a domestic (León 1989, 355). Domestics, especially live-in maids, have long work days (Paltiel 1989, 155) and the least legal protection of any workers. When they become pregnant or ill or are too old to work quickly they are turned out, swelling the population of people living on the streets (León 1989, 356, 359).

Women workers suffer pathologies that affect their reproductive organs, although the etiology is not gender specific. Women who work with farm animals can contract brucellosis, which lodges in the reproductive tract and causes tubo-ovarian and pelvic abscesses. In the apparel trades, women have higher incidence of breast, uterine, and cervical cancers because of the chemicals used in dyeing and finishing (Paltiel 1989, 148, 150). Women in those trades also have higher risk of those cancers because, as poor women, they have less access to early warning tests, such as Pap smears and mammograms. Women generally carry the water for the family, which can be an onerous task, especially for women who have had many pregnancies. Carrying water can use up 12 percent of daily caloric intake. In mountainous or arid regions, where the trek is longer, it can use up one-fourth of the woman's energy intake, aggravating malnutrition, especially for pregnant and lactating women. As water haulers and clothes washers, women have greater exposure to contaminated water. In addition to the usual risk from the whole gamut of waterborne diseases, infectious hepatitis generally is fatal during pregnancy (PAHO 1990a, 127).

Costs of Adult Ill Health

Adults are the economically active population on whom the old and young depend. Illness and disability limit the output of adults and impoverish the next generation of workers. "Inadequate health care for workers leads to low productivity and high absenteeism, early aging, a shorter active life span, and poor quality of life. These conditions affect not only the workers but also their families, contributing to increasing poverty and the worsening of the economic situation" (PAHO 1990a, 50). Illness and physical and mental disability impose costs on the individual and on society. In addition to the psychic costs for the individual and the family and friends of the person afflicted, there are direct economic costs and the opportunity cost of lost output.

Medical costs for developing countries are multiplied because of the "epidemiologic accumulation," the very high rates of infectious and parasitic diseases and unintentional injuries, and high rates of chronic noncommunicable diseases. Cardiovascular disease is the number one cause of death in thirty-one Western

Hemisphere nations, and malignant tumors are the second leading cause of death in about half the countries of the region (PAHO 1990a, 93). Since poor people fall ill with chronic diseases earlier than the affluent, they depend on expensive curative care longer. The average low- to middle-income country spends 4 percent of the central government budget on health services (with a range of 1 percent to 19 percent). (Argentina spent about 1 percent of its federal budget on health care in the comparable period of the mid-1980s.) That amounts to 1 to 2 percent of GNP as an international average, to which another 1 to 5 percent of GNP is spent on private medical care. In almost all countries, more than 50 percent of health care costs are for hospital care, and 70 percent or more of hospital costs are for adults (Over et al. 1992, 170).

Although chronic conditions constitute a large proportion of morbidity, medical training, facilities, or local practices do not permit modern cost-saving curative methods. For example, in 1987 in Argentina, there were 3,000 patients with kidney disease on dialysis, costing $45 million a year. Each dialysis patient cost $15,000 a year (Braun 1987, 40). Transplants would be cost effective, but the social climate does not foster organ donations since it involves helping strangers. Eighty percent of patients who need liver transplants and 60 percent of those who need heart transplants die while waiting for a donor. Transplants still are not a viable option in Argentina because, for patients who do receive kidney transplants, the survival rate is the lowest in the world, according to Hector Estraviz, head of the Argentine Transplant Association (*Buenos Aires Herald*, October 20, 1991, p. 4).

Accidents are a leading cause of death in many countries and cause even more cases of permanent disability. Treatment for injuries is expensive, and since young people are more prone to accidents, the costs extend over a long period of time. Prevention of accidents is barely mentioned in medical education (PAHO 1990a, 102). The direct medical costs of treating adult illness and disability are attributable largely to avoidable conditions. Child deaths have long been recognized as largely avoidable. Now it is clear that three-fourths of adult deaths in the developing world are attributable to avoidable causes (Murray et al. 1992b, 29).

The other cost of adult illness and disability is the opportunity cost of absenteeism due to illness, years of productive life lost due to premature death, the productivity loss for coworkers and family members who substitute for those out sick, and lower productivity on the job from illness, fatigue, and impairment. Quantifying the opportunity cost is complicated by a number of factors. First, the impact on productivity, household income, and national income is due not only to mortality but also to adult morbidity. The extent of adult morbidity is not known. In China, for example, where 32 percent of adults in the developing world live, there is no nationwide data collection on morbidity. A survey system covers only one out of every ten households and extrapolates national estimates (Murray et al. 1992*b*, 82–83). Even that system is probably more comprehensive than in many countries.

Lacking morbidity data, countries use mortality estimates to measure the loss of work time. Because morbidity is not necessarily proportional to mortality, its impact on adult work performance is underestimated (Murray et al. 1992*a*, 113). Parasites, such as helminths, and diseases such as malaria and Chagas', can cause death, but more often they leave the worker disabled for part or all of the year. Malaria can recur every rainy season. Injuries can leave a worker with only partial use of limbs. Furthermore, chronic conditions, endured by a large proportion of the population, often go unrecorded. People may not even recognize the toll it takes on their work performance because they cannot picture what the counterfactual would be. Since everybody is ailing, they cannot imagine nor can they measure a well person's potential output. To construct a test of the output loss, what would be the control group? Where would you find someone without worms? There are, nevertheless, important output-dampening effects of morbidity, even though it is part of people's everyday lives.

Early attempts to measure productivity loss from poor health (Gwatkin 1983) were inadequately specified. Instead of throwing out the implausible results and starting over, Gwatkin concluded that it was not possible to confirm a link between good health and greater productivity and wealth. In 1988, Andreano and Helmeniak came to the same conclusion, but they inferred that results so obviously counterintuitive must suggest that households and firms cope with illness and disability, somehow compensating for productivity losses. Coping imposes costs, which are multiplied as each person in the circle of family and friends adapts work output, study, leisure, food intake, or land purchases in the face of an illness or death.

The inadequacies of the earlier models were addressed in a study for the World Bank (Over et al. 1992). The study concluded that, in countless ways, firms and households do bear the cost of illness and disability in lower consumption, investment, production, and earnings. When children miss school to take over household tasks or to care for adults, their future contribution is diminished. When family members and coworkers compensate by working harder, that diminishes the other work they would have done on the job or at home. The advantages of specialization are lost when one person must do two jobs. Anticipating illness, employers build slack into production schedules or require less specialization of employees (Over et al. 1992, 161–162).

Coping among farm workers takes various forms. In a Sudanese study, each household lost, on average, forty work hours per year from malaria alone. Families self-insure, in the absence of disability insurance or sick pay. In the Sudan study, other families members worked harder but were able to make up only 68 percent of the lost output. "When illness strikes, an individual's lost output and earnings often go undetected in economic statistics because they are borne by the household" (World Bank 1993, 18). In the Sudan, those affected by malaria could not work for 22 percent of the year (*World Health* 1997, 50(1): 28). In another type of coping, farmers in Paraguay grew crops of lower value because they could be grown outside the malaria season (World Bank 1993, 18). That was a sensible, but not optimal, solution. Such coping behavior is exactly what was practiced at the University of Dar es Salaam, Tanzania, when I taught there in 1984 and 1985. The certainty of malaria is such that employers must allow for frequent absences when they plan their hiring. The economics department left two faculty members without course assignments each semester. Those two would fill in for professors who fell ill during the semester. Each course was divided into topics that were distributed among the staff to allow greater flexibility in substitutions. The prediction was correct: during the year, every Tanzanian professor fell ill. The coping mechanism for the university was expensive, but the planned output was maintained.

Other significant costs to society were documented by the World Bank study. Infant and child survival is greatly reduced by a maternal death. Some of the increase in child mortality is due to postnatal transmission of maternal disease to the child, as in tuberculosis; some is through congenital transmission, as in malaria, herpes, toxoplasmosis, or syphilis; and some is due to the malnutrition that provoked the mother's death as well. But much of the increased infant and child mortality is due to the central role of mothers in ensuring child survival. The death of any adult, but especially the death of a woman, affects sanitation, water supply, food, and affective support. In Bangladesh, the death rate of male children doubled with a mother's death, and deaths of daughters tripled. Adult morbidity also is harmful to household members. Each year of living with a TB-infected person generates a 30-percent risk of infection and a 1- to 2-percent risk of active disease (Over et al. 1992, 164–167).

Another inefficient outcome of adult ill health is the loss of productive assets. The poor use up all their liquid assets in a major illness and then sell their land. After that wealth is used up, treatment stops. In Thailand, 60 percent of all involuntary land sales are due to ill health; in Kenya, 24 percent of land transactions are due to ill health (Over et al. 1992, 187–188). The entire household loses its source of employment and income due to the illness of an adult member.

In calculating the costs of adult illness, another opportunity cost should be kept in mind. Because much of adult ill health is noncommunicable and caused by consumption or overconsumption of noxious substances, the cost of diverting scarce national resources to their production is not a small issue in very poor countries. The production of refined sugars, refined grains, alcohol, tobacco, and high-fat foods allocates resources to products that produce chronic disease and imposes double costs on society (Campbell and Chen 1994, 68).

Other infectious and parasitic diseases, such as guinea worm and onchocerciasis, take a heavy toll on workers and on their productivity. River blindness, as onchocerciasis is called, has left huge areas of West Africa uninhabited. The most fertile, well-watered areas, ideal for agriculture, are uninhabited because of that scourge. In recent years, tremendous progress has been made in eradicating river blindness, thanks to the recognition of the effects of blindness on production and the donation of the drug ivermectin by its manufacturer, Merck. Half a million people have been spared from blindness as a result of the campaign, at a cost of less than one dollar per person per year. Twenty-five million hectares (more than sixty million acres) of land have been reopened to settlement because the disease is being eliminated (World Bank 1993, 19). Since the onchocerciasis control program began, more that 1.7 million additional years of productive labor have been made available (*World Health* 1997, 50(1): 28). The forest strain of onchocerciasis, which does not lead to blindness, has been relatively neglected. Now health workers are recognizing the burden caused by the incessant itching and disfiguring lesions that lead to ostracism. The lesions dampen productivity by depriving people of work and limit their ability to work when they do have jobs (Leary 1995).

Nutritional deficiencies, which may be difficult to measure directly, can be evaluated from the increase in output that results from supplementing nutrition. Iron supplements increased productivity even in short-run trials. In long-run studies in the United States, Sri Lanka, and Indonesia, sustained nutritional supplementation increased work capacity (Over et al. 1992, 184). In a study of latex workers, iron supplements increased work by approximately 20 percent. The benefit-cost ratio of the experiment was 260:1 (Read 1977, 104).

Rehabilitative services are not common in developing countries; therefore, people have less opportunity to contribute to family income after an illness or injury. Only 4 percent of Argentine hospitals have rehabilitative services. Of countries surveyed by PAHO, the best services were in Chile and Colombia, each with about 14.5 percent of hospitals having rehabilitative services (PAHO 1990a, 113). When the lack of rehabilitation is combined with social or cultural attitudes that stigmatize families with a disabled member, the person's contribution is completely lost. The disabled person is confined at home and never interacts in society. PAHO estimates that 10 percent of the population in any country have some kind of disability. In the United States, 14 percent of the population are limited in activity due to chronic health conditions (PAHO 1990a, 112). In Mexico alone, there are 600,000 paraplegics (Crossette 1996, A7). Worldwide, the loss of productive input of less than fully able, employable adults is enormous. The loss of their social interaction is tragic.

Illness and disability of adults impose heavy costs on developing countries. Adults suffer the chronic burden of childhood afflictions and new injuries and illnesses from work, motherhood, poor diet, and lack of medical care and leisure. Adult illness leads to high medical costs and reduced productivity during the most productive years. Communities, families, and employers cope with illness by compensatory behavior that entails significant cost. The loss of output for the hundreds of millions of people who will never be able to work to their potential is unmeasured. As hard as they work, they have so little to enjoy. Illness exacerbates fatalism and passivity, stifling democracy and development.

It would be useful to have more studies that quantify the effect of ill health on work performance. But we do not need to wait until those studies are completed to begin to remedy the situation. If we wish to know if development is held back by disease and disability, we only have to consider the obvious. Does it affect a woman's agricultural work output to be afflicted with the discomfort of a reproductive tract infection? Does it rob her of incentive to work hard in the fields when she knows that her infertility, once discovered, will cause her husband's family to throw her out? What is the productivity loss from blindness in a rural worker? What does the community lose when one-fourth of the adult population is mentally impaired due to iodine deficiency, a condition that can be prevented for pennies a year? What kind of workers do young people make when they have spent their teen years sniffing glue and eating from garbage cans? How much productivity is lost when a farm worker loses a hand to an unguarded threshing machine? How much more difficult is it to fetch water when a fractured bone is not set? Do hungry workers work energetically? Do workers with no upper teeth obtain the necessary nutrients to fuel a good day's work? Poor people often do not have just one disabling condition. How much does productivity falter when a field worker has three reproductive tract infections, two parasites, an unset fracture, and no upper teeth? That is the health status of a significant proportion of the world's work force. Can we calculate the GDP loss when a third of the population suffers from a combination such as malaria, guinea worm, hepatitis B, a toothache, *and* clinical depression? It simply is common sense to recognize the enormous waste of human potential and common decency to correct it.

Part V

Prospects for National Development

Thirteen

Healthy Development

This book has had three goals: to describe the living conditions of poor people in developing countries; to show that poverty and poor health undermine a nation's economy; and to offer reasonable, and often low-cost, ways to solve the problems of poor health and underdevelopment.

What I hope this book has conveyed is the inexorable bleakness that life can mean for the poor. That is not to say that poor people enjoy none of life's pleasures—love, humor, children, friendship. But the environment in which those pleasures are enjoyed is relentlessly daunting. To be poor is not like going on a rainy backpacking trip, then home to a dry, warm house with flush toilets. The bugs never go away. The smell never goes away. There is never enough privacy. There is never warm water at the turn of a faucet.

The discouraging web of poverty and ill health robs poor people of the chance to use their full energy, intellect, strength, flexibility, and creativity and robs the nation of their contribution. Many of the health problems of the poor have well-known, even simple, solutions. Each solution helps people overcome a dispiriting obstacle to well-being. The cumulative effect of these microsolutions contradicts fatalism and enables people to change their lives.

The environment of poverty invades every area of life—housing, sanitation, food, work, health care, sex. Home should provide shelter, comfort, respite, tranquility. Drafty, leaky shacks with dirt floors or tenements, sharing bath and kitchen with other households, are not very comforting. There is a constant tension keeping a shanty warm without having the house and its occupants go up in flames. Sleep provides little rest if thousands of bugs crawl out of the walls and roof and swarm over the inhabitants. When every night is a face-off with death from malaria-carrying mosquitoes, it is hard to wake up refreshed.

Water is essential and so difficult to obtain. After being hauled a great distance, the water likely will be contaminated, if not at the source, then in the house. Every sip adds more microbes to already compromised digestive systems. The cycle of contamination recurs in streams and groundwater fouled by human waste. Increasingly, the water people drink is not only biologically contaminated but also poisoned by heavy metals and chemical waste. Toxic industrial and hospital waste make it unhealthy for people to utilize the enormous quantity of discarded materials to be found in landfills. Even without such hazards, living off the dumps is a demoralizing existence because of the smell and the filth.

When people buy food at the local store, it might be contaminated. They line up for buses at five in the morning to fight for a handle on the outside of the bus as it hurtles along in the dark, cold gloom before dawn. At work, they are insulted and endangered. They have no protection from acids, fumes, shards, and poorly designed machinery.

If they are injured or their children are sick, they stand for hours in waiting rooms that are too cold or too hot, with no bathrooms. What should and can be a delightful experience, bearing children, many women face with dread, knowing that their chance of dying or being gravely disabled is high.

Each poor person confronts not just one hazard, but a whole grab bag of them. Men and women enter old age early, battered by life, in an environment that may deny them even one day of really good health. That they go on working, with intestinal parasites, reproductive tract infections, unhealed fractures, hemiplegic, anemic, and depressed, is testament to their indomitable humanity.

The question is often asked: "Why are these countries not developing?" Considering the condition of life for the majority of the people, we might ask instead, "How did these countries get this far?" The answer is that people are resourceful and devise remarkable ways of surviving. The outcome, however, is not optimal. The vast intelligence, strength, flexibility, and creativity of the population are squandered. The resources of the nation are thrown away.

This book is about the entire developing world, using Argentina as a case study. The extent and the degree of poverty vary greatly between the poorest of sub-Saharan and South Asian countries and the middle-income countries of Latin America. A larger proportion of Asian and African people live in conditions of extreme poverty. Different regions have different endemic pathologies—Chagas' disease in the Americas, yaws in Asia, onchocerciasis in Africa. Life expectancy also varies greatly, from thirty-nine years in Sierra Leone to seventy-six years in Costa Rica. The cause of death for women in Africa and South Asia is much more likely to be childbearing, and in Latin America, an undiagnosed cancer. For men, the cause of death or disability in South Asia or Africa could be snake bite or farm accident, and in Latin America, a bus accident. In spite of the differences, the similarities are numbing. Living near a chemical plant in Bhopal, India, *maquiladoras* along the U.S. border in Mexico exposes people to lethal industr toxins that cause blindness or anencephalic babies or leukemia.

The similarities of living in poverty around the world are reflected in every topic addressed by the present study, from housing to occupational injury, from oversight to repression. For every situation cited here for Argentina, countless more examples can be found in other countries. In Johannesburg, 250,000 people are homeless or live as squatters downtown, near highways, in garbage dumps, and in flood zones (Daley 1996b, A10). Throughout the Americas, eighteen million people are infected with Chagas' disease. In Africa, another trypanosome causes sleeping sickness and 200,000 deaths per year in Zaire alone (*Economist*, May 20, 1995, p. 15). Malaria is endemic in almost 100 countries and is spreading into areas in which it was previously unknown.

Argentina ranks as the twelfth-worst country in the world for rural access to clean water, sharing that rank with Afghanistan, Laos, Mozambique, and Zaire. But scores of other countries fail to provide decent water or sanitation for the urban and rural populations. About one-fourth of the world's population is without safe water and sanitation (Lean and Hinrichsen 1992, 31). In India, 700 million of the 930 million people have no toilets, and so either defecate into buckets or on open land. In Bangladesh, over 100 million people, about 90 percent of the population, do not have any sanitary means of disposing of excreta (Griffin and McKinley 1994, 48). Cholera, typhoid, and hepatitis A are widespread in Asia, Africa, and Latin America.

Contaminated food due to lax regulation is a threat to health in most countries. In India, at least fifty-two people died in one outbreak of food poisoning (Burns 1996, A3). Bus accidents are common because of poor maintenance and lack of inspection. One bus accident in Zimbabwe caused seventy-nine deaths in 1990, and another killed eighty-nine people the following year (Swaney 1995, 167). In island and coastal countries, ferry disasters are a repeated occurrence. In part due to weak oversight and cultural factors, AIDS is soon to be a universal threat. Wherever there is industry, there are accidents and industrial contaminants, not because such things are inevitable, but because little value is placed on the safety of workers and the health of the environment. Pesticides are used excessively and carelessly across the globe. Chronic underdevelopment and the inadequate government oversight associated with political underdevelopment leave the population unprotected.

The lack of medical care or the difficult circumstances of obtaining medical care are experienced by poor people everywhere. Reports from Nicaragua repeat what is seen in so many other places. People line up at hospital emergency rooms, avoiding peripheral health centers. Clinical histories are not maintained.

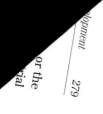
ts to a few minutes in a crowded room shared with other
little information or health education from physicians"

s reports demonstrating the greater efficacy of preventive
ealth spending in all countries still goes to expensive, high-
based care. The greatest proportion of money is spent on
the la~~ ours of life rather than on a healthy first five, or fifteen, or
seventy-five years. Even public health expenditure benefits chiefly the middle
and upper classes (Akin 1987). The outcomes for poor people are similar, although varying in degree. Infant death, childhood stunting, maternal mortality,
premature aging, death from curable diseases, and unnecessary disability because of lack of rehabilitative facilities are the common lot of poor people
throughout the developing world.

Another common thread in the developing world is the implementation of
structural adjustment programs to correct the weaknesses of earlier economic
plans. The oil price shocks of the 1970s exposed the shortcomings of economies
based on protection, rent seeking, and privilege for a small circle. When the
International Monetary Fund (IMF) first imposed conditionality on countries
needing balance of payments relief, it specifically excluded health and welfare
concerns from its analysis. The primary objectives were the restoration of balance of international payments, productivity, and inflation control, excluding con-
sideration of income distribution, employment, poverty, health, and nutrition.
"The basic assumption is that short-term belt-tightening is a necessary precon-
dition for long-term economic health. The problem with this approach is that the
poor, and poor women and children in particular, do not have the reserve for
short-term belt-tightening" (Chen 1988, 300).

The setbacks for health and education mean lower achievements in long-term
growth, even narrowly defined as an increase in GDP. What is needed is a strategy for sustainable development that not only protects natural resources from
plunder for debt servicing but also protects and enhances labor resources. By
cutting spending on health and education, structural adjustment plans trade long-
term development for short-term cost saving. When the IMF and the World
Bank recognized that health and education were not appropriate targets for government cutbacks, countries like Argentina did not heed their warnings. They
continue to impose the burden of adjustment on the most vulnerable members of
society.

Cuts in public health spending and sanitation have been shortsighted. The
avoidable disease outbreaks of the 1990s include equine encephalitis, malaria,
dengue, tuberculosis, measles, and the return of cholera in the Western Hemisphere. These diseases with well-known methods of control or cure reemerged
because prevention was neglected (Morse 1995). The 1995 outbreak of equine

encephalitis that infected 55,000 people in Colombia and Venezuela and caused about 350 deaths was 100-percent preventable, according to an epidemiologist from the U.S. Centers for Disease Control. "The technology existed first to prevent the outbreak, then to limit its spread, and finally, to avoid human deaths" (Schemo 1995, A1, A10).

In the 1950s and 1960s, *Aedes aegypti* mosquito populations were reduced or eradicated, and dengue disappeared in many locations in the Americas. Control programs were not sustained, however, and the mosquito reinfested all of Latin America, except Chile and Uruguay. Dengue is on the rise and, with it, dengue hemorrhagic fever and urban yellow fever (Brandling-Bennett and Pinheiro 1996). The cholera epidemic, which has now gained a foothold in almost every country in the Americas, was completely preventable. Maintenance and expansion of water and sanitation systems, accepted since the nineteenth century as a necessary role of government, have been abandoned.

Worsening income distribution, cutbacks, and even collapse of public services also are affecting the transition economies. The breakdown of civil order in the former Soviet Union has created a severe health crisis there. Regions that had well-established health-delivery systems are facing the specter of cholera, dysentery, diphtheria, polio, hepatitis A, measles, and tetanus (Erlanger 1995, 3). Mortality has been rising at an astounding rate in Russia. In 1993, mortality from all causes increased over 12 percent, including an 18-percent increase in deaths from infectious diseases. Between 1990 and 1994, male life expectancy in Russia fell six years; adult mortality is 10 percent higher than in India (World Bank 1996, 128). A 1994 World Bank report stated that the health crisis in Eastern Europe was making those economies uncompetitive in world markets (Perlez 1994, 10). In Eastern Europe, nutritional deficiencies are becoming critical. Bulgarians have as high a prevalence of goiter (iodine deficiency) as central Africans, and 30 percent of pregnant women in Georgia suffer from anemia (UNDP 1996, 19).

In every chapter in this book, it has been clear that shameful parallels to the conditions described for poor countries exist in the United States. The magnitude of the problem is less than in poor countries, but poverty and poor health still diminish productivity and limit future growth. Living conditions for the very poor in the United States are not so different from those in the developing world. People live in shanties without water and sanitation along the Rio Grande in Texas, in firetrap tenements in New York, and out on the street in most large American cities (Myerson 1995, F1, F4). Access to medical care is as distant for expectant mothers in parts of Mississippi as in Buenos Aires Province. Black baby boys in the United States have a life expectancy 5.5 years less than white baby boys (Firestone 1996, 29). They cannot expect to live as long as a boy from Honduras or Nicaragua. Over six thousand workers die in job site accidents in the United States each year.

Cutbacks in health spending and lack of access to care threaten to provoke epidemics of intractable diseases in a world increasingly interdependent. Hundreds of millions of people worldwide are infected with tuberculosis, and there are three million deaths a year from the disease. Spending in New York on tuberculosis fell from $40 million in 1968 to $2 million in 1989. By 1991, half of New York TB cases were drug resistant. Cost cutting saved the United States $200 million at most. The cost of treating patients and preventing the spread of drug-resistant strains of TB from 1989 to 1994 was at least one billion dollars (*Economist*, May 20, 1995, p. 15).

Even the capacity to fight disease through research and surveillance is under attack. Budget cuts and downsizing threaten the capacity, as well as the job safety of scientists, at the Centers for Disease Control and other infectious disease research centers (Altman 1995*b*, 9). It is hard to think of anything the government is doing that is more important than advancing or at least maintaining the health of the public. Research, surveillance, and epidemiology are critically important in maintaining public health and safety in rich and poor countries alike.

The economic problem—how a society allocates its resources to the satisfaction of human wants—is clear in these examples from the United States, as well as from Argentina and around the world. The resources for sustainable human development are available. The choices being made, however, are based on short-term cost and profit and are worsening the prospects for long-term development. The evidence mounts decade by decade that old theories of economic development based on skewed income distribution and "trickle-down" are wrong. Countries have had plenty of time to try vicious policies, and they have not worked. The countries with the best record of economic growth over the past thirty years are those that have done the most for basic education and health. Economic growth also supports human development. Growth provides the means to invest in people; stagnation creates conflict over limited output. (The relationship of human development and economic growth is well documented in the UNDP *Human Development Report 1996.*)

For nearly fifty years, Argentine workers have been losing ground. The decline is not just the result of successive governments having made a shambles of the economy. The declining purchasing power, health care, education, and nutrition also are the causes of the decline of the economy. The assault on the Argentine worker has been an assault on Argentine growth. Poor countries with work forces that are hungry cannot compete in a world market dominated by well-fed Americans and Germans. Every birth with injury to mother or child, every low-weight baby, every twelve-year-old girl taken out of school to keep house or to marry, every worker who loses an eye or a hand reinforces the poverty and guarantees it for the next generation. Human development requires solutions at the macroeconomic level and solutions to specific health and education problems.

National development policies should support growth, employment, and a better distribution of income. Particular solutions are easier to implement in that context. Some countries have achieved high human development in the absence of growth, but the gains have been difficult to maintain.

Microsolutions

As profound as the problems are, there are simple, common-sense solutions to many of them. For some problems, all it takes is looking at how things are done and asking if the method serves the goals of the health care center or other unit. Other problems are more difficult to solve because they are deeply rooted in the fatalism produced by faith in the unfettered operation of market forces. A culture of hatred for the poor, for the disabled, for women, for people of different racial, religious, or ethnic backgrounds also poses a more difficult challenge. Those things, too, can be changed. Education and the expansion of democracy to all citizens are long-term strategies. In the meantime, steps can be taken to directly attack prejudice and the health and development problems it causes. For every country, there are thousands of solutions to health and human development problems. All I can do here is suggest a few ideas in each area to indicate the possibilities for progress.

One of the first steps to take is to look at how human development programs are evaluated and how the costs and benefits of social infrastructure are valued. We need a strategy of what to attack first and how to proceed. Although we should not surrender our moral judgment to cost-benefit analysis, it can help us decide what programs help people most and how to go about them. Human development projects need broader cost-benefit accounting because many of the costs of continuing without services are underestimated, and many of the benefits are interdependent, having a synergistic effect. Water, drainage, garbage collection, and health clinic construction all improve health. In almost all housing projects, there has been a sharp reduction in gastrointestinal and respiratory disease, but it is hard to trace the results to a specific intervention (Laquian 1983, 140). In evaluating projects that help women, benefits can be understated because women's work is not valued in the market. For example, in estimating the costs and benefits for a water delivery system, if women's work has no market price, then the benefit of not having to haul water is undervalued. The opportunity cost of women's time is overlooked (Griffin and McKinley 1994, 13). If synergistic effects are ignored, an individual project in housing or health care is undervalued and, consequently, will not be undertaken. When the health center at Las Heras, Mendoza, was built, water lines were laid and neighborhoods along the way were connected. Gastrointestinal diseases, a major source of illness for the community, virtually disappeared. If the economy is viewed as one body, and all benefits and costs are acknowledged, a pipeline's contribution to productivity

and school performance would be part of the accounting. Devising a new accounting system is complex but not insurmountable. The following microsolutions generally follow the organization of the chapters of this book. The
macrosolutions necessary to permit these small changes are discussed at the end.

Housing

Important changes in housing and credit markets already are widely
recognized as ensuring healthier shelter for the poor. It is *not* necessary for the
government to finance a major construction program. What is necessary is for
the government to allow people to build their own houses. Title to the land and
access to credit are the help people need. People who have title to their land improve their housing, without any other assistance. Microloans, as pioneered by
the Grameen Bank in Bangladesh, enable people to improve their houses or start
small businesses with very little assistance. In rental units, the government can
lower inspection costs by encouraging and acting on reports of housing violations from the tenants.

- Construction extension services (similar to agricultural extension services)
  would enable one skilled worker to teach safe construction of cesspools, grad-
  ing and soil conservation, plumbing, wiring, and other skills to entire neighborhoods. Children can be included through 4H-type clubs or in shop classes
  at school. In combination with microloans for supplies, extension services
  would be an inexpensive way to help people build safe, protective housing.
- Testing soil for toxic elements can be inexpensively incorporated into public
  or private university course work and research. Students and teachers take a
  public bus to the area, collect some dirt, and take it back to the lab for analysis. The practical experience provides better training for scientists to contribute to national development.
- Scrap materials suitable for housing construction should be dumped in areas
  separate from regular domestic, industrial, and hospital waste. The location of
  dumps for building materials should be well advertised for the convenience of
  both dumpers and scavenger-builders. Posters in the neighborhood can warn
  people about dangerous materials, such as creosote-soaked wood and barbed
  wired.
- The government and private firms can sponsor design contests to develop
  housing styles and heating and cooking technology that use locally available
  fuels in ways that produce less indoor air pollution. The contests should be
  run in conjunction with educational campaigns to encourage cooking outside
  on porches and covered patios to avoid lung ailments and nerve damage from
  particulate pollution and carbon monoxide poisoning.
- Public buildings and institutions that serve poor people should be attractive,

well maintained, and clean. Degrading conditions in public buildings reinforce the idea that poor people deserve nothing better. Pleasant facilities encourage people to make their own homes nicer, to the extent that their budgets allow. When Padre Tomás Llorente built a school for 1,500 very poor children in Manuel Alberdi (Pilar) on the outskirts of Buenos Aires, he paid particular attention to the bathrooms. They are nothing ornate, just clean and tiled, but they stand in stark contrast to the outhouses and hand pumps in the properties around the school.

- In rural areas, the plague of the *vinchuca* can be controlled. Redesign of the house-corral unit is possible without completely altering the domestic economy. Patching walls and roofs can help to keep the bugs at bay. Home improvement, combined with spraying, can be effective in reducing infection in domestic pets, which act as host reservoirs of the parasite.
- Reforestation not only would help soil conservation but might also attract *vinchucas* and other pests back into their forest niche.
- In the absence of home improvements, even along with them, an extremely cost-effective method of protecting people from insect vectors of disease is the use of bed nets. Bed nets can reduce child mortality 25 percent overall and prevent at least 50 percent of malaria deaths of children and pregnant women. Bed nets cost only about $5 to $10 and retreatment with insecticide costs about fifty cents twice a year (Leary 1996, A13).
- Making a bed net can be part of the primary school curriculum, developing sewing skills and raising awareness of preventive health measures.
- To improve the environment of the whole neighborhood, community groups can serve as vehicles for participation. Volunteer fire fighters can play an important role in safety, sanitation awareness, and community spirit, especially among men and boys, since community health workers generally are women. The community groups should protect play areas for children and adults. They can sponsor inexpensive recreation for families, plan neighborhood walks and runs, soccer teams, and other group activities. They also can plant trees as a community activity and clean up the area to improve morale.
- On a citywide basis, the municipal government should identify areas that can be used as parks and enlist the aid of local or international firms in developing and maintaining parks. To protect the parks and provide comfort for the residents, it is simple and inexpensive to install and maintain portable toilets in recreation areas.

Water, Waste, and Garbage

In urban and suburban areas, there is no alternative to water and sanitation systems, but there are innovative designs, and international finance is available from the regional development banks and the World Bank. Smaller-scale water systems might make more sense than one system serving ten million people. Maintenance is as important as construction, since we have seen that more than half the treated water can be lost through main breaks. The costs and benefits of sanitary systems need to be reevaluated. In most basic housing supported by the World Bank, about three-fourths of the cost is for water and sanitation. Lenders require that the systems be of the best quality, which generally is better than in the rest of the city. Good sewer systems protect the whole city (Laquian 1983, 80–81). The calculation of benefits should include the externalities for the rest of the city along with health effects for the inhabitants of the housing project. For suburban and rural areas, safe well and cesspool construction is essential. There, too, the calculated benefits of the excavation need to include health effects. A primary health care program in Mali eradicated guinea worm disease in one village simply by digging a well with a cemented collar (Gray et al. 1990, 33).

- Educational campaigns in schools and neighborhoods are needed to teach people how to protect water supplies in the home and to promote basic hygiene. Hand washing is the simplest life-saving technique and is a good example of a small step that educates people and transfers to them some degree of responsibility for, and hence control over, their own health.
- Municipal garbage pits should separate reusable items from wastes that threaten public health. Public or private entities can establish good, safe reduce-reuse-recycle systems. The city should not interfere with people making a living from collecting recyclables. Recycling should be broadly defined to keep usable items out of the dump.
- The city of Curitiba, Brazil, has taken a creative approach to recyclable waste. The city trades one kilo of food for every four kilos of waste people bring in. The fruits and vegetables are purchased at market prices from small farms in the area. The city recycles the waste, saves over $100,000 a month in collection costs, and keeps waste out of streams. The city also traded with schoolchildren: waste for entrance to a Shakespeare festival (Rocha 1996, 12).
- In Barbados, the L. T. Gay Memorial Primary School initiated a recycling program that integrated all school subjects. The aim was to reduce the amount of garbage in dumps because it provides breeding areas for mosquitoes that spread dengue. After learning about the transmission cycle of dengue, the children became active health inspectors, searching the neighborhood for breeding areas (Beckles 1996, 19).
- Firms must bear the costs of their waste. Dumping into streams and along highways can be prevented. Incineration of hospital waste is important. Industry can be made to clean up and recycle chemicals rather than dump them. Firms often find, after being coerced, that reusing chemicals saves them money.

- The enforcement of hydatid-control regulation removes a serious public health hazard. It obviously is a matter of government lack of will when one province has up to 80 percent of animals carrying worms, and the next province, in the same ecological setting (Mendoza), has eliminated infestation. Requiring abattoirs to dispose of offal, rather than just leave it outside the plant, is a simple matter.
- Construction of surface water drainage reduces breeding areas for disease vectors and can protect road surfaces. Drainage construction can be less expensive than one year's application of pesticide to control mosquito populations (WHO 1991*d*, 6).

Government Oversight

The norms of government oversight of food, pharmaceuticals, automobiles, buses, elevators, syringes, and blood supplies are well established. The costs to the government and to the firms are insignificant compared to the saving in the health and safety of the population. Protection of food supplies, ensuring the safety of pharmaceutical exports, and other oversight functions are the normal business of modern governments. A government that effectively oversees health and safety establishes itself as serious in the eyes of the citizens. That perception builds confidence in the government and in the progress that the society as a whole is making. The situation is akin to the important issue of secure property rights. People will not invest capital if they have little confidence that they will see the fruits of their efforts. People will not invest themselves in the development of a country in which nothing works, in which nothing is safe, in which eating, drinking, taking elevators, and riding buses are all elements of a lunatic farce.

Several important considerations emerge from Chapter 6, on government regulation, and are highlighted here.

- From the very earliest years in school, the educational system needs to combat demeaning stereotypes of people with physical and mental disabilities, people of minority ethnic and religious groups, and people who are in other ways different from the majority. A lack of sensitivity toward any of those people not only is unjust, it also undermines democracy and the sense of shared humanity necessary for human development, both individual and national. Rehabilitation, job training, and programs of inclusion in social life are important for developing the full potential of disabled and other marginalized people.
- Occupational safety and health protection should be recognized as basic rights of workers. No country is so poor that it has the right to ask workers to risk their lives for a day's work. And none of the workers is paid enough for employers to have that right.

- Traffic safety programs can be modeled after those of the developed countries and should include mandatory seat belt and child safety seat use, enforcement of speed limits and driving-under-the-influence laws, and vehicle inspections. If a vehicle is essential to a person's business, a way will be found to bring it up to safety standards, or an alternative vehicle, such as horse and cart, can be used.
- One way to decrease the cost of government oversight is to educate the public, shifting the burden of regulation to firms themselves. "Because street vendors are responsive to customer demand, teaching consumers to look for street vendors that are visibly practicing better hygiene may reinforce more hygienic conditions" (Tauxe et al. 1995).

The Health Care System

The provision of better housing, clean water, and adequate nutrition is the basis of good health. An effective health care system complements those necessities. The momentum in most developing countries in the early 1990s was toward privatization of health services, modeling medical care on that of the United States. The United States, however, has had very poor performance in health compared to the level of spending and the level of per capita GDP. In developing countries, too, market-driven medical care is unlikely to provide the services needed by the population because of insufficient effective demand, supplier-induced demand, and vulnerable population groups. Besides emphasizing curative, *ex post* medicine, the allocation of resources among competing uses in private, market-oriented medical care is driven by profit. Skills and facilities will be used for liposuction and breast implants, rather than rehabilitation and Pap smears, if the profit is to be made in the former. The major health gains in developing countries in recent decades have been achieved by government health programs. Continuing improvement in national health depends on the public sector, not private medical care (Roemer and Roemer 1990, 1188–1192).

- In Argentina, the *obras sociales* should be eliminated. In other countries, if the system of union health and pension plans is working, it can be maintained but should not be subsidized by the government. In most developing countries, the proportion of the work force in stable wage employment, especially unionized labor, is very low. Broad health care provision cannot be achieved in an *obras sociales* system where formal-sector employment is limited. In Argentina, the system is so corrupt that it is a drain on both workers and business firms. It also subsidizes a private health care system that makes access to health care more unequal. For wage and salary workers and formal-sector self-employed, the government should continue the payroll tax on workers and employers, but the funds should be used to rebuild a public system for everyone.

- The private sector should not receive subsidies from public hospitals or from the government in general. When the private sector loses its support from the *obras sociales*, the government will have to monitor private providers to ensure that they do not increase the level of iatrogenic illness with supplier-induced demand for invasive procedures and unnecessary hospitalizations. The government could help ease the transition in the short to the medium term by paying private hospitals to provide services, such as reconstructive surgery and rehabilitation, that the public sector is not prepared to offer.
- The public system needs to decentralize decision making, supply systems, and organization, but it cannot expect every unit to be self-supporting. In poor areas, user fees cannot cover expenses.
- Each area should have a base hospital that supports satellite health posts.
- Public health needs to incorporate epidemiology, the only field that evaluates overall needs of the population. Without such criteria, the distribution of resources and the development of services usually depend on political considerations (Alderslade 1990, 274–275).

Primary Health Care

Primary health care is the basis of a rational health care system. It does not make sense to let people get sick and then try to cure them through expensive means. To be most effective, adapting national health programs to preventive care will need to occur at the ministerial level. Individual health centers have proved that it is possible to provide quality care, but national improvement will require national commitment. Otherwise, there will be isolated examples of primary care only where there are individual practitioners who possess the galaxy of talents necessary to invent a primary care system in the face of great odds. The individual would have to possess unusual organizational talent and be creative, determined, and of unflagging energy. In a system geared toward discouragement, there just are not enough people around who possess all those traits.

The nature of medical education also has to change to emphasize prevention, surveillance, and epidemiology. The training of a public health doctor must include statistics collection, epidemiological analysis, health education, and sanitation, all of which are lacking in hospital-trained physicians (Brockington 1985, 57, 66).

If the suburban health center, the rural health post, or the small hospital is the outcast zone, it undermines primary health care. Staff morale is lowest at the entry point to the entire system (Quirno Costa 1987, 67). To recruit doctors to work in remote areas with problems that are not very glamorous, with people they have not grown up respecting will require several steps. Medical education has to stress the primary importance of health posts. Pay should be higher in less comfortable posts, and doctors and nurses must be provided with enough simple equipment to do their jobs.

• One way to raise the prestige, attractiveness, and visibility of primary health care posts while improving the flow of epidemiological information to medical schools and practitioners is through medical journals. It is a step that involves only a few people on the editorial boards of the journals, can be instituted immediately, and costs nothing to implement. The respected journals should invite articles from doctors in peripheral health centers, small hospitals, and rural health posts. They can let it be known that, initially, narrative or descriptive articles will be welcome. That begins the process of epidemiological data gathering in the remote posts and informs the urban medical scholars of what the diseases of their country really are. As the quantity and quality of epidemiological research increases, the articles can be expected to be more analytical and scientific. That provides the information the country needs, improves the critical thinking of doctors in remote posts, and raises morale and quality of care in primary centers.

• Medical school education also would benefit from bringing in visiting lecturers from a variety of health posts around the country. For example, Neuquén and Río Negro have the highest rates of hydatid infestation in Argentina, and Argentina is one of the most infested countries in the world. Doctors from that region have learned that every shadow on a lung x-ray and every abdominal tumor is an hydatid cyst until proved otherwise. But they learned nothing of this in medical school at the University of Buenos Aires (Quirno Costa 1987, 65).

• Community participation is an important avenue. Community leaders should avoid endless meetings and getting bogged down in the polemics of participation, which just wears people down. Good health results are an appropriate guide.

• Community participation will raise the morale of doctors and nurses, who no longer need to feel the heavy burden of the people's suffering as something only they can solve.

Elements of Primary Health Care

Health care must be defined broadly to achieve the goals of primary care. It includes not only prenatal care, breastfeeding, oral rehydration therapy, and vaccinations, which are the basics of the *Health for All* agenda, but also disease surveillance, vector-control campaigns, testing of water quality and of the effectiveness of sewage disposal, and monitoring of housing conditions and food handling (Cumper 1991, 385).

- In regular well-baby checks, growth monitoring and other developmental measures are essential for early warning of health problems. The health center can provide nutritional supplements, such as iodine, iron, and calcium.
- Vaccinations are inexpensive preventive measures and should not be restricted to children. Booster programs for tetanus, yellow fever, and other inoculations are cost effective because they impart immunity for at least ten years.
- Primary health care should include classes for men and women. It is easy to overestimate how much information people have. At one health center, the nurses found that people do not return for treatment if they are told that their lab tests were "positive," since positive connotes something good (visit to Del Viso Maternity Hospital, September 3, 1992).
- Educational campaigns in the community and through various media about alcohol, AIDS, brucellosis, cholera, diabetes, E. coli, fertility, gonorrhea, hepatitis, infant feeding, job skills, literacy, voting rights, and so on are essential to primary care and well-being.
- Screening for adult diseases such as cervical and breast cancers, diabetes, cardiovascular disease, hypertension, vision problems, dental caries, and gum disease also is necessary.
- Oral health programs modeled after those in industrialized countries are difficult to implement where there is little capital and often no electricity. A low-cost alternative in Thailand and Zimbabwe uses only nonmotorized excavation equipment, a new filling material, and battery-operated head lamps and has been very successful (Frencken and Makoni 1994, 15–17).
- Primary health care workers should identify diseases that can be eradicated through a combination of treatment and education, eliminating the cost to the community permanently. Diseases with certain characteristics can be eliminated. For example, dracunculiasis, or guinea worm disease, can be eradicated because beyond the one-year incubation, there is no human carrier; there is no known animal reservoir; it is easy to detect since the worms protrude from the skin and transmission occurs only after protrusion; transmission is seasonal; methods for controlling transmission are simple; and the local population recognizes the disease (Ruiz-Tiben et al. 1995)
- Because of the importance of data collection, a simple method of recording incidence and prevalence must be devised for overworked doctors and nurses. Simple forms that permit the practitioner (or, better yet, a community health worker) simply to check off information can be tallied at the end of the week. One afternoon a week can be dedicated to discussing the caseload of the week and tallying the types of conditions.
- Another way of helping the health centers, while at the same time giving practical experience to students, would be to make it part of a computer

class in data entry to come to the center regularly and tabulate and enter data.

Operating a Health Center

The strategy of the *Health for All* program has to be one that succeeds in getting health services out to people in a systematic way. A person who is malnourished and living in a shack needs a different kind of medical practice from that given someone not at risk. Primary health care for the poor cannot assume that everything else in a person's life is normal and the doctor is just treating a cold or a stomach bug. The risk posed by a cold or diarrhea in an environment of need is much greater.

- The center and the area served should be small enough to ensure an ongoing relationship between the workers and the patients. Clinical history and the doctor-patient relationship are the keys to good diagnosis and attention.
- The center should have a plan with clearly enunciated goals and standards of performance. The center's layout, use of space, and procedures should be evaluated for accordance with the goal of quality, respectful patient care. That means the center must have clean waiting areas and clean bathrooms. Standard equipment should include a chair for the patient and a companion, and a private room or at least a screen for privacy.
- The plan will need to specifically mandate good manners, the use of polite forms of address particular to the region, and eye contact with patients and parents. Patients should feel they are important to the center's work, rather than barely tolerated. Using space efficiently and practicing good manners do not cost any money.
- The system of queuing should not be tiresome, anxiety producing, or competitive. There never should be a need for people to line up at four in the morning for attention. The best method is to have the center open all day for all specialties and to guarantee that everyone who shows up will be seen.
- A triage nurse can determine if the condition warrants a doctor, a nurse, a community health worker, or a class. The nurse or a volunteer can distribute numbers so people can find a comfortable place to rest or entertain children or do some shopping while they wait. Scarce resources, such as doctors, are better used and people get more of what they need when education is substituted for brief visits with a harried professional.
- While people are waiting, the time can be filled with classes in health topics or general information, such as crop rotation, geography, voter information, literacy games, or shopping for nutrition values.
- In areas where the high school runs on double shifts, half the students would be available at all times to help with the classes. The teaching opportunity would effectively double the learning time students have.

User Fees and Utilization Rates

There is a great deal of concern in the literature about people overusing health centers if there are no fees. The level of health and health knowledge in the population is such that one should not be concerned with so-called overuse. In Las Heras (Mendoza), the doctors told me that, because of the attention they receive at the health post, people come in just to talk. Especially if the equipment at a health post is basic and the personnel are not highly paid specialists, the marginal cost of attending to people's emotional needs is low. Inadequate treatment, on the other hand, can generate substantial costs. The balance should be weighted in favor of encouraging the use of health facilities. If user charges are used to generate income, they should not be barriers that keep people away (Bloom 1993, 221).

- In some neighborhoods, it is perfectly feasible to charge user fees. In Guaymallén (Mendoza), for example, there was an optional payment of one dollar, which most people paid.
- In other neighborhoods, like that of Center Number 6, it makes no sense to ask for donations. The administrative costs exceed the revenue generated in an extremely poor neighborhood.
- The centers cannot all be self-financing. That would lead to centers in poor areas like La Matanza having little or no funds for services and those in rich areas like Barrio Norte offering face lifts.
- Overuse of health centers should be seen as an opportunity, not a problem. What better could happen than that the health center become the hangout, the social spot. It is a far more wholesome scene than under the bridge, where kids are shooting up.
- The health center can encourage this "overuse" by having gatherings that are informative as well as social.
- Another way to encourage people to frequent the health center and to promote hygiene is to have community showers at the center. They need not be expensively designed but should not be degrading. There should be privacy, and the showers should be maintained. If people can afford to pay a small fee, that can be used to pay the salary of a cleaning person.
- The health center can also have a basketball hoop and other inexpensive recreational facilities.
- It is important to use every opportunity at the health center for education, shifting the burden of prevention to the people themselves.
- The idea of a community center is important, and ways should be found to hire as many local people as possible in the operation of the center.
- The answer to crowding is to give everyone a task, such as handing out information, reading instructions to nonliterate patients, organizing games for children, holding babies for mothers who are patients. That takes some

organizing at first, but it can get to be a system. It relieves the boredom, isolation, and feeling of helplessness of hours of waiting and can give children things to do.

Community Health Workers

The way to use people's time well and move them in and out of the center productively is to involve community health workers. Women already do most of the elements of primary health care, so health centers need only improve the resources (informational and material) at their disposal to make them community health workers. Having them perform immunizations and treat common diseases and injuries is a small step to creating an effective labor force of community health workers (Leslie et al. 1988, 309).

- Women who are recruited in the neighborhood to be community health workers should be paid. They should take their own small children around with them so as not to create their own child care problems and as an example to others.
- Community health workers can start with one type of job and then move on to other functions by incremental training (WHO 1991c, 238). In Jamkhed, community workers sought new jobs as they became proficient in the old ones.
- Health problems that can be solved with simple surveillance are those with easily identified symptoms and long incubation. Drs. Mabelle and Raj Arole trained uneducated people to be leprosy-control officers. A community health worker canvasses every house for people with numbness, which suggests leprosy, or persistent cough, for TB. Suspected cases can be referred for diagnosis and treatment. At every door, the community health worker is educating people about what to look for.
- The center needs to move out into the community and bring health-promoting services to the places where people live and work. Realistically, people are busy. For simple preventive care, most facilities should be portable or at least mobile. A baby scale can be carried from door to door or from one community center to the next. There is nothing demeaning to the poor in this approach. If milk and bread can be delivered to the door, why not health services?
- Public health workers can be very effective in workplace education and medical attention. A program funded by InterAmerican Development Bank in Haiti combined literacy training for factory workers with education in family health and planning, STD prevention, and services such as Pap smears (Sánchez 1994, 3).
- Blood pressure screening, oral health screening, eye tests, and hygiene classes are all possible in the community or the workplace.
- Schools are ideal settings for extension of health services. The children are a captive audience and would enjoy the break in the school routine, just as they

enjoy a fire drill or a goat loose in the hallway. Vaccinations can be kept up to date at school. Particularly important after the usual battery of early childhood shots would be boosters for tetanus and yellow fever (where necessary). Age-appropriate information on fertility, sexually transmitted diseases, and substance use fits well into health and science classes.

- Because poetry is easier to memorize than prose and is popular in Vietnam, the national Leprosy Control Program produced educational materials written in verse. The children learn about the signs of leprosy and its treatment at school and chant the verses at home, improving detection and treatment rates (Due 1996, 23).

- Another way to involve the whole community is to plan well-baby or general wellness fairs. The city or region can be divided into fifty zones, each zone to be visited one Sunday (or whatever day people take off) of the year. The city could invest in a moon bounce or trampoline and have music and dancing to attract crowds. Children's games and contests should test fitness and agility. Various booths can offer diagnostic services and test people's health knowledge, giving prizes for right answers and reserved appointments at the health center for wrong answers. Baby weighing, vaccinations, blood pressure testing, eye testing, and other simple screening can be done.

All these ideas are just a start. Once the health administration or, failing that, individual providers, decide that health for all—genuine, respectful health for all—is their goal, there will be no shortage of ideas. Once the community is involved in the process, there will be plenty of ways of making it work. This is not visionary, but it goes against inertia. Few of the suggestions presented here cost much; they just take different ways of approaching problems.

Models of Primary Health Care

Public health administrators need to identify successful primary health care providers, use them as models, and recruit them to train new staff. Existing health centers should be evaluated on the extent to which they conform to the model and rewarded accordingly.

There are successful primary health care programs. In Jamkhed (Maharashtra State, India), Dr. Mabelle Arole and Dr. Raj Arole, with a staff of nurses, developed a primary health care system that now covers 250,000 people. The Aroles have emphasized prevention, education, participation, and raising the status of women in their families and communities. They have trained over five hundred nonliterate and "untouchable" caste women to be community health workers, conquering both class and gender bias and ancient plagues with one, well-reasoned strategy. The Aroles have worked carefully and patiently to extend primary health care in remote villages of a poor rural area of India. In addition to prevention and education, they have emphasized rehabilitation. The development of the Jaipur limb, a prosthetic leg for people disabled by leprosy that is well adapted to rural conditions, was one of the accomplishments of health workers of the Jamkhed centers. Within the first ten years of the project's founding, infant mortality rates in the region dropped from 176 to 19 per 1,000 (Arole and Arole 1994; Dr. Raj Arole, March 31, 1996).

In Buenos Aires, an urban version of the Arole model is practiced by Dr. Norma Aprigliano at Center Number 6. She has trained neighborhood women to be community health workers. They use illustrated leaflets to inform people in the neighborhood about the services of the health center. They monitor children and expectant mothers. Because she has records of all the local people and what attention they need, Dr. Aprigliano also can make full use of the medical students and residents assigned a rotation to the health center.

National Education and Mobilization

Information is a valuable tool that enables people to take control of their futures. "The unmanageable universe, surrounded by suspicion, is static" (Fillol 1961, 26). Health education can be carried out effectively in the media. In the United States, it was the media that publicized epidemiological findings on the importance of serum cholesterol, untreated hypertension, and smoking. People changed their diets based on what they read in the newspaper. In ten years, there was a 25-percent decline in coronary heart disease and a 38-percent decline in stroke in the United States (Terris 1988, 818). Written media are effective in a literate population. Visual media can be used where they are readily accessible. Where the facilities are inadequate for television and radio campaigns, traveling shows are an option. In the 1970s, there was a controversy in India over the suitability of spending millions of dollars on a satellite communication system. The cost effectiveness of a national telecommunications system for health is, in fact, great in a country of almost one billion people in hundreds of thousands of villages. It also shows people what the rest of the world is like and breaks the barriers of their limited experience. It can be a tool for national unity in a country of diverse cultural and religious groups.

- Where local practices are health promoting, educational campaigns should publicize them. In the Amazon, the practice of adding citrus juice to water to improve its taste protected people from the cholera outbreak because the acid in the fruit killed the *vibrio*. An inexpensive emergency control measure was immediately available (Tauxe et al. 1995).
- The sides of buses, trash cans, and buildings are all highly visible places to promote hand washing and keeping dirty hands out of drinking water.
- It is imperative to discourage smoking through education and heavy taxes.

Use of the media should also be particularly effective, since cigarette smoking is, to a great extent, a media-produced addiction.

- Other suitable topics for media campaigns are alcohol abuse, sexually transmitted diseases, family violence, early cancer screening, oral health, sanitation, food adulteration, family planning, breastfeeding, and safe use of pesticides.
- Swim lessons should be part of the school curriculum anywhere that people live near water.
- In Mali, an effective educational campaign in oral health was carried out in the schools. Children examined each other's teeth and mouths to begin their education in oral diseases and then participated in skits in which each child helped write the story and act it out (Abellard 1994, 12).
- Where the population has little access to radios, the government or private firms can promote the production of new technology, like the wind-up radios produced in South Africa. The radio's inventor was prompted by a BBC program on the difficulty of disseminating AIDS-prevention information in South Africa.
- Certain remedies are suitable for mass mobilization. A polio vaccination campaign in India, involving hundreds of thousands of volunteers on a few selected days, is bringing the country closer to its goal of eliminating polio by the year 2000. In the past twenty-five years, at least 25,000,000 people in India have been severely disabled by polio. Now it will be eliminated within a few years (Burns 1997, 3).

Public Hospitals

Hospital care is well defined and does not have to be invented in the way that primary health care does. The plan for the hospital in a primary care system is well laid out in World Health Organization publications (WHO 1992). Norms of cleanliness and standards for the use of antibiotics are essential for avoiding intrahospital infection. Certain obvious needs can be pointed out here.

- Qualified personnel should be available or on call at all times. A poorly educated, first-year resident operating on little sleep is no substitute for an experienced doctor or a well-trained nurse.
- Basic tools, including a working telephone (in urban areas) and resuscitation equipment, are a minimum for an institution to call itself a hospital. There needs to be a sink, with soap and towels, in every room. In waiting areas, toilets should be clean and in working order.
- Enormous improvement is possible with normal investment in maintenance. Janitors and maintenance workers should be made aware how critical their work is in the operation of the hospital. When the hospital is evaluated,

cleanliness and readiness of equipment are important factors. The entire staff should be recognized for their contributions.

- Supply systems need to be carefully studied for ways to avoid waste and theft. In the Hospital de Quemados, Dr. María Coruja designed a supply system that was labor intensive (ordering medicines for only two to three days at a time) but that saved on what was most scarce, funds for critically needed medicine.

- Management of human resources is important, so that doctors and nurses are not doing jobs that clerks or community health workers could do. In the case of referrals to better-equipped hospitals, for example, if a community worker made the phone calls to get patients placed, the doctors would have more time with patients. (In a system where getting patients placed depends on cronyism and calling in favors, however, it would not work to have a clerk do the job.)

- Nurses trained empirically should have their practical training supplemented with formal study on hospital time. The education must include a high level of literacy, serious hygiene training, and the elements of basic science.

- For *empíricos* who are reluctant to wash their hands, some simple science education might be useful. Viewing samples from their own unwashed hands under a microscope, along with slides taken from patients whom they know to have died from infectious disease, could be a simple but convincing exercise.

- There should be incentives for nurses to upgrade their skills. Higher levels of education should be accorded not only higher pay but also greater responsibility. To compensate for the shortage of nurses, surplus medical school graduates can be used as physician's assistants and nurse practitioners for nursing, screening, and rehabilitation. Without residencies, medical school graduates are not prepared for the tasks of a fully certified doctor.

- Hospitals must institute good recordkeeping and quality-control programs with measurable indicators, such as incidence of postoperative infections, eclampsia, sores on long-term patients, intrahospital infection, hemorrhage, rates of Caesarean sections and forceps use, and late transfer of complicated cases (WHO 1992, 31).

- In Cali, Colombia, creating intermediate health units with twenty to thirty beds, an emergency ambulance, and a two-way radio for short stays reduced crowding at the university hospital. For low-risk births, women could avoid the necessity of traveling a great distance to deliver (WHO1991c, 235). In Del Viso (Greater Buenos Aires), the maternity hospital was similarly designed for normal deliveries and emergencies but without extravagant equipment. People with special problems were referred to better-equipped hospitals.

- Linkages back to the community are important for hospitals in a primary care system to make sure that the costly investment in hospital care pays off in long-term survival. The neonatology ward of Mendoza's Lagomaggiore General Hospital has a halfway house in which mothers begin to have full care for their premature babies about to be discharged. When the babies are so tiny and have been in incubators and hooked up to tubes and wires, it is frightening for the mothers and difficult for them to bond with their babies. The inexpensive measure of providing shelter for the mother for a few days might make all the previous expenditure on the premature infant's care worthwhile, so the child is not lost due to the mother's fear, superstition, or lack of experience (Irma Bojio, October 31, 1991).

- Another important linkage is reporting births to the neighborhood health centers so they can follow up on newborns with vaccinations and well-baby visits. This hands-on approach, practiced at Center Number 6 in Buenos Aires, is what is needed when people are poor and marginalized. Getting started making a success of their lives is very difficult without some assistance.

These are but a few solutions, suggestive of the possibilities for a program of human development. They take an interventionist approach, but it is not patronizing to recognize the obstacles that people face in organizing healthy lives for themselves and their families. It is compassionate, and it is good resource management. It has to be easy for people to enter the system, because too many factors—time, money, fatigue, lack of information, and discouragement—conspire against good health.

Macrosolutions

For all these microchanges to take place, each as simple as it is, requires change at the macroeconomic or macrosocial level. Human development is not the direction in which most countries, from Sierra Leone to the United States, are headed. Human development is a moral decision, but it is also a pragmatic choice that furthers long-term economic growth. Three key areas affect the possibility for human development: democracy, the status of women, and the role of the market.

Freedom not only is part of the definition of human development, it also is a means. Without political freedom, human development is held back. If people have to divert energy to protecting themselves from arbitrary arrest, they cannot be as productive. If creativity is dangerous and initiative is subversive, passivity seems like a safe, indeed the only, option. A free press is fundamental to achieving the goals of human development. It informs the people of corruption, the failure of government oversight, and the plight of their neighbors.

One of the most important steps in advancing human development and health in particular is raising the status of women. Human development is held back by the role of women as chattel, *de jure* or *de facto*. Not only do women hold up half the sky, they do almost all the raising of children, a large proportion of the farm work, most of the family health care and domestic education, and, where they are permitted, significant work in all other fields as well. The education of girls has a profound impact on family life, reducing infant mortality, even without increases in household income. Falling infant mortality, higher wages outside the home, and greater power within the home lead to low fertility rates and slower rate of population growth. When women achieve mastery over subjects in school, they have a different sense of their own capacity to change their environment. They also learn that there are places to look for information and help for most difficulties. They can teach their children how to shape their lives rather than be molded by external forces.

Because the oppression of women is deeply rooted in most societies, it will take the concerted effort of community groups, government, and nongovernmental organizations to improve women's position in society. Religious groups especially, if they are at all interested in the temporal well-being of the people, should concentrate on truly elevating the status of women in the family. In particular, if religious groups do not like the direction taken by other groups that speak for women, they need to lead in materially changing women's lives and challenging men to change their behavior.

The movement to raise the status of women must have a broad focus. Education for girls, access to clean water supplies, availability of fuel supplies, some control over family finances, and protection from spousal abuse are all ways in which women's health (and the population's general health) can be improved. Women's rights need to be seen in a broad context of social justice and human rights. To emphasize *women's* rights does not mean to narrow development policy to the issues of population or reproduction. A women's movement should not reduce women's issues to reproduction or women to their reproductive potential. Such a focus reinforces sexist notions of the role of women.

In some countries, the focus of the women's movement has been narrowed even further (or at least has been construed as such) to the sole issue of abortion. It may be easier to organize for abortion because it is something men can support even if, or especially if, they have no interest in changing social roles. Abortion makes absolutely no demands on men to change their behavior or the way they relate to women and abandons women to a world in which fundamentally little has changed. Of course, none of that is to say that women should not be provided with the information and support they need to plan their fertility in a healthy way. Human development requires that women can look forward to pregnancy as a blessing, not a curse.

Women are more than half of humanity; women do more than half the work; women raise the next generation. Development is empty of meaning if its benefits flow to the minority alone.

The other big challenge is whether economies will be in the thrall of the market or harness it as a tool. In certain areas, the market has worked extremely well. In developed countries, deciding how many boxes of each kind of cereal to have on supermarket shelves, rationing luxury cars, luring capital into financial investments are all ways in which markets work. The inputs and outputs, or investment and returns, are well specified.

In many other areas, market failure abounds. The market system depends on prices as signals to buyers and sellers. A high price for oil, for example, is a signal to firms to look for alternative energy sources. Prices are the key to markets; flexible prices allow markets to adjust quickly to changing circumstances. The problem in relying exclusively on the market is that many inputs and outputs are not accurately priced or have no price at all. Clean air and water had no price in most economies until at least the 1970s. They still are inaccurately priced to maintain them as a resource. Consequently, firms dump toxic wastes into the air and water.

Prices are inadequately assigned in health because property rights in one's person are insufficiently specified. What is the price of a baby lost to a mother's uterine infection? What is a hand crushed in a thresher worth? It is not very comfortable, or probably even suitable, to assign prices in such cases. Unfortunately, in a market system, things that do not have prices are taken as free goods. To rely solely on the market requires us to price every imaginable thing, if we are to claim that it honestly allocates resources to the satisfaction of human wants.

The obstetrician charges $70 for a visit. The bus costs $2. The vitamins cost $10. The woman makes $3.50 a day. All these things have prices. The woman wants to have a baby, but she keeps miscarrying because of toxic exposure at work. How much did each lost baby cost? Was the value of each baby included in the $3.50-a-day wage? Does the fifty cents a day wage for an agricultural worker include a payment for the disabling effects of schistosomiasis or the discounted future value of work time lost to injury? We cannot put prices on everything, but where prices are not assigned, the market does not work.

Even where prices reflect the opportunity cost of inputs, the most basic problem of reliance on an unfettered market is that the allocation of resources depends on effective demand, which is based on a preexisting distribution of income. Prices are determined by supply and demand, and demand depends, in part, on a person's income. The world's 385 billionaires are not just another 385 households in the circular flow. Their combined worth is equal to the total annual incomes of countries with 45 percent of the world's population. The influence of persons with significant purchasing power defines the market. The distribution of goods and services is determined by the rationing mechanism of prices. Even more significantly, the preexisting distribution of income determines *what goods and services* will be produced. The distribution of income dictates how the resources of the economy are allocated. Consequently, $3 million houses are built while people live on heating grates. Fresh bread is flown in from Paris each morning to the capital of Ivory Coast, while the infant mortality rate there is 90 per 1,000. The market allocates resources in response to price signals based on the distribution of income. The market is said to be operating efficiently.

This is a fundamental obstacle to human development in a market economy. It perpetuates poverty because people with little purchasing power have little influence in the market. Affordable housing, wholesome cheap food, and accessible preventive health care are produced in insufficient quantities. Shortages exist, but they are not registered in the market. When there is not enough affordable housing, people do not line up outside the few inexpensive apartments with cash in hand, waiting for the occupants to move out. When food is too expensive, bakeries do not have queues of 100,000 people waiting for a five-cent roll. People experiencing shortages of food, clothing, shelter, clean water, and safe jobs do not show up in the market. They turn up on heating grates and in garbage dumps, hospitals, and morgues.

Relying on the market as though it relieves us of the burden of moral judgment or political choices is escapist. No-work solutions do not exist. The issue is not whether to use the market. It is whether it will be the master and all other considerations ignored. This is not just a muddle that capitalism has gotten itself into, that with a little tinkering we can fix. This requires a fundamentally different look at the role of the market.

It is possible that capitalism is not equal to the task of human development, but I do not think we need to be defeatist. If people decide they have the energy and the confidence to shape the world with its enormous potential for human development, they can use the market mechanism to make it work. But that means harnessing the market, making it a tool, not submitting to it as an all-powerful genie. We should not rely on magic, on the alchemy of the invisible hand, any more than we should fear the evil eye. Superstition and the belief in magic make people powerless and fatalistic, whether they are peasants or economists.

Fatalism defeats human development. If we do not want to live in a world where people suffer in the midst of plenty, we have to view the market as a tool that we can wield constructively. We are not at the mercy of an impersonal, all-powerful market. We are masters of our fate.

Notes

One The Plague of Poverty

1. Many of the data in subsequent chapters are aggregated using the categories of structural, or chronic, poverty and the newly impoverished.

Two Argentine History and Society

1. Argentina claims a sector of Antarctica and the Islas Malvinas (Falkland Islands).
2. For a detailed description of the resources and level of development of the regions of the Argentine interior, see Sawers 1996.
3. New copper mines became economically viable in the 1990s, when government regulations were relaxed.
4. It is striking how much these ideas conflict with the tenets of Christianity and the Judeo-Christian tradition. From the beginning in the Jewish law, people were liberated from irrational and multiple gods and had control over their lives because what people do matters (Eban 1984, 49). That was reaffirmed in Christianity. Argentina is considered a very Catholic country, but the notion of being at the whim of fate belies a pre-Judeo-Christian Mediterranean culture. Some Christian denominations went back to the notion of fate, of places in paradise being allocated *a priori*, but it is not part of Catholicism. Argentines and other Latin peoples (Hispanics and Italians) have combined their Christianity with pre-Christian superstition. For some, every statement that includes any hint of future tense must conclude with the phrase *Si Dios quiere*, "if God wills it."
5. After paying a $7,500 hookup charge, customers still had to wait ten years for installation. The phone system was so bad that one never had to fulfill social or business obligations, because an excuse that the phone was not working was always plausible.
6. Self-employment is not necessarily indicative of underdevelopment. In the United States, many doctors, lawyers, writers, computer software inventors, and consultants are self-employed.
7. The World Bank and the IMF respond to public outrage by writing reforms into their

subsequent reports. They are to be credited for learning from criticism, even if the reports read as though the new ideas originated at the Bank or the IMF.

Three   Housing and Health

1. I spent many days in the Retiro *villa* in the winter and spring of 1992. Each day I would find another block of hurriedly erected structures in the neighborhood called Autopista. The older residents said that the new people were coming from other parts of Greater Buenos Aires to erect houses in the path of the new highway, hoping to be relocated by the city government when the *villa* was ultimately demolished.
2. Two types of institutions in which crowding is a serious problem are nursing homes and prisons. Investigators found as many as 500 unlicensed and overcrowded nursing homes in Greater Buenos Aires serving spoiled food and failing to meet basic hygiene standards (*Buenos Aires Herald*, May 16, 1993, p. 4). An overburdened and grossly inefficient court system has resulted in serious jail crowding. Riots among detainees and convicts have resulted in numerous deaths on repeated occasions in Argentina. In March and April 1996, 6,000 prisoners in several jails around the country rioted, leaving an indeterminable number dead. The jails involved held 50 percent more prisoners than their maximum capacity. Seventy percent of those held had not been tried after one to two years in detention (*Buenos Aires Herald*, April 7, 1996, pp. 1, 13). In 1993, rioting by 500 detainees in Catamarca held in a space intended for 100 resulted in at least twelve deaths. In 1990, rioting led to thirty-six deaths in Olmos prison, and in 1978, seventy were dead after riots in Villa Devoto jail in Buenos Aires (*Buenos Aires Herald*, November 25, 1993, p. 10).
3. In comparison, in the United States (population 250 million), which also has a serious TB epidemic, there are about 25,000 new cases per year. The annual case load in the United States had declined every year until 1985, when it reached 22,000. From that time, the number of new cases has increased due to the AIDS epidemic.
4. Because humans are the only known reservoir for leprosy, it is possible that with commitment to a public health program based on multidrug therapy, transmission could be stopped and the disease eradicated, as was the case for smallpox (Noordeen 1992, 301).

Five   Water, Waste, and Garbage

1. For the poor, it is also an economic problem because of its expense. In 1992, it cost $40 to $50 per visit; disposal companies do not lower their prices on combined trips to one poor neighborhood.
2. We were lucky. In our house, only large frogs came out of the toilet and the floor drain.

Six   The Underdeveloped State

1. Where more than one item came from the same source, the citation follows all items from that source.
2. Automobile inspections were initiated in the United States in 1929, in Germany in 1954, in Japan in 1980, and in Spain in 1985.

Seven   Divided Economy, Divided Medicine

1. In the United States, there are 126 medical schools, with an average of 820 full-time professors (including researchers) for every 1,000 students. In Canada, with sixteen medical schools, there are 600 full-time professors for every 1,000 students (Etcheverry 1987, 190).
2. I worked forty hours a week for six weeks in the pediatrics ward of Clínicas Hospital in 1992 and two weeks in 1993 at the kind invitation of Dr. Carlos Ray, First Chair in Pediatrics of the Faculty of Medicine of the University of Buenos Aires.
3. This is not, however, the case in good residencies. In pediatrics in Clínicas, the chief of residents, Dr. Ana Bernard, and the First Chair in Pediatrics, Dr. Carlos Ray, repeatedly sent the residents to the library to find data to help them diagnose conditions.

Eight   Primary Health Care

1. Reform movements are not completely lacking, but they are few and have tended to be isolated, such as the cooperative groups of Jewish settlers in Santa Fe and Entre Ríos.
2. *Salita* is the term used almost universally in Argentina for peripheral health center or primary care facilities outside of hospitals. In Florencio Varela, however, *salita* is considered undignified, and the term *centro de salud* (health center) is used.
3. Late vaccination for measles is particularly dangerous because it is in children under two that the most deaths from complications occur. It probably is a waste to vaccinate children over three because they likely have had measles by that age. In developing countries, it makes sense to inoculate children earlier than they are in developed countries. Malnourished children apparently metabolize the passively acquired maternal antibodies to preserve their own protein stores. Vaccination campaigns protect both the vaccinated and the unvaccinated. If a high proportion of the population is protected, children are less likely to be exposed until they are older, when they are better able to survive the disease and its complications, in particular anorexia in the malnourished child. In many countries, it has been observed that the average age of measles infection increased after vaccination programs (Halsey 1983, 7, 11).
4. For the immediate future, Argentina needs to maintain a hospital or residence for lepers, who have reason to believe that they would not be accepted in society.

Nine   Public Hospitals

1. In Argentina, *hospital* refers to a public hospital. A private hospital is called a *clínica* or a *sanatorio*.
2. The practice in pediatrics throughout the country is that a family member stays in the ward to take care of all the child's needs. In Hospital de Clínicas in Buenos Aires, this was sometimes fathers, although generally mothers. In Mendoza, only mothers could stay with the children, because most of the family companions would be mothers and the presence of a man overnight would give rise to scandal.
3. For the patient, living in the hospital has some pleasant advantages. The room is free, dry, and reasonably clean. The food is free and usually clean. In their absence, the patients' makeshift homes may have been carried off. A patient's whole family may move into the hospital out of the weather.
4. Quemados was the hospital I was determined not to visit because I thought it would be a very sad place. Dr. Pablo Muntaabski persuaded me to go, and I did not regret it. The

hospital is full of spirit. The nurses' office was exploding with life, and the determination of the staff to save their patients gives everyone the opportunity to fully exploit their intellect and generosity. With another director, would Quemados be Montes de Oca?

5. In fact, San Justo was the only place, of the scores of hospitals and health centers that I visited in Argentina, in which the behavior among the staff was so unpleasant.

6. Only bacterial infections are treatable with antibiotics. Viruses are not treated with antibiotics.

Ten Infant and Child Mortality

1. Quoted in Battellino and Bennun 1991, 45.

2. The figures have to be evaluated in light of the deterioration of vital statistics in Argentina and the role of cronyism in public administration. According to the National Director for Maternal and Child Health in the Ministry of Health and Social Action (1991), Dr. Eduardo Duro, the actual numbers and rates of infant mortality are not known. Some provinces do not count births, let alone neonatal deaths. The infant mortality rate is a political variable that in many jurisdictions is lowered during election campaigns. Decreases from 45 to 30 per 1,000 in some jurisdictions have no valid explanation other than that the data were released in an election year (Duro 1991, 271).

3. Another way of looking at the improvement in infant and child mortality is the increase in life expectancy for the population. So much greater are the differences in risks for infants and young children that, once the hurdle of the first five years is passed, life expectancy is much more uniform among different populations. There still are significant differential risks for the poor, but they are not so extreme as those for the youngest poor. Consequently, the improvements in child survival account for most of the increase in life expectancy. In 1959–1961, residents of the Federal Capital could expect to live twenty-one years longer than those of Jujuy (seventy-one years and fifty years, respectively). In the period 1980–1981, the gap in life expectancy between the two areas had diminished to 8.5 years (OPS 1989, 30).

4. Some higher rates were recorded but in categories in which deaths (and births) were so few as to be statistically invalid. Considering the disaggregation of the data, that is not surprising. There would be very few women in rural areas with more than twelve years of education whose husbands were at the lowest occupational rank. Similarly, very few women in large urban areas whose husbands are of the highest occupational class would have fewer than seven years of schooling.

5. Some data for postneonatal mortality are based on the period one to eleven months and for child mortality on eleven months to four years inclusive.

6. Where there are high rates of infant mortality, there also usually are high proportions of unknown causes. Typical are Santiago del Estero and Jujuy, where more than 30 percent of infant and child deaths are from unknown causes. The Federal Capital is atypical because it has very high rates of mortality from unknown causes but the lowest rates for neonatal and postneonatal mortality (Mychaszula and Acosta 1990, 61, 62).

7. Some congenital factors are genetically determined and unavoidable. Some congenital injuries are caused by environmental factors, such as tobacco, alcohol, exposure to toxic substances, and rubella and are avoidable.

8. Similar results were obtained in numerous studies in Mexico, where the incidence of low birth weight is 15 percent and is determined much more by social conditions than

by biological factors. Lack of prenatal control increased the risk of having a low-birth-weight child eighteen times. If the father was a worker or a peasant or had not finished primary school, if the mother had not finished primary school, if they lived in a rural or a periurban area, and if they had a monthly salary below the minimum wage, there was a relative risk of producing a low-birth-weight child 320 times that of parents in the upper social strata, who had better jobs, education, locations, and salaries (Avila-Rosas et al. 1988, 51, 52).

9. There were also three sites each in Colombia and Brazil and one each in Jamaica, Mexico, El Salvador, Bolivia, Chile, Canada, and the United States.

Eleven   Stunted Development in Children and Adolescents

1. In the developed countries, especially in the United States, excess food intake and the consumption of low-quality, high-fat refined and processed foods contribute to the high rates of obesity, metabolic disorders, heart disease, hyperactivity, and numerous other conditions. Such so-called overnutrition also is a problem for some developing countries, but it is not the kind of malnutrition with which we are primarily concerned here.

2. In an extremely small percentage of cases, a mother's milk would be harmful to the infant. When mothers have very high levels of toxic chemicals or heavy metals in their systems, the fat in breast milk carries those toxins to the infant. Mothers with AIDS also can pass the infection to their children through breast milk.

3. There is a debate among nutritionists in public health. Some say stunting is a useful adaptation because the stunted child needs less food. Studies show that stunted children, in terms of work capacity per unit of body weight, are equal to or more capable than children of the same age who are taller or heavier; in absolute terms, however, they may be at a disadvantage (Waterlow 1987, 46).

4. Genetic differences between ethnic groups account for little variation in average weight and height. "In favorable conditions of nutrition and health, the growth potential of the human race is considered similar. . . . the maximum difference in height in the ages five to seven years that can be imputed to genetics is about 3.5 cm [1.37 inches]. However, poverty produces populations of heights of 12 cm [4.68 inches] or more below the 50th percentile of the standards" (UNICEF 1990*b*, 76).

5. The Food and Agriculture Organization of the United Nations recommends per capita daily consumption of 2,250 calories. In the Americas, Argentina's consumption is exceeded only by Canada (3,425 calories per person per day) and the United States (3,642 calories per person per day).

6. Numerous acquaintances told me that they had given up eating breakfast and lunch because it was healthier. I was not convinced of their reason for doing so.

7. This reinforcement of the greater natural strength of females makes even more remarkable the excess female mortality from malnutrition, and from diseases directly linked to malnutrition, discussed in Chapter 10.

Twelve   The Debilitated Work Force

1. This tendency is counteracted somewhat in Argentina for women workers because they are in charge of family health and so much of their own health has to do with children. Women's social and biological role permits, even compels, them to be open to physical and sensory concerns. "Men, on the other hand, resist assuming the role of

the sick person, since virility is identified in our culture with physical and psychic health. The role of principal provider for the family's support accentuates this resistance" (Prece and Schufer de Paikin 1991, 28). In some poor countries, however, the privilege of seeking medical attention goes to those who enjoy the other privileges in society. In Mali, it was the men who used the services of the primary health care centers, although the children and pregnant women were at highest risk (Gray et al. 1990, 34).

2. This is true not only for the poor but also for the middle and upper classes. Recall that Menem appointed his tarot card reader's son to a judgeship (Cooper 1994, 14).

3. The only clearly discriminatory factor was the very high proportion of the people who disappeared who were Jewish. In a population that is less than 1 percent Jewish, one-third of the disappeared persons were Jewish.

4. This is an enormous field. I direct those who can face the implications of torture to the literature, including the collection by Eric Stover and Elena Nightingale (1985).

5. One cause of death that is less a hazard for poor women is that of unnecessary Caesarean sections. Because poor women have less access to hospital births, the abuse of C-sections falls more heavily on women in *obras sociales* and private hospitals. In three of the five census cities, the rate of C-sections for poor women was about 60 percent that for nonpoor women. In the two poorest of the provincial cities surveyed, the difference was even greater. In Posadas, nonpoor women had more than three times the rate (47 percent) of C-sections as poor women (14 percent). In Santiago del Estero, the rate for poor women was 22 percent and for nonpoor women was 53 percent (INDEC 1990, 223).

6. By comparison, 1.2 percent of Canadian women of that age group and 2.7 percent of U.S. women, both countries where abortion is legal, had abortions each year in the same time period (Brooke 1994, C5).

7. It is hard to imagine how a sexually transmitted disease could have such a high prevalence or how vaccination could do any good in that case, since hepatitis B is also transmitted from mother to child.

8. Surveys of army conscripts in Thailand in 1993 found that 96 percent had used a prostitute. While government education campaigns seem to have had some effect, 85 percent of conscripts still were reporting prostitute use in 1995 (Wheeler 1996, A9).

9. Even in the United States, with a well-understood toxic effect, the problem goes unrecorded if ongoing exams of former workers are not made, as was the case with chronic beryllium disease (Meier 1996, 8).

10. Easy access to pesticides facilitates suicides. Fourteen percent of all deaths from injury in the villages in the Indian study were suicides, all of which were due to ingestion of pesticides (Mohan 1993, 12).

11. Even in the otherwise very good British Hospital in Buenos Aires, I had to be extremely firm with the radiology technician to get a lead apron for my twelve-year-old daughter, who was having her wrists x-rayed.

Glossary

cardiomyopathy: disorder of the heart muscle

cephalopelvic disproportion: inability of the baby's head to pass through the birth canal; in malnourished mothers results from inadequate development of the pelvis

changas: odd jobs secured by a shape-up

cuentapropista: self-employed

eclampsia: a severe, often fatal, form of toxemia in pregnancy

endemic: a disease that is always present in the locality

epidemiology: the study of diseases, especially those of greatest significance in a community

etiology: how a disease is transmitted and progresses

helminths: worms

hydatids: cysts of tapeworms, which, in humans, tend to be found in the liver and the lungs

iatrogenic: caused by medical intervention

incidence: frequency of new cases

macroadjustment: changes in economic policy intended to correct problems that affect the economy as a whole, such as inflation or unemployment

morbidity: sickness

oral rehydration therapy: a life-saving solution for dehydration due to diarrhea and vomiting

pandemic: outbreak of a disease in many locations at the same time

periurban: around the perimeter of a city, called *suburban* in the United States

prevalence: how common a disease is in a community, how many cases at any one time

Proceso: Process of National Reorganization, Argentine military regime of 1976 to 1983

rent seeking: attempting to gain profit from holding an advantage. Rent, in economics, is the payment to a factor in fixed supply (such as land). For example, a person who seeks to profit, not by investment, but by access to friends in positions of power or by tariffs that impart differential benefit to some firms is rent seeking.

serological: from blood tests

seropositive: having a positive blood test

T. cruzi: parasitic protozoa that causes Chagas' disease

vectors: carriers of a disease, such as mosquitoes, *vinchucas*, or rats

villas: shantytowns of Argentina; *villas miseria*, towns of misery

vinchuca: a reduvid bug that is a vector of Chagas' disease in South America

Bibliography

Numerous articles cited in the text from Argentine newspapers, even quite lengthy feature articles involving considerable research, were published anonymously. The libel laws in Argentina are such that any comment that could cast a public figure, in particular the President, in an unattractive light, can lead to imprisonment. The climate for journalists during the Menem presidency has been hostile, with numerous beatings, death threats, at least one death, and the attempt to silence criticism with new libel legislation. Anonymous articles are cited in full in the text but are not listed in the bibliography.

In a few cases, I have withheld the name of the person interviewed because I thought that the person's safety or career could be in jeopardy. Hundreds of nurses, doctors, social workers, patients, journalists, and *villeros* gave generously of their time and spoke openly and honestly. I worked with staff under their normal conditions. They did not hide from me the deficiencies in their service, nor did they shrink from disagreements among themselves when I was present. No one ever asked me not to use his or her name or to conceal any information, but I do not want the fact that people felt comfortable speaking with me to have effects they did not anticipate.

To make it easier for the reader to distinguish between citations to English-language publications of the Pan American Health Organization and those that are in Spanish, I have cited the Spanish texts by the Spanish acronym OPS, for Organización Panamericana de la Salud, and those in English by PAHO. Some of the publications listed in Spanish also exist in English versions, although I used the Spanish version. All translations are my own.

The following newspapers, magazines, and scholarly journals are cited in the text.

American Journal of Medicine
American Journal of Public Health
American Journal of Tropical Medicine and Hygiene
Annals of Tropical Medicine and Parasitology
Archivos Argentinos de Pediatría, Buenos Aires
Boletín de la Oficina Sanitaria Panamericana, Buenos Aires
Boletín Epidemiológico Nacional, Buenos Aires
Boletín Informativo Techint
Buenos Aires Herald
Circulation
Clarín, Buenos Aires
Cuadernos Médico Sociales, Rosario, Santa Fe, Argentina
Desarrollo de Base
Desarrollo Económico, Buenos Aires
Diario de Cuyo, Mendoza, Argentina
Entrerriano, Concordia, Entre Ríos, Argentina
Epidemiologic Reviews
Estudios, Córdoba, Argentina
Health Policy and Planning
Journal of Commerce, New York
Journal of the American Medical Association
Journal of Public Health Policy
Medicina, Buenos Aires
Medicina y Sociedad, Buenos Aires
The New York Times
Norte, Resistencia, Chaco
Noticias de la Semana, Buenos Aires
Salud Pública de México
Salud y Sociedad, Córdoba
Transactions of the Royal Society of Tropical Medicine and Hygiene
The Wall Street Journal
World Journal of Surgery

Books and Articles

Abalo, Carlos. 1989. "Deuda externa y deuda sanitaria." In *III Jornadas de Atención Primaria de la Salud*, pp. 59–96. Buenos Aires.

Abba, Artemio, Gustavo Dardik, and Ana María Facciolo. 1986. "Diagnóstico de la situación habitacional de los sectores carenciados de la Capital Federal." In Nora Clichevsky et al., eds., *Habitat popular: Experiencias y alternativas en países de América Latina*, pp. 57–76. Buenos Aires: Centro de Estudios Urbanos y Regionales.

Abellard, Jacques. 1994. "Oral Health in Mali's Schools." *World Health* 47 (no. 1): 12.

Accinelli, M. M., and M. S. Müller. 1978. *Un hecho inquietante: La evolución reciente de la mortalidad en la Argentina.* Buenos Aires: Centro de Estudios de Población.

Acquatella, H., F. Catalioti, J. R. Gómez-Mancebo, V. Davalos, and L. Villalobos. 1987. "Long-Term Control of Chagas Disease in Venezuela: Effects on Serologic Findings, Electrocardiographic Abnormalities, and Clinical Outcome." *Circulation* 76 (no. 3): 556–562.

Agrest, Alberto. 1988. "Errores de diagnóstico: análisis prospectivo de sus causas." *Medicina* 48 (no. 1): 99–100.

———. 1990. "Problemas de la investigación clínica." *Medicina* 50 (no. 6): 557–562.

Aguirre, Patricia. 1991. "Hiperinflación-estabilización en las estrategias domésticas de consumo de familias en situación de extrema pobreza." *Cuadernos Médico Sociales* (no. 57): 13–33.

Akin, John S. 1987. *Financing Health Services in Developing Countries: An Agenda for Reform.* Washington, D.C.: World Bank.

Albiano, Nelson. 1991. "Ecología y salud." In *V Jornadas de Atención Primaria de la Salud,* pp. 117–144. Buenos Aires.

Alderslade, Richard. 1990. "La gestión de la salud pública en la era de salud para todos." *Foro Mundial de la Salud* 11 (no. 3): 271–275.

Allodi, Federico, G. Randall, E. Lutz, J. Quiroga, M. Zunzunegui, C. Kolff, A. Deutsch, and R. Doan. 1985. "Physical and Psychiatric Effects of Torture: Two Medical Studies." In Eric Stover and Elena Nightingale, eds., *The Breaking of Bodies and Minds: Torture, Psychiatric Abuse, and the Health Professions,* pp. 58–78. New York: W. H. Freeman.

Alonso, Héctor O. 1990. "El clínico, el generalista y la economía." *Medicina* 50 (no. 6): 566–567.

Alonso, J. M., A. Risso, M. Mangiaterra, C. Guillerón, and J. Gorodner. 1987. "Prevalencia de dengue en una área de riesgo en la Argentina." *Medicina* 47 (no. 5): 551.

Alvarez, Rubén, and Ana Alvarez. 1992. "Los nuevos rostros de la pobreza." *Clarín*, second section, June 7, pp. 6–7.

Altman, Lawrence K. 1995*a*. "Ebola Virus Cases Expected to Rise." *New York Times*, May 16, p. C3.

———. 1995*b*. "U.S. Agency on Front Line of Disease War: Crowded, Understaffed and Overwhelmed." *New York Times*, May 20, p. 9.

———. 1995*c*. "Vitamin A Deficiency Linked to Transmission of AIDS Virus from Mothers to Infants." *New York Times*, February 3, p. A17.

Andreano, R., and T. Helmeniak. 1988. "Economics, Health, and Tropical Diseases: A Review." In A. N. Herrin and P. L. Rosenfield, eds., *Economics, Health and Tropical Diseases.* Manila: School of Economics, University of the Philippines.

Anigstein, Carlos, M. Fradusco, and L. Mazzonelli. 1987. "Fallas en la técnica de preparación del biberón con leche en polvo entera." *Archivos Argentinos de Pediatría* 85 (no. 4): 318–324.

Arce, Hugo. 1988. "Argentina: Diagnóstico sanitario sintético." *Medicina y Sociedad* 11 (no. 4): 102–106.

Arce, Hugo, and Aquiles Roncoroni. 1987. "Acerca del histórico fatalismo de los hospitales públicos." *Medicina y Sociedad* 10 (no. 1/2): 33–37.

Arias, Daniel. 1992. "Este mismo gobierno fue el que degradó a la oficina que controlaba los medicamentos." *Clarín*, August 23, pp. 36–37.

Arole, Mabelle, and Rajanikant Arole. 1994. *Jamkhed: A Comprehensive Rural Health Project.* London: Macmillan.

Aulicino, Jorge. 1992. "¿Qué remedios toman los Argentinos?" *Clarín*, second section, November 1, pp. 1–5.

Avila-Rosas, H., E. Casanueva, A. Barrera, I. Cruz, and M. C. Rojo. 1988. "Algunos determinantes biológicos y sociales del peso al nacer." *Salud Pública de México* 30 (no. 1): 47–53.

Baccaro, Diana. 1992. "Las madres niñas." *Clarín*, January 12, pp. 32–33.

Badhwar, Inderjit. 1994. "The Emperors of Garbage." *New York Times*, November 5, p. 23.

Balcazar, H., and J. D. Haas. 1991. "Retarded Fetal Growth Patterns and Early Neonatal Mortality in a Mexico City Population." *Bulletin of the Pan American Health Organization* 25 (no. 1): 55–63.

Bangdiwala, Shrikant I., and Elías Anzola-Pérez. 1987. "Accidentes de tránsito: Problema de salud en paises en desarrollo de las Américas." *Boletín de la Oficina Sanitaria Panamericana* 103 (no. 2): 130–139.

Barri, Horacio. 1991. "¿Estamos avanzando?" *Salud y Sociedad* 8 (no. 21): 37–39.

Battellino, Luis. 1988. "Políticas sobre tecnología y medicamentos: Situación actual y posibilidades futuras." In *II Jornadas de Atención Primaria de la Salud*, pp. 471–474. Buenos Aires.

Battellino, Luis, and Fernando Bennun. 1991. "Niveles, tendencias y estructura de la mortalidad infantil en la provincia de Córdoba (Argentina)." *Cuadernos Médico Sociales* (no. 56): 45–58.

Beck, Melinda. 1991. "State of Emergency." *Newsweek*, October 14, pp. 44–45.

Becker, David. 1985. "Políticas sanitarias para el control de la enfermedad de Chagas." In Rodolfo Carcavallo et al., *Factores biológicos y ecológicos en la enfermedad de Chagas*, vol. 2, pp. 305–308. Washington, D.C.: Centro Panamericano de Ecología Humana y Salud, Organización Panamericana de la Salud.

Beckles, Verity. 1996. "Children Versus Mosquitoes." *World Health*, 49(4): 19.

Belizán, J., J. Nardín, G. Carroli, and L. Campodónico. 1989. "Factores de riesgo de bajo peso al nacer en un grupo de embarazadas de Rosario, Argentina." *Boletín de la Oficina Sanitaria Panamericana* 106 (no. 5): 380–388.

Belmartino, Susana. 1991. "Políticas de salud en Argentina: perspectiva histórica." *Cuadernos Médico Sociales* (no. 55): 13–33.

———. 1992. "El sistema de salud en Argentina: perspectivas de reformulación." *Cuadernos Médico Sociales* (no. 61): 1–5.

Belmartino, Susana, Carlos Bloch, M. I. Carnino, and A. V. Persello. 1991. *Fundamentos históricos da la construcción de relaciones de poder en el sector salud. Argentina 1940–1960*. Buenos Aires: Organización Panamericana de la Salud.

BEN (Boletín Epidemiológico Nacional). 1990a. "Lepra: Situación nacional." 1 (no. 1): 60–64.

———. 1990b. "Los accidentes de tránsito de la República Argentina." 1 (no. 1): 35–38.

———. 1990c. "Sarampión en la Argentina." 1 (no. 2): 32–38.

———. 1990d. "Tétanos del recién nacido." 1 (no. 2): 39–43.

Berg, Alan. 1973. *The Nutrition Factor*. Washington, D.C.: The Brookings Institution.

Bergel, Rúben. 1989. "Atención primaria o primitiva de la salud: ¿Qué pasa en Argentina hoy?" In *III Jornadas de Atención Primaria de la Salud*, pp. 15–58. Buenos Aires.

Bloom, Gerald. 1993. "Managing Health Sector Development: Markets and Institutional Reform." In Christopher Colclough and James Manor, eds., *States or Markets? Neoliberalism and the Development Policy Debate*, pp. 214–237. Oxford: Clarendon.

Bobadilla, J. L., P. Cowley, P. Musgrove, and H. Saxenian. 1994. "Design, Content and Financing of an Essential National Package of Health Services." In C.J.L. Murray and A. D. Lopez, *Global Comparative Assessments in the Health Sector: Disease Burden, Expenditures and Intervention Packages*, pp. 171–180. Geneva: World Health Organization.

Boyer, Mario, H. Jouval, R. Tafani, and C. Vidal. 1989. *Informe final. Taller sobre economía y financiamiento de salud.* Buenos Aires: Organización Panamericana de la Salud.

Brandling-Bennett, David, and Francisco Pinheiro. 1996. "Infectious Diseases in Latin America and the Caribbean: Are They Really Emerging and Increasing?" *Emerging Infectious Diseases* 2 (no. 1).

Braun, Rafael. 1987. "La ética médica y la atención primaria." *Medicina y Sociedad* 10 (no. 1/2): 38–40.

Brenner, Rodolfo R., and Angel de la Merced Stoka, eds. 1987. *Chagas' Disease Vectors*, vol. 1. Boca Raton, Fla.: CRC Press.

British Medical Association. 1991. *Hazardous Waste and Human Health.* Oxford: Oxford University Press.

Brockington, Fraser. 1985. *The Health of the Developing World.* Lewes, Sussex: Book Guild Limited.

Brody, Jane. 1991. "To Preserve Their Health and Heritage, Arizona Indians Reclaim Ancient Foods." *New York Times*, May 21, p. C21.

———. 1996. "Life in Womb May Affect Adult Heart Risk." *New York Times*, October 1, pp. C1, C6.

Brooke, Elizabeth. 1994. "Latin America May Outpace U.S. in Abortions." *New York Times*, April 12, p. C5.

Brown, Lester, C. Flavin, and L. Starke, eds. 1996. *State of the World 1996.* New York: W. W. Norton.

Brunstein, Fernando. 1986. "Población de bajos ingresos y agua potable en Argentina: Un aspecto poco tratado de la acción del Estado sobre el habitat." In Nora Clichevsky et al., *Habitat popular: Experiencias y alternativas en paises de América Latina*, pp. 147–162. Buenos Aires: Centro de Estudios Urbanos y Regionales.

———, ed. 1988. *Crisis y servicios públicos: Agua y saneamiento en la región metropolitana de Buenos Aires.* Buenos Aires: Centro de Estudios Urbanos y Regionales.

Brunstein, Fernando, S. Grisotto, and G. Peirano. 1988. "Saneamiento hídrico en el Gran Buenos Aires: Límite de la precariedad." In Fernando Brunstein, ed., *Crisis y servicios públicos: Agua y saneamiento en la región metropolitana de Buenos Aires*, pp. 5–41. Buenos Aires: Centro de Estudios Urbanos y Regionales.

Burke, Mary. 1979. "Inter-American Investigation of Mortality in Childhood: Report on a Household Sample." In Mary Burke et al., *Inter-American Investigation of Mortality in Childhood: Report on a Household Survey.* Scientific publication no. 386, pp. 1–54. Washington, D.C.: Pan American Health Organization.

Burke, Mary, Marjorie York, and Innis Sande. 1979. *Inter-American Investigation of Mortality in Childhood: Report on a Household Sample.* Scientific publication no. 386. Washington, D.C.: Pan American Health Organization.

Burns, John. 1996. "Accident or Mass Murder? India's Food-Poisoning Mystery." *New York Times*, August 19, p. A3.

———. 1997. "Vaccine War Emboldens India as It Weakens Polio." *New York Times*, January 26, p. 3.

Bustelo, Eduardo. 1989. "Deuda externa y deuda sanitaria." In *III Jornadas de Atención Primaria de la Salud*, pp. 59–96. Buenos Aires.

Bustelo, Eduardo, and Ernesto Isuani, eds. 1990. *Mucho, poquito o nada: Crisis y alternativas de política social en los '90.* Buenos Aires: UNICEF.

Calvert, Susan, and Peter Calvert. 1989. *Argentina: Political Culture and Instability.* Pittsburgh: University of Pittsburgh Press.

Calvo, Elvira, E. Abeyá, A. Masautis, N. Gnazzo, I. Steinel, M. Baiocchi, E. Sosa, S. González, and R. Tassara. 1989. "Evaluación del estado nutricional y prevalencia de anemia en una población de alto riesgo." In Alfredo Lattes et al., *Salud, enfermedad y muerte de los niños en América Latina*, pp. 131–157. Buenos Aires: Consejo Latinoamericano de Ciencias Sociales.

Campbell, T. Colin, and Junshi Chen. 1994. "Diet and Chronic Degenerative Diseases." In Norman Temple and Denis Burkitt, eds., *Western Diseases: Their Dietary Prevention and Reversibility*, pp. 67–118. Totowa, N.J.: Humana.

Camps, Sibila. 1992*a*. "El juez ecologista." *Clarín*, May 3, second section, p. 12.

————. 1992*b*. "La bacteria que causa el brote de meningitis es la más agresiva y provendría del sur del Brasil." *Clarín*, September 20, pp. 40–41.

Canepa, María. 1991. "Fight to Prevent Caesarean Abuse." *Buenos Aires Herald*, September 29, p. 18.

Carbonara, María F. 1991. "Efectos adversos de los plaguicidas sobre la salud de los conductores que transportan cereales y sobre la comunidad." *Cuadernos Médico Sociales* (no. 56): 69–86.

Carcavallo, Rodolfo, J. Rabinovich, and R. Tonn, eds. 1985. *Factores biológicos y ecológicos en la enfermedad de Chagas*, vol. 2. Washington, D.C.: Centro Panamericano de Ecología Humana y Salud, Organización Panamericana de la Salud.

Castañaro, Atilio. 1991. "60 niños menores de un año mueren diariamente en nuestro país, la mitad por causas prevenibles. ¿Por qué?, ¿Hasta cuándo?" In *V Jornadas de Atención Primaria de la Salud*, pp. 263–287. Buenos Aires.

Castellanos, Pedro. 1984. "Principales problemas de salud en las áreas marginales." *Cuadernos Médico Sociales* (no. 29/30): 25–40.

Chafkin, Sol H. 1987. "Comments." In OPS, *Problemas nutricionales en países en desarrollo en las décadas de 1980 y 1990.* Cuaderno técnico no. 10, pp. 77–80. Washington, D.C.: Organización Panamericana de la Salud.

Chandhary, Vivek. 1992. "Salta Still Braced for Cholera." *Buenos Aires Herald*, August 30, p. 4.

Chen, Lincoln C. 1987. "Nutrición en países en desarrollo y la función de los organismos internacionales: en busca de una visión." In OPS, *Problemas nutricionales en países en desarrollo en las décadas de 1980 y 1990.* Cuaderno técnico no. 10, pp. 57–72. Washington, D.C.: Organización Panamericana de la Salud.

————. 1988. "Health Policy Responses: An Approach Derived from the China and India Experiences." In David Bell and Michael Reich, eds., *Health, Nutrition, and Economic Crises: Approaches to Policy in the Third World*, pp. 279–305. Dover, Mass.: Auburn House.

Chuit, R., E. Subias, A. C. Pérez, I. Paulone, C. Wisnivesky-Colli, and E. L. Segura. 1989. "Usefulness of Serology for the Evaluation of *Trypanosoma cruzi* Transmission in Endemic Areas of Chagas' Disease." *Revista da Sociedade Brasileira de Medicina Tropical* 22 (no. 3): 119–124.

Clichevsky, Nora, Beatriz Cuenya, and Susana Peñalva. 1986. *Habitat popular: Experiencias y alternativas en paises de América Latina.* Buenos Aires: Centro de Estudios Urbanos y Regionales.

Clivaggio, Graciela. 1991. "Una cuestión de peso." *Noticias de la Semana*, August 18, pp. 130–131.

———. 1993*a*. "Cuando los controles no son seguros." *Clarín*, September 12, p. 42.

———. 1993*b*. "El 26% de los argentinos padece de hipertensión." *Clarín*, November 28, p. 43.

Cochrane, A. L., A. S. St. Leger, and F. Moore. 1988. "Health Service 'Input' and Mortality 'Output' in Developed Countries." In Pan American Health Organization, *The Challenge of Epidemiology*, pp. 930–937. Washington, D.C.: Pan American Health Organization.

Cohen, Hugo. 1987. "Salud mental y atención primaria." In *Jornadas de Atención Primaria de la Salud*, pp. 349–408. Buenos Aires.

Confederación General del Trabajo. 1991. "Perfil del médico que necesitamos." *Salud y Sociedad* 8 (no. 21): 60–63.

Cooper, Julian. 1994. "Obsessively Thorough Verbitsky." *Buenos Aires Herald*, October 2, pp. 14–15.

Corradi, Juan. 1987. "The Culture of Fear in Civil Society." In Monica Peralta-Ramos and Carlos Waisman, eds., *From Military Rule to Liberal Democracy in Argentina*, pp. 113–129. Boulder, Colo.: Westview.

Corrales, M., G. Fronchkowsky, and T. Eiguer. 1989. "Aislamiento en Argentina de *Vibrio cholerae no 01* en líquidos cloacales." *Revista Argentina de Microbiología* 21 (no. 2): 71–77.

Cotic, Andrés, and Guillermo Dascal. 1988. "Technología y saneamiento urbano en la región metropolitana de Buenos Aires." In Fernando Brunstein, ed., *Crisis y servicios públicos: Agua y saneamiento en la región metropolitana de Buenos Aires*, pp. 109–143. Buenos Aires: Centro de Estudios Urbanos y Regionales.

Cowell, Alan. 1994. "Italy's Public Health-Care System Is Doing Poorly." *New York Times*, November 8, p. A3.

Cox, David. 1992. "Public Health School Courses Closed." *Buenos Aires Herald*, November 1, p. 4.

Cravino, Graciela. 1992. "La vida que se escapa." *Clarín*, November 8, second section, pp. 1–3.

Crivos, Marta. 1988. "Estudio antropológico de una sala de hospital." *Medicina y Sociedad* 11 (no. 5/6): 127–137.

Crossette, Barbara. 1995*a*. "Mental Illness Found Rising in Poor Nations." *New York Times*, May 16, p. C9.

———. 1995*b*. "Unicef Asks Broader Aid for Children." *New York Times*, June 12, p. 5.

———. 1996. "Noncommunicable Diseases Seen as Growing Health Problem." *New York Times*, September 16, p. A7.

Cuenya, Beatriz. 1985. *Condiciones de habitat y salud de los sectores populares: Un estudio piloto en el Asentamiento San Martín de Quilmes*. Buenos Aires: Centro de Estudios Urbanos y Regionales.

Cumper, George. 1991. "What Ever Happened to Public Health?" *Health Policy and Planning* 6 (no. 4): 384–386.

Cutait, D. E., and R. Cutait. 1991. "Surgery of Chagasic Megacolon." *World Journal of Surgery* 15 (no. 2): 188–197.

Daley, Suzanne. 1996*a*. "In Malawi, Pilgrims Throng to an AIDS Potion." *New York Times*, June 6, p. A3.

———. 1996*b*. "South Africa Losing Battle to House Homeless." *New York Times*, May 3, p. A10.

Darwin, Charles. 1958. *The Voyage of the Beagle*. New York: Bantam Books.

De Genaro, Víctor. 1989. "Las condiciones de trabajo y su relación con el proceso salud-enfermedad." In *III Jornadas de Atención Primaria de la Salud*, pp. 240–245. Buenos Aires.

de Kantor, I., L. Barrera, V. Ritacco, and I. Miceli. 1991. "Utilidad del enzimoinmunoensayo en el diagnóstico de la Tb." *Boletín de la Oficina Sanitaria Panamericana* 110 (no. 6): 461.

Del Rey, Eusebio Cleto, and M. A. Basombrío. 1992. "Costos y beneficios de la prevención del mal de Chagas. Una aproximación metodológica." *Estudios* Enero/Marzo: 3–12.

Denny, Floyd, and F. A. Loda. 1986. "Acute Respiratory Infections Are the Leading Cause of Death in Children in Developing Countries." *American Journal of Tropical Medicine and Hygiene* 35 (no. 1): 1–2.

DeParle, Jason. 1994. "Census Sees Falling Income and More Poor." *New York Times*, October 7, p. A16.

de Sarasqueta, Pedro. 1987. "Relato de la experiencia en el control de la mujer embarazada en el barrio de San Pedro, La Matanza (Pcia. de Bs. As.)." In *Jornadas de Atención Primaria de la Salud*, pp. 545–557. Buenos Aires.

———. 1988. "Significado, dilemas y dificultades de la atención primaria de la salud." In *II Jornadas de Atención Primaria de la Salud*, pp. 52–56. Buenos Aires.

———. 1990. "58 menores de un año mueren diariamente en nuestro país, la mitad por causas prevenibles. ¿Por qué?" In *IV Jornadas de Atención Primaria de la Salud*, pp. 721–752. Buenos Aires.

———. 1991. "60 niños menores de un año mueren diariamente en nuestro país, la mitad por causas prevenibles. ¿Por qué?, ¿Hasta cuándo?" In *V Jornadas de Atención Primaria de la Salud*, pp. 263–287. Buenos Aires.

de Sarasqueta, Pedro, and Graciela Basso. 1988. "Mortalidad postneonatal en la ciudad de Buenos Aires en 1987." *Archivos Argentinos de Pediatría* 86: 327–333.

de Sarasqueta, Pedro, C. Díaz, A. Schwarcz, R. Guntin, S. Marzo, and R. Morresi. 1988. "Análisis de los factores gestacionales y del parto relacionados con la mortalidad perinatal en el Hospital 'Diego Paroissien', La Matanza, Provincia de Buenos Aires." *Archivos Argentinos de Pediatría* 86: 193–198.

Dias, João Carlos Pinto. 1985. "Aspectos socio-culturales y económicos relativos al vector de la enfermedad de Chagas." In Rodolfo Carcavallo et al., *Factores biológicos y ecológicos en la enfermedad de Chagas*, vol. 2, pp. 289–304. Washington, D.C.: Centro Panamericano de Ecología Humana y Salud, Organización Panamericana de la Salud.

———. 1987. "Epidemiology of Chagas' Disease in Brazil." In R. R. Brenner and A. de la M. Stoka, eds., *Chagas' Disease Vectors*, vol. 1, pp. 57–84. Boca Raton, Fla.: CRC Press.

Digregorio, Jorge, H. Sexer, M. de los A. López, and P. de Sarasqueta. 1988. "Estudio de la predicción clínica de la prematurez y el retardo de crecimiento intrauterino por factores de riesgo de la embarazada." *Archivos Argentinos de Pediatría* 86: 17–21.

Dillon, Sam. 1991. "Argentina's Privatization Efforts Bog Down in Controversy." *Journal of Commerce*, March 7, p. 10A.

di Tella, Guido. 1986. "Economic Controversies in Argentina from the 1920s to the 1940s." In Guido di Tella and D.C.M. Platt, eds., *The Political Economy of Argentina*, pp. 39–59. London: Macmillan.

di Tella, Guido, and Rudiger Dornbusch, eds. 1989. *The Political Economy of Argentina*, 1946–1983. Pittsburgh: University of Pittsburgh Press.

di Tella, Guido, and D.C.M. Platt, eds. 1986. *The Political Economy of Argentina*. London: Macmillan.

Dolkart, R. H. 1969. *Manuel A. Fresco, Governor of the Province of Buenos Aires, 1936–1940: A Study of the Argentine Right and Its Response to Economic and Social Change.* Ph.D. dissertation, University of California at Los Angeles.

Douglas, David. 1990. "Tras la estela del buque: El Decenio del Agua y su legado." *Desarrollo de Base* 14 (no. 2): 2–11.

Downes, Patricio, Marina García, and Stella Bin. 1993. "El 5% de los argentinos nunca fue a la escuela." *Clarín*, December 12, Educación, pp. 1–4.

Due, Le Kinh. 1996. "Overcoming the Stigma." *World Health* 49(3): 22–23.

Duro, Eduardo. 1991. "60 niños menores de un año mueren diariamente en nuestro país, la mitad por causas prevenibles. ¿Por qué?, ¿Hasta cuándo?" In *V Jornadas de Atención Primaria de la Salud*, pp. 263–287. Buenos Aires.

Eban, Abba. 1984. *Heritage: Civilization and the Jews.* New York: Summit Books.

ECLA (Economic Commission for Latin America). 1969. *Economic Development and Income Distribution in Argentina.* New York: United Nations.

Enria, Graciela. 1991. "Proceso de salud-enfermedad y condiciones de pobreza. Rosario 1981." *Cuadernos Médico Sociales* (no. 56): 59–68.

Epelman, Mario. 1988. "Salud y trabajo." In *II Jornadas de Atención Primaria de la Salud*, pp. 359–388. Buenos Aires.

———. 1991. "Ecología y salud." In *V Jornadas de Atención Primaria de la Salud*, pp. 117–144. Buenos Aires.

Erlanger, Steven. 1995. "In Fallen Chechen Capital, Medical Care Is in Ruins." *New York Times*, April 9, p. 3.

Escudé, Carlos Andrés. 1989. "Health in Buenos Aires in the Second Half of the Nineteenth Century." In D.C.M. Platt, ed., *Social Welfare, 1850–1950: Australia, Argentina and Canada Compared*, pp. 60–70. London: Macmillan.

Escudero, José Carlos. 1987. "Corrientes de pensamiento en la salud pública argentina." In *Jornadas de Atención Primaria de la Salud*, pp. 521–532. Buenos Aires.

Etcheverry, Guillermo. 1987. "La facultad de medicina en la formación del pregrado." In *Jornadas de Atención Primaria de la Salud*, pp. 181–196. Buenos Aires.

Faber, Daniel. 1993. *Environment under Fire: Imperialism and the Ecological Crisis in Central America.* New York: Monthly Review Press.

Feachem, Richard, T. Kjellstrom, C. Murray, M. Over, and M. A. Phillips, eds. 1992. *The Health of Adults in the Developing World.* New York: Oxford University Press.

Fernández Guinti, Daniel. 1992. "Los ribereños no quieren irse." *Clarín*, June 7, p. 40.

Ferrer, Aldo. 1967. *The Argentine Economy.* Berkeley: University of California Press.

Ferrero, Hilario. 1987. "Experiencia de A.P.S. en Ingeniero Juárez." In *Jornadas de Atención Primaria de la Salud*, pp. 167–179. Buenos Aires.

FIEL (Fundación de Investigaciones Económicas Latinoamericanas).1988. *Regulaciones y estancamiento: El caso argentino.* Buenos Aires: Ediciones Manantial.

Fiennes, Richard N. T-W-. 1978. *Zoonoses and the Origins and Ecology of Human Disease.* London: Academic Press.

Fillol, Tomás Roberto. 1961. *Social Factors in Economic Development: The Argentine Case.* Cambridge: MIT Press.

Firestone, David. 1996. "Life Span Dips for Men Born in New York." *New York Times*, April 27, pp. 25, 29.

Fodor, Jorge. 1975. "Perón's Policies for Agricultural Exports 1946–1948: Dogmatism or Common Sense?" In David Rock, *Argentina in the 20th Century*, pp. 135–161. Pittsburgh: University of Pittsburgh Press.

———. 1989. "Argentina's Nationalism: Myth or Reality?" In Guido di Tella and Rudiger

Dornbusch, eds., *The Political Economy of Argentina, 1946–1983*, pp. 31–57. Pittsburgh: University of Pittsburgh Press.

Fontán, Marcelino. 1991. "Política sanitaria y diferentes alternativas." *Salud y Sociedad* 8 (no. 21): 33–35.

Foster, Phillips. 1992. *The World Food Problem: Tackling the Causes of Undernutrition in the Third World.* Boulder, Colo.: Lynne Rienner.

Fraker, P. J., R. Caruso, and F. Kierszenbaum. 1982. "Alteration of the Immune and Nutritional Status of Mice by Synergy between Zinc Deficiency and Infection with *Trypanosoma cruzi.*" *Journal of Nutrition* 112 (no. 6): 1224–1229.

Franco Agudelo, Saúl. 1988. "Crisis y salud en América Latina." In *II Jornadas de Atención Primaria de la Salud*, pp. 177–192. Buenos Aires.

———. 1989. "Viejos y nuevos problemas en epidemiología." In *III Jornadas de Atención Primaria de la Salud*, pp. 299–326. Buenos Aires.

Frencken, Jo, and Fiona Makoni. 1994. "A Treatment Technique for Tooth Decay in Deprived Communities." *World Health* 47 (no. 1): 15–17.

Friedman, Herbert. 1985. "The Health of Adolescents and Youth: A Global Overview." *World Health Statistical Quarterly* 38 (no. 3): 256–266.

García Díaz, C. J. 1990. "Plétora de especialistas." *Medicina y Sociedad* 13 (no. 5/6): 15–16.

Gardner, Gary. 1996. "Preserving Agricultural Resources." In Lester Brown, C. Flavin, and L. Starke, eds., *State of the World 1996*, pp. 78–94. New York: W. W. Norton.

Gaslonde, Santiago. 1975. "Studies in Fertility and Abortion in Asunción, Bogotá, Buenos Aires, Lima, and Panama City." In Pan American Health Organization and Transnational Family Research Institute, *Epidemiology of Abortion and Practices of Fertility Regulation in Latin America: Selected Reports*, pp. 9–25. Washington, D.C.: Pan American Health Organization.

Gatto, Francisco. c1982. "Características de las economías provinciales y de las disparidades regionales." In Felipe González Arzac and Alfredo Calcagno, eds., *El desarrollo regional argentino: los espacios susceptibles de tratamiento especializado.* Buenos Aires: CFI.

Gené, R., J. A. Mazzei, and C. R. Posse. 1989. "Mortalidad por asma en la Argentina. ¿Por qué es tan alta?" *Medicina* 49 (no. 5): 545–546.

Germani, Gino. 1955. *La estructura social de la Argentina.* Buenos Aires: Raigal.

Giménez, Estela. 1991. "Ecología y salud." In *V Jornadas de Atención Primaria de la Salud*, pp. 117–144. Buenos Aires.

Giojalas, L. C., S. S. Catala, S. N. Asin and D. E. Gorla. 1990. "Seasonal Changes in Infectivity of Domestic Populations of *Triatoma infestans.*" *Transactions of the Royal Society of Tropical Medicine and Hygiene* 84 (no. 3): 439–442.

Giubellino, Gabriel. 1992. "Pettigiani: 'Ahora matan por placer.'" *Clarín*, January 19, p. 32.

Golden, Tim. 1994. "Health Care, Pride of Cuba, Is Falling on Tough Times." *New York Times*, October 30, pp. 1, 8.

Goñi, Uki. 1992*a*. "Thames to Run into River Plate?" *Buenos Aires Herald*, August 28, p. 5.

———. 1992*b*. "The Week in Business." *Buenos Aires Herald*, December 6, p. 2.

———. 1993*a*. "Measuring Poverty." *Buenos Aires Herald*, September 7, p. 5.

———. 1993*b*. "The Week in Business." *Buenos Aires Herald*, December 12, p. 2.

———. 1994. "The Week in Business." *Buenos Aires Herald*, January 2, p. 2.

González García, Gines, Pablo Abadie, Juan José Llovet, and Silvina Ramos. 1987. *El gasto en salud y en medicamentos: Argentina, 1985.* Buenos Aires: Centro de Estudios de Estado y Sociedad.

González Toro, Alberto. 1992. "Villa Retiro: El duro oficio de vivir." *Clarín*, second section, May 31, pp. 6–7.

Gorban, Marcos. 1993. "Ratas: ¿La batalla perdida?" *Clarín*, second section, November 28, pp. 8–9.

Goyoaga, Beatriz. 1990. "Chagas Disease Infects 2,500,000." *Buenos Aires Herald*, January 7, p. 10.

Gradizuela, Eduardo. 1991. "Residuos domiciliarios: un diagnóstico." *Entrerriano*, October 5, p. 21.

Graham-Yooll, Andrew. 1995. "The Argentine Church's Dirty War Record." *Buenos Aires Herald*, July 16, p. 13.

Gray, Clive, J. Baudouy, K. Martin, M. Bang, and R. Cash. 1990. *Primary Health Care in Africa: A Study of the Mali Rural Health Project*. Boulder, Colo.: Westview.

Greene, Lawrence. 1977. "Hyperendemic Goiter, Cretinism and Social Organization in Highland Ecuador." In Lawrence Greene, ed., *Malnutrition, Behavior, and Social Organization*, pp. 55–94. New York: Academic Press.

Griffin, Keith, and Terry McKinley. 1994. *Implementing a Human Development Strategy*. New York : St. Martin's Press.

Gualtieri, J. M., M. Nelson, and J. A. Cichero. 1985. "Presente y perspectiva del control químico." In Rodolfo Carcavallo et al., *Factores biológicos y ecológicos en la enfermedad de Chagas*, vol. 2, pp. 319–330. Washington, D.C.: Centro Panamericano de Ecología Humana y Salud, Organización Panamericana de la Salud.

Guerberoff, Simon. 1989. "Argentina: Muddling through Is Not Fine." In F. Desmond McCarthy, ed., *Developing Economies in Transition. Vol. 2: Country Studies*, pp. 13–48. Washington, D.C.: World Bank.

Gürtler, R. E., F. Kravetz, R. Petersen, M. Lauricella, and C. Wisnivesky-Colli. 1990. "The Prevalence of *Trypanosoma cruzi* and the Demography of Dog Populations After Insecticidal Spraying of Houses: A Predictive Model." *Annals of Tropical Medicine and Parasitology* 84 (no. 4): 313–323.

Gwatkin, D. R. 1983. "Does Better Health Produce Greater Wealth? A Review of the Evidence Concerning Health, Nutrition, and Output." Overseas Development Council. (August). Unpublished paper.

Halperín, Tulio. 1986. "The Argentine Export Economy: Intimations of Mortality, 1894–1930." In Guido di Tella and D.C.M. Platt, eds., *The Political Economy of Argentina*, pp. 39–59. London: Macmillan.

Halsey, Neal. 1983. "The Optimal Age for Administering Measles Vaccine in Developing Countries." In Neal Halsey and Ciro de Quadros, coordinators, *Recent Advances in Immunization: A Bibliographic Review*, pp. 1–17. Scientific publication no. 541. Washington, D.C.: Pan American Health Organization.

Harpham, Trudy, and Carolyn Stephens. 1991. "Urbanization and Health in Developing Countries." *World Health Statistical Quarterly* 44 (no. 2): 62–69.

Heise, Lori. 1993. "Violence against Women: The Missing Agenda." In Marge Koblinsky, J. Timyan, and J. Gay, eds., *The Health of Women: A Global Perspective*, pp. 171–196. Boulder, Colo.: Westview Press.

Higa de Landoni, Julia. 1991. "Contaminación: Impacto sobre la salud humana." In INTA (Instituto Nacional de Tecnología Agropecuaria), *Juicio a nuestra agricultura: Hacia el desarrollo de una agricultura sostenible*, pp. 161–179. Buenos Aires: Hemisferio Sur.

Hill, Austin Bradford. 1992. "Ambiente y enfermedad: ¿Asociación o causación?" *Boletín de la Oficina Sanitaria Panamericana* 113 (no. 3): 233–242.

Horwitz, Abraham. 1987. "Introducción." In OPS, *Problemas nutricionales en países en desarrollo en las décadas de 1980 y 1990*. Cuaderno técnico no. 10, pp. 1–3. Washington, D.C.: Organización Panamericana de la Salud.

Hospital Fernández. n.d. *Area de Riesgo Villa Numero 31—Villa Retiro*. Buenos Aires.

Huttly, Sharon. 1990. "The Impact of Inadequate Sanitary Conditions on Health in Developing Countries." *World Health Statistical Quarterly* 43, pp. 118–126.

INDEC (Instituto Nacional de Estadística y Censos) n.d. *Anuario Estadístico de la República Argentina, 1983–1986*. Buenos Aires.

———. 1985. *La juventud de la Argentina*. Buenos Aires.

———. 1989. *La pobreza en el conurbano bonaerense*. Buenos Aires.

———. 1990. *La pobreza urbana en la Argentina*. Buenos Aires.

———. 1991*a*. *Censo nacional de población y vivienda 1991. Resultados provisionales*. Buenos Aires.

———. 1991*b*. *Conurbano bonaerense: Aproximación a la determinación de hogares y población en riesgo sanitario a través de la encuesta permanente de hogares*. Buenos Aires.

Irigoyen, Dr. 1987. "Experiencia en la Provincia de Neuquén." In *Jornadas de Atención Primaria de la Salud*, pp. 61–87. Buenos Aires.

Isuani, Ernesto, and Hugo Mercer. 1986. "La fragmentación institucional del sector salud en la Argentina: ¿pluralismo o irracionalidad?" *Boletín Informativo Techint* (no. 244): 9–40.

Ives, Jane. 1985. "The Health Effects of the Transfer of Technology to the Developing World: Report and Case Studies." In Jane Ives, ed., *The Export of Hazard*, pp. 172–192. Boston: Routledge and Kegan Paul.

Jacobson, Jodi. 1992. "The Other Epidemic." *World Watch* 5 (no. 3): 10–17.

Johnson, Allie. 1995. "Greens See Red over Plans for Parks." *Buenos Aires Herald*, October 1, pp. 1, 13.

Karasek, Robert, and Tores Theorell. 1990. *Healthy Work: Stress, Productivity, and the Reconstruction of Working Life*. New York: Basic Books.

Katz, Jorge. 1988. "La salud y la crisis económica." In *II Jornadas de Atención Primaria de la Salud*, pp. 151–175. Buenos Aires.

———. 1989. "Deuda externa y deuda sanitaria." In *III Jornadas de Atención Primaria de la Salud*, pp. 59–96. Buenos Aires.

Katz, Jorge, and Daniel Maceira. 1990. "Mortalidad infantil y el funcionamiento de los mercados de atención neonatal. Un examen del caso argentino." *Desarrollo Económico* 30 (no. 118): 173–198.

Katz, Jorge, and Alberto Muñoz. 1988. *Organización del sector salud: Puja distributiva y equidad*. Buenos Aires: Centro Editor de América Latina.

Kifner, John. 1994. "'Nothing to Build On': Haiti Starting at Zero." *New York Times*, December 4, pp. 1, 26.

Kirchhoff, L. V., A. A. Gam, and F. C. Gilliam. 1987. "American Trypanosomiasis (Chagas' Disease) in Central American Immigrants." *American Journal of Medicine* 82 (no. 5): 915–920.

Kjellstrom, Tord, J. Koplan, and R. Rothenberg. 1992. "Current and Future Determinants of Adult Ill-Health." In Richard Feachem et al., eds., *The Health of Adults in the Developing World*, pp. 209–259. New York: Oxford University Press.

Koblinsky, Marge, J. Timyan, and J. Gay, eds. 1993. *The Health of Women: A Global Perspective*. Boulder, Colo.: Westview Press.

Kolata, Gina. 1994. "Study Says Many of Tiniest Babies Will Have Learning Problems." *New York Times*, September 22, p. A25.

Kreplak, Enrique. 1991. "Los hospitales y la gente." *Salud y Sociedad* 8 (no. 21): 31–32.

Lacayo, Richard. 1991. "Death on the Shop Floor." *Time*, September 16, pp. 44–45.

Lamazares, Silvina. 1992. "Por qué se matan los jubilados." *Clarín*, October 18, pp. 42–43.

———. 1993a. "Buenos Aires, líder del mundo." *Clarín*, August 29, p. 44.

———. 1993b. "'Es un síntoma de la sociedad.'" *Clarín*, August 29, p. 45.

———. 1993c. "Las muertes por accidentes de tránsito en la Capital aumentaron un 55 por ciento." *Clarín*, August 29, pp. 44–45.

Lattes, Alfredo, Mark Farren, and Jane MacDonald, eds. 1989. *Salud, enfermedad y muerte de los niños en América Latina*. Buenos Aires: Consejo Latinoamericano de Ciencias Sociales.

Laquian, Aprodicio. 1983. *Basic Housing: Policies for Urban Sites, Services and Shelter in Developing Countries*. Ottawa, Canada: International Development Resource Center.

Laurelli, Elsa. 1988. "Sistema real de decisiones en la productividad y accesibilidad de servicios de agua y saneamiento." In Fernando Brunstein, ed., *Crisis y servicios públicos: Agua y saneamiento en la región metropolitana de Buenos Aires*, pp. 43–83. Buenos Aires: Centro de Estudios Urbanos y Regionales.

Lauricella, M. A., A. J. Sinagra, I. Paulone, A. R. Riarte, and E. L. Segura. 1989. "Natural *Trypanosoma cruzi* Infection in Dogs of Endemic Areas of the Argentine Republic." *Revista do Instituto de Medicina Tropical* (São Paulo) 31 (no. 2): 63–70.

Lauro, Adriana. 1992. "Para los pobres." *Clarín*, September 20, Economía, p. 24.

———. 1993. "Radiografía de la desocupación." *Clarín*, August 22, Economía, pp. 22–23.

Lean, Geoffrey, and Don Hinrichsen. 1992. *Atlas of the Environment*. 2d ed. New York: HarperCollins.

Leary, Warren. 1995. "River Blindness Disease Has 2d Devastating Side." *New York Times*, March 28, p. C7.

———. 1996. "U.N. Says Mosquito Netting Could Save 500,000 Lives in Africa." *New York Times*, April 4, p. A13.

Lejarraga, Horacio, E. Abeyá G., J. Andrade, and H. Boffi. 1991. "Evaluación del peso y la talle en 88.861 varones de 18 años de la República Argentina (1987). *Archivos Argentinos de Pediatría* 89: 185.

Lejarraga, Horacio, O. Meletti, S. Biocca, and V. Alonso. 1986. "Peso y talla de 15.214 adolescentes de todo el país. Tendencia secular." *Archivos Argentinos de Pediatría* 84: 219–235.

Lejarraga, Horacio, and Gerardo Orfila. 1987. "Estandares de peso y estatura para niños argentinos desde el nacimiento hasta la madurez." *Archivos Argentinos de Pediatría* 85: 209–222.

León, Magdalena. 1989. "The Invisible Worker: Health Conditions of the Domestic Worker in Colombia." In PAHO, *Midlife and Older Women in Latin America and the Caribbean*, pp. 354–366. Washington, D.C.: Pan American Health Organization.

Leowski, Jerzy. 1986. "Mortality from Acute Respiratory Infections in Children under 5 Years of Age: Global Estimates." *World Health Statistical Quarterly* 39 (no. 2): 138–144.

Leslie, Joanne, M. Lycette, and M. Buvinic. 1988. "Weathering Economic Crises: The Crucial Role of Women in Health." In David Bell and Michael Reich, eds., *Health, Nutrition, and Economic Crises: Approaches to Policy in the Third World*, pp. 307–348, Dover, Mass.: Auburn House.

Llovet, Juan José. 1984. *Servicios de salud y sectores populares: Los años del Proceso.* Buenos Aires: Estudios CEDES.

Llovet, Juan José, and Silvina Ramos. 1988. *La práctica del aborto en las mujeres de sectores populares de Buenos Aires.* Buenos Aires: Centro de Estudios de Estado y Sociedad.

Londres, Albert. 1928. *The Road to Buenos Ayres.* New York: Blue Ribbon Books.

Looney, Robert. 1987. "Impact of Increased External Debt Servicing on Government Budgetary Priorities: The Case of Argentina." *Socio-Economic Planning Sciences* 21 (no. 1): 25–32.

Loterszpil, Jaime, and Mario Loterszpil. 1988. "Saneamiento hídrico: Aspectos económico-financieros." In Fernando Brunstein, ed., *Crisis y servicios públicos: Agua y saneamiento en la región metropolitana de Buenos Aires*, pp. 85–108. Buenos Aires: Centro de Estudios Urbanos y Regionales.

Lumi, Susana. 1990. "Restricciones y posibilidades de la política habitacional argentina." In Eduardo Bustelo and Ernesto Isuani, eds., *Mucho, poquito o nada: Crisis y alternativas de política social en los '90*, pp. 183–222. Buenos Aires: UNICEF.

Lunven, Paul. 1987. "Comments." In OPS, *Problemas nutricionales en países en desarrollo en las décadas de 1980 y 1990.* Cuaderno técnico no. 10, p. 84. Washington, D.C.: Organización Panamericana de la Salud.

Maguire, J. H., R. Hoff, A. C. Sleigh, and K. E. Mott. 1986. "An Outbreak of Chagas' Disease in Southwestern Bahia, Brazil." *American Journal of Tropical Medicine and Hygiene* 35 (no. 5): 931–936.

Mahler, Halfdan T. 1987. "Perspectivas de una nutrición mejor mediante la atención primaria de salud." In OPS, *Problemas nutricionales en países en desarrollo en las décadas de 1980 y 1990.* Cuaderno técnico no. 10, pp. 7–13. Washington, D.C.: Organización Panamericana de la Salud.

Mallon, Richard, and Juan Sourrouille. 1975. *Economic Policymaking in a Conflict Society: The Argentine Case.* Cambridge: Harvard University Press.

Manterola, Alberto, A. S. de Gentile, F. Di Gregorio, and I. Lamela. 1987. "Riesgo de sarampión en la ciudad de Buenos Aires según grupos sociales." *Archivos Argentinos de Pediatría* 85 (no. 1): 44–53.

Manterola, Alberto, A. S. de Gentile, C. Wainstein, R. Ruvinsky, and M. Szeffner. 1989. "Estudio de prevalencia de infección hospitalaria." *Archivos Argentinos de Pediatría* 87 (no. 1/2): 19–28.

Manzanal, Mabel, and Alejandro B. Rofman. 1989. *Las economías regionales de la Argentina: Crisis y políticas de desarrollo.* Buenos Aires: Centro de Estudios Urbanos y Regionales.

Marconi, Elida, I. Moreno, M. de la M. Méndez Alonso, M. C. Uthurralt, and W. Zipper. 1990. "La mortalidad en áreas urbanas carenciadas." *Cuadernos Médico Sociales* no. 54: 43–50.

Martorell, R. 1987. "Comentario." In OPS, *Problemas nutricionales en países en desarrollo en las décadas de 1980 y 1990.* Cuaderno técnico no. 10, p. 53. Washington, D.C.: Organización Panamericana de la Salud.

Maxwell, Simon. 1992. "The Forgotten Human Cost of Hunger." *Buenos Aires Herald*, January 20, p. 4.

Mazzei, J. A., C. Riva Posse, and R. Gené. 1988. "Mortalidad por asma en la Argentina. ¿Por qué es tan alta?" *Medicina* 48 (no. 6): 714–716.

McCarthy, F. Desmond, ed. 1989. *Developing Economies in Transition. Vol. 2: Country Studies.* Washington, D.C.: World Bank.

McDermott, Jeanne, M. Bangser, E. Ngugi, and I. Sandvold. 1993. "Infection: Social and

Medical Realities." In Marge Koblinsky, J. Timyan, and J. Gay, eds., *The Health of Women: A Global Perspective*, pp. 91–104. Boulder, Colo.: Westview Press.

Medina, Ernesto, and Ana M. Kaempffer 1991. "Tabaquismo y salud en Chile." *Boletín de la Oficina Sanitaria Panamericana* 111 (no. 2): 112–121.

Medina, Romeo. 1992a. "Choque de criterios." *Clarín*, Economía, May 3, p. 23.

———. 1992b. "La concentración." *Clarín*, Economía, August 2, pp. 20–21.

Meier, Barry. 1996. "The Dark Side of a Magical Metal." *New York Times*, section 3, August 25, pp. 1, 8.

Mellor, John W. 1987. "Producción y suministro de alimentos y estado nutricional." In OPS, *Problemas nutricionales en países en desarrollo en las décadas de 1980 y 1990*. Cuaderno técnico no. 10, pp. 23–37. Washington, D.C.: Organización Panamericana de la Salud.

Mera, Jorge. 1988. *Política de salud en la Argentina: La construcción del Seguro Nacional de Salud*. Buenos Aires: Hachette.

———. 1990. "Política de recursos humanos de salud." *Medicina y Sociedad* 13 (no. 4): 38–42.

Mercer, Hugo. 1990. "La atención a la salud infantil: Un espacio para el cambio." In Eduardo Bustelo and Ernesto Isuani, eds., *Mucho, poquito o nada: Crisis y alternativas de política social en los '90*, pp. 183–222. Buenos Aires: UNICEF.

Mesa-Lago, Carmelo. 1978. *Social Security in Latin America: Pressure Groups, Stratification, and Inequality*. Pittsburgh: University of Pittsburgh Press.

Messi, Virginia. 1992. "Las farmacias acusan al Estado de las muertes por el propóleo." *Clarín*, August 16, p. 2.

Miceli, Isabel. 1990. "Meningitis tuberculosa en niños de 0 a 4 años." *Boletín Epidemiológico Nacional* 1 (no. 1): 29–34.

Michaels, David, C. Barrera, and M. Gacharna. 1985. "Occupational Health and the Economic Development of Latin America." In Jane Ives, ed., *The Export of Hazard*, pp. 94–114. Boston: Routledge and Kegan Paul.

Míguez, Daniel. 1992. "Secuestran 600 jeringas descartables." *Clarín*, August 29, pp. 32–33.

Mohan, Dinesh. 1993. "Avoidable Dangers on the Farm." *World Health* 46 (no. 1): 12–13.

Morasso, María del Carmen, and Horacio Lejarraga. 1984. "Estado nutricional en la Argentina: Perspectiva del sector salud." Mimeo. Ministerio de Salud y Acción Social.

Moreno, Liliana. 1992. "En el país no existe un plan de salud." *Clarín*, August 23, pp. 38–39.

Morse, Stephen. 1995. "Factors in the Emergence of Infectious Diseases." *Emerging Infectious Diseases* 1 (no. 1).

Moscona, Rafael, Pedro de Sarasqueta, and Luis Prudent. 1985. "Estudio de la mortalidad neonatal en la ciudad de Buenos Aires en 1984." *Archivos Argentinos de Pediatría* 83: 307–312.

Müller, María. 1984. *Mortalidad infantil y desigualdades sociales en Misiones*. Buenos Aires: Centro de Estudios de Población.

Murdock, Deroy. 1995. "Pussyfooting around Patent Piracy." *Wall Street Journal*, June 30, p. A15.

Murray, Christopher, R. Feacham, M. Phillips, and C. Willis. 1992a. "Adult Morbidity: Limited Data and Methodological Uncertainty." In Richard Feachem et al., eds., *The Health of Adults in the Developing World*, pp. 113–160. New York: Oxford University Press.

Murray, Christopher, G. Yang, and X. Qiao. 1992b. "Adult Mortality: Levels, Patterns, and Causes." In Richard Feachem et al., eds., *The Health of Adults in the Developing World*, pp. 23–111. New York: Oxford University Press.

Mychaszula, Sonia, and Luis Acosta. 1990. *La mortalidad infantil en la Argentina, 1976–1981.* Buenos Aires: Centro de Estudios de Población.

Myerson, Allen. 1995. "This Is the House That Greed Built." *New York Times*, April 2, pp. F1, F14.

Neffa, Julio. 1986. *El trabajo temporario en el sector agropecuario de América Latina.* Geneva: International Labor Office.

Neri, Aldo. 1982. *Salud y política social.* Buenos Aires: Hachette.

——. 1987. "Sostén económico de las estrategias de salud para todos." *Medicina y Sociedad* 10 (no. 5): 178–183.

Noguero, Bernardo. 1988. "El hospital público y la actividad extramural: Objetivos, dificultades y resistencias." In *II Jornadas de Atención Primaria de la Salud*, pp. 495–500. Buenos Aires.

Nogues, Julio. 1989. "Commment." In F. Desmond McCarthy, ed., *Developing Economies in Transition. Vol. 2: Country Studies*, pp. 49–51. Washington, D.C.: World Bank.

Noordeen, Shaik. 1992. "Where Are We Now?: Leprosy." *Health Policy and Planning* 7 (no. 3): 299–304.

Nordheimer, Jon. 1996. "One Day's Death Toll on the Job." *New York Times*, December 22, pp. F1, F10, F11.

Novik, Marta. 1988. "Salud y trabajo." In *II Jornadas de Atención Primaria de la Salud*, pp. 359–388. Buenos Aires.

Nowikowski, Frank. 1992. "Mould Suspected as Child Killer." *Buenos Aires Herald*, February 25, p. 9.

Núñez Urquiza, Rosa María. 1988. "La placenta de madres desnutridas." *Salud Pública de México* 30 (no. 1): 54–67.

Olivier, Margaret C., L. J. Olivier, and D. B. Segal. 1972. *A Bibliography on Chagas' Disease (1909–1969).* Washington, D.C.: U. S. Government Printing Office.

OPS (Organización Panamericana de la Salud). 1987. *Problemas nutricionales en países en desarrollo en las décadas de 1980 y 1990.* Cuaderno técnico no. 10. Washington, D.C.

——. 1988. *Los servicios de salud en las Américas. Análisis de indicadores básicos.* Cuaderno técnico no. 14. Washington, D.C.

——. 1989. *Argentina: Condiciones de salud, 1985–1988.* Buenos Aires.

——. 1992a. "Temas de Actualidad." *Boletin de la Oficina Sanitaria Panamericana* 113 (no. 3): 256–258.

——. 1992b. "Tipo de tabaco y crecimiento fetal." *Boletin de la Oficina Sanitaria Panamericana* 113 (no. 3): 255.

Over, Mead, R. Ellis, J. Huber, and O. Solon. 1992. "The Consequences of Adult Ill-Health." In Richard Feachem et al., eds., *The Health of Adults in the Developing World*, pp. 161–207. New York: Oxford University Press.

Oya-Sawyer, Diana, R. Fernandez-Castilla, and R. de Melo Monte-Mor. 1987. "The Impact of Urbanization and Industrialization on Mortality in Brazil." *World Health Statistical Quarterly* 40: 84–95.

Page, Joseph. 1983. *Perón: A Biography.* New York: Random House.

PAHO (Pan American Health Organization). 1981. *Hospitals in the Americas.* Scientific publication no. 416. Washington, D.C.

——. 1984. *Development and Implementation of Drug Formularies.* Scientific publication no. 474. Washington, D.C.

——. 1989. *Midlife and Older Women in Latin America and the Caribbean.* Washington, D.C.

———. 1990*a*. *Health Conditions in the Americas. Vol. 1.* Scientific publication no. 524. Washington, D.C.

———. 1990*b*. *Health Conditions in the Americas. Vol. 2.* Scientific publication no. 524. Washington, D.C.

Palomino, Héctor. 1987. *Cambios ocupacionales y sociales en Argentina 1947–1985.* Buenos Aires: Centro de Investigaciones Sociales sobre el Estado y la Administración.

Paltiel, Freda. 1989. "Occupational Health of Midlife and Older Women in Latin America and the Caribbean." In Pan American Health Organization, *Midlife and Older Women in Latin America and the Caribbean*, pp. 142–158. Washington, D.C.

Pampliega, Eneas. 1989. "Las leyes del mercado y la atención de la salud." *Medicina y Sociedad* 12 (no. 1/2): 21–27.

———. 1991. "Costos y ética en atención médica." Paper delivered at III Seminario Internacional de Economía Médica, Universidad Argentina de la Empresa, September 16–18.

Pampliega, Eneas, Sergio Muszkats, and Graciela Eleta. 1990. "Demanda de atención médica por edad y sexo en una obra social." *Medicina y Sociedad* 13 (no. 5/6): 42–43.

Pasqualini, R. Q. 1988. "Cómo mueren los Institutos." *Medicina* 48 (no. 1): 107–108.

Pazos, Luis. 1992. "Porqué es tan complicado donar órganos en la Argentina." *Clarín*, November 29, p. 41.

Pazos, Luis, and Adrián van der Horst. 1993. "Los que viven en la calle." *Clarín*, August 15, p. 44.

Pear, Robert. 1994. "Health Insurance Percentage Is Lowest in 4 Sun Belt States." *New York Times*, October 7, p. A16.

Peralta-Ramos, Monica, and Carlos Waisman, eds. 1987. *From Military Rule to Liberal Democracy in Argentina.* Boulder, Colo.: Westview.

Pérez Arias, Elsa, and Jorge Feller. 1990. "Estudio de la población médica de la Provincia de Buenos Aires." *Medicina y Sociedad* 13 (no. 5/6): 17–24.

Perlez, Jane. 1994. "East Europe Health Care, Out of Cash, Has Relapse." *New York Times*, November 23, p. A10.

Peto, Richard, A. Lopez, J. Boreham, M. Thun, and C. Heath Jr. 1994. *Mortality from Smoking in Developed Countries 1950–2000.* Oxford: Oxford University Press.

Pfefferman, Guy, and Charles Griffin. 1989. *Nutrition and Health Programs in Latin America: Targeting Social Expenditures.* Washington, D.C.: World Bank.

Phillips, Margaret A., R. Feachem, and J. Koplan. 1992. "The Emerging Agenda for Adult Health." In Richard Feachem et al., eds., *The Health of Adults in the Developing World*, pp. 261–294. New York: Oxford University Press.

Piccinini, Alberto. 1988. "Salud y trabajo." In *II Jornadas de Atención Primaria de la Salud*, pp. 359–388. Buenos Aires.

Piesman, J., I. A. Sherlock, E. Mota, and C. W. Todd. 1985. "Association between Household Triatomine Density and Incidence of *Trypanosoma cruzi* Infection during a Nine-Year Study in Castro Alves, Bahia, Brazil." *American Journal of Tropical Medicine and Hygiene* 34 (no. 5): 866–869.

Pignotti, Carmen. 1992*a*. "AIDS—Some Myths of Prevention." *Buenos Aires Herald*, June 7, p. 17.

———. 1992*b*. "Birth Control Promotion Still Taboo." *Buenos Aires Herald*, May 31, p. 17.

———. 1992*c*. "Speaking Loud and Clear on AIDS." *Buenos Aires Herald*, December 1, p. 9.

———. 1993. "Day of Reckoning for Riachuelo." *Buenos Aires Herald*, October 2, p. 4.

Pogoriles, Eduardo. 1992. "El país de los autos eternos." *Clarín*, May 3, pp. 40–41.

———. 1993. "Avellaneda: Respirar con miedo." *Clarín*, October 24, pp. 48–49.

Poletto, L., and J. C. Morini. 1990. "Cancer Mortality and Some Socio-Economic Correlates in Rosario, Argentina." *Cancer Letter* 49 (no. 3): 201–205.

Portantiero, Juan Carlos. 1989. "Political and Economic Crises in Argentina." In Guido di Tella and Rudiger Dornbusch, eds., *The Political Economy of Argentina, 1946–1983*. Pittsburgh: University of Pittsburgh Press.

Prece, Graciela, and Marta Schufer de Paikin. 1991. "Diferente percepción de enfermedad y consulta médica según niveles socioeconómicos en las ciudades de Buenos Aires y San Salvador de Jujuy." *Medicina y Sociedad* 14 (no. 4): 27–30.

Programa Nacional de Investigaciones de Enfermedades Endémicas. 1980. *Contribución a la bibliografía argentina sobre enfermedad de Chagas y fiebre hemorrágica argentina*. Buenos Aires.

Quirno Costa, Dr. 1987. "Experiencia en la Provincia de Neuquén." In *Jornadas de Atención Primaria de la Salud*, pp. 61–87. Buenos Aires.

Quistgard, Kaitlin. 1994. "AIDS Cases Rising." *Buenos Aires Herald*, May 29, p. 4.

Rabinovich, J. E., C. Wisnivesky-Colli, N. D. Solarz, and R. E. Gurtler. 1990. "Probability of Transmission of Chagas Disease by *Triatoma infestans (Hemiptera: Reduviidae)* in an Endemic Area of Santiago del Estero, Argentina." *Bulletin of the World Health Organization* 68 (no. 6): 737–746.

Read, Merrill. 1977. "Malnutrition and Human Performance." In Lawrence Greene, ed., *Malnutrition, Behavior, and Social Organization*, pp. 95–107. New York: Academic Press.

Renshaw, John, and Daniel Rivas. 1991. "A Community Development Approach to Chagas' Disease: The Sucre Health Project, Bolivia." *Health Policy and Planning* 6 (no. 3): 244–253.

Rocha, Jan. 1996. "Let Them Eat Cake." *Guardian Weekly*, June 16, p. 12.

Rock, David. 1975. "The Survival of Peronism." In David Rock, ed., *Argentina in the 20th Century*, pp. 179–222. Pittsburgh: University of Pittsburgh Press.

———. 1985. *Argentina 1516–1982*. Berkeley: University of California Press.

Rodríguez, Carlos. 1988. "Salud y trabajo." In *II Jornadas de Atención Primaria de la Salud*, pp. 359–388. Buenos Aires.

Rodríguez, Julio. 1990. "58 Menores de un año mueren diariamente en nuestro país, la mitad por causas prevenibles. ¿Por qué?" In *IV Jornadas de Atención Primaria de la Salud*, pp. 721–752. Buenos Aires.

Roemer, M. I., and R. Roemer. 1990. "Global Health, National Development, and the Role of Government." *American Journal of Public Health* 80 (no. 10): 1188–1192.

Rofman, Alejandro. 1992. "Vivimos juntos, pero peleados." *Clarín*, November 4, pp. 20–21.

Rofman, Alejandro, and Nora Marqués. 1988. *Desigualdades regionales en la Argentina: Su evolución desde 1970*. Buenos Aires: Centro de Estudios Urbanos y Regionales.

Rojas, J. C., E. Malo, E. Espinoza-Medinilla, and R. Ondarza. 1989. "Sylvatic Focus of Chagas' Disease in Oaxaca, Mexico." *Annals of Tropical Medicine and Parasitology* 83 (no. 2): 115–120.

Romero, Remigio. 1987. "El hospital deseable en Río Negro." *Medicina y Sociedad* 10 (no. 6): 223–227.

Roncoroni, A. J. 1989. "Mortalidad por asma en la Argentina. ¿Por qué es tan alta?" *Medicina* 49 (no. 5): 544–545.

Roncoroni, A. J., G. García Damiano, H. M. Bianchini, and J. Smayevsky. 1987. "Faringoamigdalitis estreptocóccica. ¿Otro indicador de pobreza en la Argentina?" *Medicina* 47 (no. 4): 443.

Ronderos, Ricardo, and Juan Schnack. 1987. "Ecological Aspects of Triatominae in Argentina." In R. Brenner and A. de la M. Stoka, eds., *Chagas' Disease Vectors*, vol. 1, pp. 85–97. Boca Raton, Fla.: CRC Press.

Ruiz-Tiben, Ernesto, D. Hopkins, T. Ruebush, and R. Kaiser. 1995. "Progress Toward the Eradication of Dracunculiasis (Guinea Worm Disease): 1994." *Emerging Infectious Diseases* 1 (no. 2).

Rutledge, Ian. 1975. "Plantations and Peasants in Northern Argentina: The Sugar Cane Industry of Salta and Jujuy, 1930–1943." In David Rock, ed., *Argentina in the 20th Century*, pp. 88–113. Pittsburgh: University of Pittsburgh Press.

Ryan, Frank. 1993. *The Forgotten Plague: How the Battle against Tuberculosis Was Won— and Lost.* Boston: Little Brown.

Sai, Fred T. 1984. "The Priority of Nutrition in a Nation's Development." In Pradip K. Ghosh, ed., *Health, Food and Nutrition in Third World Development.* Westport, Conn.: Greenwood Press.

Sainz, Carola. 1992a. "El bacilo ataca." *Clarín,* second section, October 18, p. 19.

———. 1992b. "Queréme así, piantao." *Clarín,* second section, August 16, p. 11.

Salvaneschi, J. P., B. Salvaneschi, A. Moralejo, and J. García. 1991. "La endemia bociogena en la República Argentina." *Medicina* 51: 99–105.

Sánchez, Jane. 1994. "Programs to Meet Real Needs." *IDB EXTRA: Reproductive Health,* p. 3.

Sánchez, Matilde. 1992. "Viaje a la locura: La increíble historia de la colonia Montes de Oca." *Clarín,* second section, February 23, pp. 1–5.

Sande, Innis. 1979a. "Products of Pregnancy and Their Survival Related to the Characteristics of Mothers." In Mary Burke et al., *Inter-American Investigation of Mortality in Childhood: Report on a Household Survey,* scientific publication no. 386, pp. 115–145. Washington, D.C.: Pan American Health Organization.

———. 1979b. "Social and Economic Characteristics of Mothers." In Mary Burke et al., *Inter-American Investigation of Mortality in Childhood: Report on a Household Survey,* scientific publication no. 386, pp. 95–114. Washington, D.C.: Pan American Health Organization.

Sandiford, Peter, P. Morales, A. Gorter, E. Coyle, and G. D. Smith. 1991. "Why Do Child Mortality Rates Fall? An Analysis of the Nicaraguan Experience." *American Journal of Public Health* 81: 30–37.

Santhia, Miguel, M. Liborio, Z. Torres de Quinteros, B. Perez, and E. Rondelli. 1990. "Estudio de la población atendida en el subsector público de la ciudad de Rosario." *Medicina y Sociedad* 13 (no. 5/6): 31–35.

Sawers, Larry. 1996. *The Other Argentina: The Interior and National Development.* Boulder, Colo.: Westview Press.

Schemo, Diana. 1995. "A Latin Epidemic Spreads Horror, and Questions." *New York Times,* October 26, pp. A1, A10.

Schwarcz, Alberto. 1987. "Relato de la experiencia en el control de la mujer embarazada en el barrio de San Pedro, La Matanza (Pcia. de Bs. As.)." In *Jornadas de Atención Primaria de la Salud,* pp. 545–557. Buenos Aires.

———. 1988. "El hospital público y la actividad extramural: Objetivos, dificultades y resistencias." In *II Jornadas de Atención Primaria de la Salud,* pp. 500–502. Buenos Aires.

———. 1989. "Atención primaria o primitiva de la salud: ¿Qué pasa en Argentina hoy?" In *III Jornadas de Atención Primaria de la Salud*, pp. 15–58. Buenos Aires.

Scobie, James. 1988. *Secondary Cities of Argentina: The Social History of Corrientes, Salta, and Mendoza, 1850–1910*. Palo Alto, Calif.: Stanford University Press.

Seia, Héctor. 1991. "La historia no se repite." *Salud y Sociedad* 8 (no. 21): 39–40.

Sen, Amartya K. "The Economics of Life and Death." *Scientific American*, May 1993: 40–47.

Shneour, Elie. 1974. *The Malnourished Mind*. Garden City: Anchor/Doubleday.

Shostak, Arthur. 1980. *Blue-Collar Stress*. Reading, Mass.: Addison-Wesley.

Siglioccoli, Alberto. 1992. "Las cifras del deterioro." *Clarín*, suplemento económico, May 31, p. 9.

Simons, Marlise. 1996. "H.I.V. Virus Still Spreading Rapidly, U.N. Says." *New York Times*, June 7, p. A3.

Sims, Calvin. 1995*a*. "Argentina Gets Tough on Drivers." *New York Times*, February 8, p. A11.

———. 1995*b*. "Menem Complains, But Press Has Turned President to 'Star.'" *New York Times*, May 25, p. A16.

———. 1996. "On Every Argentine Cellblock, Specter of AIDS." *New York Times*, March 22, p. A4.

Skolnick, Andrew. 1989. "Does Influx from Endemic Areas Mean More Transfusion-Associated Chagas' Disease?" *Journal of the American Medical Association*, September 15, p. 1433.

———. 1991. "Deferral Aims to Deter Chagas' Parasite." *Journal of the American Medical Association*, January 9, p. 173.

Slater, R. Giuseppi. 1989. "Reflections on Curative Health Care in Nicaragua." *American Journal of Public Health* 79 (no. 5): 646–651.

Smith, Gordon S., and Peter Barss. 1991. "Unintentional Injuries in Developing Countries: The Epidemiology of a Neglected Problem." *Epidemiologic Reviews* 13: 228–266.

Solberg, Carl. 1987. *The Prairies and the Pampas: Agrarian Policy in Canada and Argentina, 1880–1930*. Palo Alto, Calif.: Stanford University Press.

Solo, Tova M., P. Gutman, and G. Dascal. 1990. *Las aguas bajan turbias: Technologías alternativas para el saneamiento en el Gran Buenos Aires*. Buenos Aires: Centro de Estudios Urbanos y Regionales.

Soltys, Michael. 1993*a*. "Politics and Labour." *Buenos Aires Herald*, March 7, pp. 3, 18.

———. 1993*b*. "Politics and Labour." *Buenos Aires Herald*, April 4, pp. 3, 17.

———. 1994*a*. "Politics and Labour." *Buenos Aires Herald*, January 2, pp. 3, 26.

———. 1994*b*. "Politics and Labour." *Buenos Aires Herald*, February 6, p. 3.

———. 1995. "Politics and Labour." *Buenos Aires Herald*, January 22, p. 3.

Spector, Paul. 1994. "Failure, by the Numbers." *New York Times*, September 24, p. 19.

Spinelli, Hugo. 1991. "Ajuste y salud." *Salud y Sociedad* 8 (no. 21): 29–31.

Spinelli, Oscar. 1992. "Mala praxis." *Clarín*, second section, August 16, pp. 1–5.

Stanbury, John. 1977. "The Role of the Thyroid in the Development of the Human Nervous System." In Lawrence Greene, ed., *Malnutrition, Behavior, and Social Organization*, pp. 39–54. New York: Academic Press.

Stover, Eric, and Elena Nightingale. 1985. *The Breaking of Bodies and Minds: Torture, Psychiatric Abuse, and the Health Professions*. New York: W. H. Freeman.

Styblo, Karel, and Annik Rouillon. 1991. "Where Are We Now?: Tuberculosis." *Health Policy and Planning* 6 (no. 4): 391–397.

Swaney, Deanna. 1995. *Zimbabwe, Botswana, and Namibia.* Hawthorn, Australia: Lonely Planet Publications.

Tafani, Roberto. 1989. "Dinámica morfológica y órgano de conducción del sector salud." Mimeo. Buenos Aires.

Tauxe, Robert, E. Mintz, and R. Quick. 1995. "Epidemic Cholera in the New World: Translating Field Epidemiology into New Preventive Strategies." *Emerging Infectious Diseases* 1 (no. 4).

Temple, Norman, and Denis Burkitt, eds. 1994. *Western Diseases: Their Dietary Prevention and Reversibility.* Totowa, N.J.: Humana.

Tenti, Emilio. 1990. "Escuela y equidad: Criterios de políticas." In Eduardo Bustelo and Ernesto Isuani, eds., *Mucho, poquito o nada: Crisis y alternativas de política social en los '90*, pp. 183–222. Buenos Aires: UNICEF.

Terris, Milton. 1988. "Health Services and Health Policy: Discussions." In Pan American Health Organization, *Challenge of Epidemiology*, pp. 809–827. Washington, D.C.: Pan American Health Organization.

———. 1991. "The Health Situation in the Americas." *Journal of Public Health Policy* 12 (no. 3): 362–377.

Tietze, C., and M. C. Murstein. 1975. "El aborto inducido, compendio de datos, 1975." *Informes sobre población/planificación familiar*, no. 14.

Tonn, Robert J. 1985. "Problemas e implicaciones del control integrado de la enfermedad de Chagas." In Rodolfo Carcavallo et al., *Factores biológicos y ecológicos en la enfermedad de Chagas*, vol. 2, pp. 331–338. Washington, D.C.: Centro Panamericano de Ecología Humana y Salud, Organización Panamericana de la Salud.

Torrado, Susana. 1986. *Salud-enfermedad en el primer año de vida: Rosario, 1981–1982.* Buenos Aires: Centro de Estudios Urbanos y Regionales.

Torres, Aída, C. de Fischer, S. Aulet, S. de Moreno, N. Fernández, S. M. Fernández, M. Silman, A. de Trejo, and A. de Merchan. 1990. "Evaluación de los programas para el control de la infección hospitalaria y utilización de antibióticos en un hospital pediátrico de Tucumán, Argentina." *Archivos Argentinos de Pediatría* 88 (no. 1): 37–44.

Tozer, Nicholas. 1993a. "Politics and Labour." *Buenos Aires Herald*, February 28, pp. 3, 18.

———. 1993b. "Politics and Labour." *Buenos Aires Herald*, October 3, pp. 3, 22.

Tucker, Bonnie. 1993. "Fines for B.A. Trash Offenders?" *Buenos Aires Herald*, April 18, p. 6.

———. 1995. "More Than Stench Rotten in Dock Sud." *Buenos Aires Herald*, July 30, p. 13.

Tulchin, Joseph. 1986. "The Relationship between Labor and Capital in Rural Argentina, 1880–1914." In Guido di Tella and D.C.M. Platt, eds., *The Political Economy of Argentina*, pp. 19–39. London: Macmillan.

Tyler, Patrick. 1996. "China Confronts Retardation of Millions Who Lack Iodine." *New York Times*, June 4, pp. A1, A10.

Ugalde, Antonio. 1985. "The Integration of Health Care Programs into a National Health Service." In Carmelo Mesa-Lago, ed., *The Crisis of Social Security and Health Care: Latin American Experiences and Lessons*, pp. 111–142. Pittsburgh: University of Pittsburgh Press.

Ulanovsky Sack, Daniel. 1993. "En el sida, discriminar es escupir hacia el techo." *Clarín*, September 19, pp. 20–21.

UNDP (United Nations Development Program). 1995. *Human Development Report.* New York.

———. 1996. *Human Development Report.* New York.

UNICEF. n.d. *Salud materno-infantil en cifras*. 2d ed. Buenos Aires.

———. 1990*a*. *Infancia y pobreza en la Argentina*. Buenos Aires.

———. 1990*b*. *Piden pan . . . y algo más: Un estudio sobre crecimiento y desarrollo infantil*. Buenos Aires.

———. 1991. *Estado mundial de la infancia 1991*. New York.

———. 1996. *The Progress of Nations*. New York.

United Nations. 1984. *Transnational Corporations in the Pharmaceutical Industry of Developing Countries*. New York.

Uribe Vázquez, Griselda, J. C. Ramírez, L. G. Romero, and N. C. Gutiérrez de la Torre. 1991. "El trabajo femenino y la salud de cuatro grupos de mujeres en Guadalajara, México." *Boletín de la Oficina Sanitaria Panamericana* 111 (no. 2): 101–110.

Valdés, J. M., R. de Silberber, and C. Farías. 1986. "Epidemiología de la tuberculosis en el grupo etario de 13 a 18 años en la Provincia de Córdoba." *Archivos Argentinos de Pediatría* 84 (no. 5): 321–325.

van der Horst, Adrián. 1992*a*. "Lo que hicieron en seis meses." *Clarín*, October 11, p. 40.

———. 1992*b*. "SIDA: Una campaña cuestionada." *Clarín*, October 11, pp. 40–41.

Veltri, Patricia. 1992. "Duhalde promete pagar los trasplantes de los bonaerenses sin recursos." *Clarín*, August 29, pp. 32–33.

Verbitsky, Horacio. 1993. *Robo para la corona*. Buenos Aires: Planeta.

Vidal, Armando. 1992. "No es bueno que un chico esté solo." *Clarín*, second section, October 25, pp. 6–7.

Viladrich, Anahí. 1990. "Maternidad y servicios de salud." *Medicina y Sociedad* 13 (no. 1/2): 22–27.

Villa, Pedro. 1991. "El hospital público: Su situación en el marco de la crisis." In *V Jornadas de Atención Primaria de la Salud*, pp. 75–116. Buenos Aires.

Vinocur, Pablo. 1991. "60 niños menores de un año mueren diariamente en nuestro país, la mitad por causas prevenibles. ¿Por qué?, ¿Hasta cuándo?" *V Jornadas de Atención Primaria de la Salud*, pp. 263–287. Buenos Aires.

Wainerman, Catalina, and Rosa Geldstein. 1990. *Condiciones de vida y de trabajo de las enfermeras en la Argentina*. Buenos Aires: Centro de Estudios de Población.

Ward, Peter. 1986. *Welfare Politics in Mexico: Papering over the Cracks*. London: Allen and Unwin.

Warr, Peter. 1987. *Work, Unemployment, and Mental Health*. Oxford: Clarendon Press.

Waserstreguer, Silvia, V. Bollini, J. Arazi, E. Farfallini, M. Rodríguez, M. Taboadella, and F. Boente. 1987. "Detección de los factores de riesgo y características de la población que se interna en el Hospital de Niños de San Isidro." *Archivos Argentinos Pediatría* 85: 190–197.

Waterlow, John C. 1987. "Prioridades que surgen en las ciencias de la nutrición." In OPS, *Problemas nutricionales en países en desarrollo en las décadas de 1980 y 1990*. Cuaderno técnico no. 10, pp. 41–52. Washington, D.C.: Organización Panamericana de la Salud.

Weber, Peter. 1992. "A Place for Pesticides?" *World Watch* 5 (no. 3): 18–25.

Wells, Stuart, and Steven Klees. 1980. *Health Economics and Development*. New York: Praeger.

Werthein, Leonardo. 1989. "Viejos y nuevos problemas en epidemiología." In *III Jornadas de Atención Primaria de la Salud*, pp. 299–326. Buenos Aires.

———. 1990. "Usos de la epidemiología." In *IV Jornadas de Atención Primaria de la Salud*, pp. 629–659. Buenos Aires.

———. 1991. "Los indicadores de la crisis." *Salud y Sociedad* 8 (no. 21): 27–29.

Wheeler, David. 1996. "North Americans Join Thais in the Fight against AIDS." *The Chronicle of Higher Education*, April 12, p. A9.

WHO (World Health Organization). 1990. "World Malaria Situation, 1988." *World Health Statistical Quarterly* 43: 68–79.

———. 1991*a*. *Control of Chagas' Disease: Report of a WHO Expert Committee*, WHO/TRS/811. Geneva.

———. 1991*b*. *Environmental Health in Urban Development: Report of a WHO Expert Committee*, WHO/TRS/807. Geneva.

———. 1991*c*. "Improving Urban Health Systems." *World Health Statistical Quarterly* 44: 234–244.

———. 1991*d*. *Surface Water Drainage for Low-Income Communities*. Geneva.

———. 1991*e*. "Urbanization and the Urban Environment." *World Health Statistical Quarterly* 44: 198–203.

———. 1992. *The Hospital in Rural and Urban Districts: Report of a WHO Study Group*, WHO/TRS/819. Geneva.

World Bank. 1987*a*. *Argentina: Population, Health and Nutrition Sector Review*. Washington, D.C.

———. 1987*b*. *World Development Report 1987*. New York: Oxford University Press.

———. 1988. *Argentina: Social Sectors in Crisis*. World Bank Country Study. Washington, D.C.

———. 1991. *World Development Report 1991*. New York: Oxford University Press.

———. 1993. *World Development Report 1993*. New York: Oxford University Press.

———. 1995. *World Development Report 1995*. New York: Oxford University Press.

———. 1996. *World Development Report 1996*. New York: Oxford University Press.

World Resources 1994–1995. 1994. New York: Oxford University Press.

Wright, Amaranta. 1995. "Argentines Cut a Fine Figure." *Guardian Weekly*, December 3, p. 5.

Wright, Angus. 1990. *The Death of Ramón González: The Modern Agricultural Dilemma*. Austin: University of Texas Press.

York, Marjorie. 1979. "Growth Curves and Nutritional Status of Children in Selected Study Areas of Latin America." In Mary Burke et al., *Inter-American Investigation of Mortality in Childhood: Report on a Household Survey*, scientific publication no. 386, pp. 115–145. Washington, D.C.: Pan American Health Organization.

Zaragoza, Norma, C. Drangosch, and S. González. 1991. "Control de embarazo en sectores populares." Unpublished paper presented to *V Jornadas de Atención Primaria de la Salud*. Buenos Aires.

Zicolillo, Jorge. 1992. "Las tentaciones peligrosas." *Clarín*, June 28, *Revista*, pp. 8–9.

Zwi, Anthony, and Antonio Ugalde. 1991. "Political Violence in the Third World: A Public Health Issue." *Health Policy and Planning* 6 (no. 3): 203–217.

Visits

Barrio Autopista and Barrio Comunicaciones, Villa de Retiro, Buenos Aires, with student nurses, July 1 and 2, 1992.

Barrio Autopista, Villa de Retiro, Buenos Aires, with nurses from Hospital Italiano, September 8, 1992.

Health Center in Guaymallén, Mendoza, November 1, 1991.

Health Center in Las Heras, Mendoza, November 1, 1991.

Health Center Number 149, Godoy Cruz, Mendoza, November 1, 1991.

Hospital de Clínicas General San Martín, Pediatrics, September 28 to November 11, 1992; August 23 to 31, 1993.

Hospital de Niños Emilio Civit, Mendoza, October 31, 1991.

Hospital de Niños San Justo, September 2, 1992.

Hospital Fernández, Buenos Aires, September 9, 1992.

Hospital General Lagomaggiore, Mendoza, October 31, 1991.

Hospital Materno-infantil Del Viso, Greater Buenos Aires, September 3, 1992.

Hospital Materno-infantil Gregorio La Ferrere, La Matanza, November 2, 3, 4, 6, 11, 1992.

Hospital Materno-infantil Umberto, Mendoza, October 31, 1991.

Hospital *Mi Pueblo*, Florencio Varela, Greater Buenos Aires, September 7, 1993.

Hospital Municipal de Niños Ricardo Gutiérrez, Buenos Aires, numerous visits in 1991, 1992.

Hospital Municipal de Quemados, Buenos Aires, September 16, 1992.

Interviews

Aprigliano, Dra. Norma. At Health Center Number 6, Villa Soldati, Villa Fátima, Buenos Aires, September 24, 1991.

Bojio, Irma. At Hospital General Lagomaggiore, Mendoza, October 31, 1991.

Coruja, Dra. María. At Hospital Municipal de Quemados, September 16, 1992.

de Sarasqueta, Dr. Pedro. At Hospital Nacional de Pediatría Dr. Garrahan, September 25, 1991; June 9, 1992.

Fontán, Marcelino. At UNICEF, Buenos Aires, December 10, 1991.

García, Rosana. At Diego Paroissien Hospital, La Matanza, August 21, 1992.

Gutiérrez, Geraldo. At Secretariat of Health, Florencio Varela, and Health Center, Villa Mónica, Florencio Varela, September 7, 1993.

Kurlat, Dra. Isabel. At Neonatal Intensive Care Unit , Hospital de Clínicas General San Martín, August 26, 1993.

Lemus, Dr. Jorge. At Fernández Hospital, Buenos Aires, September 9, 1992.

López, Laura. At Diego Paroissien Hospital, La Matanza, August 21, 1992.

Martínez de Hoz, José. Talk given to The American University Semester in Buenos Aires, November 23, 1989, at Universidad Argentina de la Empresa.

Mele, Dr. Eduardo. At Sanitorio Anchorena, August 26, 1991.

Ménguez, Carlos. At Diego Paroissien Hospital, La Matanza, August 21, 1992.

Mercer, Dr. Raúl. At *Mi Pueblo* Hospital, Florencio Varela, August 31, 1993.

Muntaabski, Dr. Pablo. At Health Center Number 21, Villa de Retiro, Villa No. 31, Buenos Aires, June 26, 1992.

Obilla, Dra. Adriana. At Emilio Civit Children's Hospital, October 31, 1991.

Rípoli, Dr. Mario. At Health Center Number 5, so-called Ciudad Oculta, Buenos Aires, November 27, 1991.

Saracco, Dra. Lucía. At Hospital Diego Paroissien, La Matanza, Province of Buenos Aires, August 21, 1992.

Schwarcz, Dr. Alberto. At Hospital Diego Paroissien, La Matanza, Province of Buenos Aires, August 21, 1992.

Sparvoli, Jorge. At Hospital Materno-infantil Del Viso, September 3, 1992.

Spatz, Dra. Graciela. At Universidad de Palermo, Buenos Aires, December 6, 1991.

Teixidor, Dr. Roque. Interviews in Mendoza, October 31, 1991 and November 1, 1991.

Index

abattoirs. *See* slaughterhouses
abortion, 257–259
absenteeism, 267–271
accidents, 79–80, 133–136, 223–228, 269
acquired human immunodeficiency
  syndrome. *See* AIDS
AIDS, 136–141, 155, 173, 175, 181, 189, 195,
  260–261, 267; and tuberculosis, 75–76
air pollution, 73, 128, 194
alcoholism, 81, 134, 254
Alfonsín, Raúl, 39–40, 152
American trypanosomiasis. *See* Chagas'
  disease
amniotic infections, 176–177, 220
anemia. *See* iron deficiency
anthropomorphic measurement. *See* growth
  monitoring
Aprigliano de Schnitler, Norma, 174–175, 296
aranceles. See user fees
Argentine hemorrhagic fever, 265
Arole, Mabelle, 294–296
Arole, Raj, 294–296
ascorbic acid, 243
asistencialismo, 173
austerity. *See* macroeconomic adjustment
authoritarianism. *See caudillos;* military
  coup; *Proceso*
Autopista, 58, 96, 171–172
Axis powers, 31

Bangladesh, 231, 256, 271, 279
Barbados, 286
bathing facilities, 101, 293

bathrooms, 169, 171, 198, 203, 285, 292
bed crowding. *See* promiscuity
bed nets, 93, 285
begging, 17, 253
Bengal famine, 231
Bernard, Ana, 200, 305n.3
bilharzia. *See* schistosomiasis
birth defects, 264
blindness. *See* vitamin A deficiency
blood donors. *See* blood transfusions
blood transfusions, 86–88, 133, 138–140
boarding houses. *See* tenements
Bolivia, 12, 23, 84, 90, 94, 118, 179, 242, 266
boycott, 31, 33
Braulio Moyano asylum, 133
Brazil, 11, 17, 84, 86–93, 114, 150, 157, 180,
  224, 261, 263, 266, 286
breastfeeding, 86, 170, 181, 234–235
budget deficit, 9, 30, 35, 40
Buenos Aires Province, 13, 116, 118, 147,
  154, 176, 213, 266
Bulgaria, 281
bureaucracy, 250
burn hospital, 79, 155, 187
burns, 79–80, 197
bus hazards, 133–136, 279

Caesarean sections, 150, 257
calcium deficiency, 227, 243
Canada, 22, 150, 256
cancer, 260, 264–265. *See also* occupational
  hazards; radioactive waste; smoking
cardiac disease, 84, 87, 248

About the Author

Eileen Stillwaggon is an economist educated at Georgetown University, the American University, and the University of Cambridge. She has taught at Howard University, at the University of Dar es Salaam as a Fulbright Senior Scholar, at Lincoln University College in Buenos Aires, and is Assistant Professor of Economics at Gettysburg College. Her research includes work in Tanzania, in Argentina, and on the Ute reservation in Utah.

ADT - 3364   1-21-00
         Armstrong
      RA
      418.5
      P6
      574
       1998